Radiology Oral Examinations

100 Cases and Revision Notes

AF711262

Radiology Oral Examinations

100 Cases and Revision Notes

Richard White
Consultant Radiologist
University Hospital of Wales
Cardiff, UK

Robin Proctor
Consultant Radiologist
The Royal Lancaster Infirmary
Lancaster, UK

Ian Zealley
Consultant Radiologist
Ninewells Hospital
Dundee, UK

JP medical publishers

London • New Delhi

© 2026 JP Medical Ltd.

Published by JP Medical Ltd,
83 Victoria Street, London,
SW1H 0HW, UK
Tel: +44 (0)20 3170 8910
Email: info@jpmedpub.com
Web: www.jpmedpub.com

EU GPSR Authorised Representative
Logos Europe, 9 rue Nicolas Poussin
17000, La Rochelle, France
Phone: +33 (0) 6 67 93 73 78
E-mail: Contact@logoseurope.eu

The rights of Richard White, Robin Proctor, Ian Zealley to be identified as the authors of this work have been asserted by them in accordance with the Copyright, Designs and Patents Act 1988.

All rights reserved. No part of this publication may be reproduced, stored or transmitted in any form or by any means, electronic, mechanical, photocopying, recording or otherwise, except as permitted by the UK Copyright, Designs and Patents Act 1988, without the prior permission in writing of the publishers. Permissions may be sought directly from JP Medical Ltd at the address printed above.

All brand names and product names used in this book are trade names, service marks, trademarks or registered trademarks of their respective owners. The publisher is not associated with any product or vendor mentioned in this book.

Medical knowledge and practice change constantly. This book is designed to provide accurate, authoritative information about the subject matter in question. However readers are advised to check the most current information available on procedures included and check information from the manufacturer of each product to be administered, to verify the recommended dose, formula, method and duration of administration, adverse effects and contraindications. It is the responsibility of the practitioner to take all appropriate safety precautions. Neither the publisher nor the authors assume any liability for any injury and/or damage to persons or property arising from or related to use of material in this book.

This book is sold on the understanding that the publisher is not engaged in providing professional medical services. If such advice or services are required, the services of a competent medical professional should be sought.

ISBN: 978-1-78779-169-5

British Library Cataloguing in Publication Data
A catalogue record for this book is available from the British Library

Library of Congress Cataloging in Publication Data
A catalog record for this book is available from the Library of Congress

Project Manager: Bhavana Sharma

Editorial Assistant: Keshav Kumar Baghel

Cover Design: Seema Dogra

Typeset, printed and bound in India.

Preface

This book will help you to pass your final radiology viva/oral examination. Radiologists who are approaching final certification fear the oral examinations the most. But, if you are about to sit your final oral examinations then there is one thing you really do not have to worry about, and that is whether you have enough radiology knowledge. By passing the various examinations leading up to the final oral examination you have already proven that you have enough knowledge. However, what you may not be so good at is marshalling your thoughts and articulating your knowledge to successfully demonstrate to your examiners that you possess the requisite perception, interpretation and management skills to become an independent radiologist.

This book contains 100 typical cases with model answers, together with key points to think about during discussion of the case. The aim is to provide you with a store of well-worded phrases which you can learn ahead of time to allow you to suitably express yourself during the stress of the examination. Having a store of stock phrases leaves more of your brain's processing power free to concentrate on the radiological abnormalities and their interpretation, without the additional struggle of finding the right words to describe what you are seeing.

The cases have been selected by asking over 100 radiologists what types of cases they encountered in their final oral examinations, and ranking these by frequency, so the most common cases appear early in the book. We have presented a typical case in each chapter, accompanied by a comprehensive model answer which will prepare you for a much wider range of variations of the cases than could ever be covered in a single book.

In addition to the top 100 cases, we have also included an important preliminary section of preparation for the examination, developed over many years by distilling comments from past examiners and candidates. This section shows you how to make the best use of your existing radiological knowledge, e.g., by showing you how to deal with hard cases and what to do when you are completely stuck.

You can step up a gear in your performance simply by developing an examination technique and phrase bank which allows you to concentrate on the images, and without devoting unnecessary brain processing power to thinking about what you are going to say or how you are going to say it.

This book will increase your confidence going into your final oral examinations.
Good luck!

Richard White
Robin Proctor
Ian Zealley

Contents

How this book works

If you are about to sit your radiology oral examination then there is one thing you really *don't* need to worry about, and that is whether you know enough radiology. By getting to this stage, you have proven that you do.

Many candidates fear the oral examinations. Despite the solid foundation in your knowledge, what you may not be so good at is verbally articulating it in a fashion that reassures the examiners you possess the requisite perception, interpretation and management skills to be a radiologist. There is already the substantial challenge of reading and interpreting the examiners' cases in a stressful environment. In addition, there is the challenge of finding words with which to express yourself.

The goal of the 'suggested response' sections in this book is to arm you with phrases and structured responses which will allow you to devote your attention to reading the images, and not worry about what you are going to say as you discuss your findings. If you learn phrases from the scripts, you can focus on the 'working things out' bit while the eloquent descriptions flowing from you are, in fact, made up of phrases you have already learnt and rehearsed during practice sessions.

Reading this book will enable you to make the most out of what you already know. You will also learn how to avoid the terrible spiral of sequential bad cases. And if you do find yourself sinking without trace, we offer advice to help you to dig yourself out of the deepest holes.

Preparing for the examination

Senior radiology viva examinations format

Most senior radiology examinations employ a digital workstation-based format which reflects a typical working environment. A digital imaging and communications in medicine (DICOM) viewer is used, although this may be different from the radiology information system (RIS)/picture archiving and communication systems (PACS) with which you are familiar from your workplace. It is desirable that you acquaint yourself with the relevant hardware and software that will be used in your examination. You should be able to find out details about what type of workstation and what DICOM viewer software you will be using from the examining body.
On the day of the examination, you will be given instructions on how to use the equipment. Nevertheless, it would be preferable if you are already familiar with the format employed. You may find an examination preparation course which allows you to practise using the set-up used in the viva. You may be lucky enough to have workstations using the examination set-up in your own department. One way or another, you should make a concerted effort to become adept at using the prescribed DICOM viewer prior to your viva.

Despite the fact that we all use PACS-based digital images, in this book we frequently use the term 'film' to describe radiological images. This is because even in the digital era this descriptor remains in common usage. An image or film 'goes up' at the start of a case and 'comes down' at its conclusion.

Different types of examiner

You will encounter a variety of examiners in your viva. Some may appear more friendly and more talkative than others. Some will provide a lot of relevant clinical history when a new case is presented, and will indulge in discussion about the cases. Others might put films up giving little background, listen as you talk about the case and then switch to the next case while saying nothing: The dreaded 'silent' examiner. You may struggle to know what the silent examiner is thinking or wanting: Does the fact that a case is staying up mean you are completely wrong? That you have not quite got the right diagnosis. That they want another relevant comment from you, to 'earn' you the right to see the next case. You may never know. You may meet a 'hawk' who interrupts you, challenges you and seems unsympathetic or even pedantic, or you may meet a 'dove' who may smile a lot and appear friendly. The important thing is that you should expect a range of different behaviours from different examiners and not be put off by it. They will have similar pass rates regardless of their demeanour and will be assessing the same skills.

We have structured our 'suggested responses' as if being delivered to a 'silent' examiner, because this allows us to make them as comprehensive as possible. The radiological findings are presented, followed by interpretation of key points and, if relevant, a management plan. The text supplies everything you would need to achieve full marks in a situation where the examiner does not provide any relevant clinical information.

Examination set-up

Your examination may consist of one session or multiple sessions, possibly over several days. Typically, there will be two examiners in each viva room, who may take turns in acting as examiner and marker/grader or may both mark all the cases. The premise is that you are performing as a general radiologist and the examiners are assessing your ability to help clinicians who want you to help them to manage their patients effectively. Remember that these are *clinical* radiology examinations and that you are being evaluated as a *clinical* radiologist who helps clinicians to help their patients. Also, remember you are not expected to be an all-knowing expert in all sub-specialties and the examiners are not trying to catch you out, make you look foolish or prove that they are superior.

Examiners see too many candidates who switch to viva mode, with an 'eyes-ahead' demeanour. They prefer ordinary human social interaction, lightening what for them is often a long, repetitive day. If you use normal social cues then you are already ahead. Be yourself: Your ordinary, everyday body language is both appropriate and welcome. Being yourself is also the easiest way for you to behave because no rehearsal is required.

If the examination is in person, greet both examiners with a smile. When you are seated, always turn towards the examiner who is talking to you, just as you do when you are talking to people at work. One former senior examiner suggests that it is nice if candidates 'sparkle.' We accept that this is a tall order on viva day, but do try to maintain your ordinary, sociable behaviour and avoid becoming robotic and rigid.

If the examination is online then your 'point of contact' with the examiners is the tiny camera lens at the top of the screen. Clearly, this is very different from your normal working environment but as we are all becoming more used to online meetings the setup should not feel too awkward. The important point to remember is that when you are talking to the examiners (not reviewing images) you should look directly at the camera and not at the screen. From the examiners perspective this looks like you are talking directly to them and is far more 'normal' than talking downwards to your own screen (which is what you see most people doing in online meetings). So, say 'hello' looking directly into the camera, and remember to look up into the camera whenever you are engaged in dialogue with the examiners.

Adopt a neutral but positive posture. Sit upright, very slightly tilted forward. Many candidates find it helpful to have something in their hand–a pen to point with in in-person examinations and perhaps their hand resting on the computer mouse to avoid fidgeting for digital examinations. If you happen to look away from the screen or the examiners, make sure you look up and not down. Looking downwards conveys an air of defeat! Do not shut your eyes and do not groan when a difficult film goes up. Do not touch the screen; use the electronic cursor or a pen for pointing.

When you start to speak, think about your cadence; that is, the speed and rhythm of your speech. Think of the best lecturers you ever heard at medical school.

Did they speak really fast? Almost certainly not. Speaking slowly conveys an impression of thoughtfulness and consideration. In contrast, fast speech tends to sound disorganised. You can use this to your advantage: Firstly, it is relatively easy to adopt a slightly slower speaking style, giving an impression of thoughtfulness; secondly, by taking a little longer to speak you have more 'thinking time' to ensure that what you are about to say makes sense.

Practise appropriate posture and manner throughout every practice session. Ask close friends and colleagues to tell you how you come over when you present cases. In particular, ask them to point out any irritating habits or unhelpful phrases.

It is possible that you may have to sit your viva examination using an online format where your only interaction with the examiners is via video link. In this section, we suggest several behaviours for face-to-face examinations which are impossible to replicate in online examinations but there are alternative strategies which you may adopt. The main thing to remember is that when you are looking at the images on the screen you are not looking at the examiners directly. In ordinary everyday speech, people look at each other. The way to do this in an online viva is to look at the camera and not at the screen. This is very important when you want to show the examiners that you have stopped talking, and to help to initiate a dialogue between you and the examiners. So, if this is what will be happening in your viva you should practise it in your viva practice sessions. At moments when you would normally turn to the examiner and talk directly to them in a face-to-face setting, you should look up at the top edge of the screen instead and pretend you are talking to, and looking at the camera. This will look and feel very odd to you and also to your colleague who is running the viva practice session but if you explain what you are doing they will understand.

Using a structured response for each image

It helps if you stick to the same basic template when each new image goes up. Avoid complete silence. Prolonged silence in a viva is awful but we will arm you with a selection of phrases which will prevent a yawning chasm of silence from opening up in front of you. Having said that, the first step in your standard structure for reporting is a brief silence.

A brief silence

A few seconds of silence are fine. This gives you time to marshal your thoughts and will also avoid you appearing too hasty. Think of the best radiologists you know. It is far more likely that they are measured, perhaps even ponderous, in their approach to films. Be the same and consider them as role models for the examination.

Describe the image(s)

Say what the film is. In particular, repeat any clinical information which you may have been given, e.g. 'This is a frontal chest radiograph of an adult female who presents with a history of cough...'.

Repetition of any clinical information is crucially important. It shows that you were listening (which is polite) and it will also help to steer you away from false trails. If you are given any information about a film, it will be critically important to the appropriate interpretation of the findings. The information will not be deliberately deceptive. Repeating it helps you to remember what was said.

Describe any positive findings

If there is an obvious abnormality then that is the place to start, so do not spend ages seeking out further abnormalities before you start to speak. Even if you are really struggling to spot the abnormality, one excellent piece of advice is to identify *anything* on the film which is definitely not normal and start talking about that. This begins a dialogue which will hopefully steer you onto the right track. At the very least, it shows willing. If you are using a review pattern, then talk the examiners through it as you use it. Do not allow silences to build up: Keep talking, even if very slowly.

Summarise

Again, as you summarise positive findings, repeat any clinical information you were given. You will find your own form of words, but consider using a phrase such as 'So, we have...', 'To summarise, this is a...' or 'In summary...'.

After a few practice sessions, you will tire of hearing yourself repeating the same phrase, but your phrases will be new to your examiners, so this is fine. Accept that you will repeat yourself and do not waste energy trying to sound different and exciting with every new film.

State pertinent negatives if appropriate but only truly pertinent ones, e.g. 'There is subcutaneous emphysema but no pneumothorax'. For the examiners, there is nothing more dull than a list of features that are not present.

After your summary turn your body very slightly towards the examiner and face him or her (or look directly at the camera if the examination is not face-to-face), just as you would in an everyday clinical setting. This sends a very strong nonverbal cue that it is his or her turn to speak next. This sort of cue is almost irresistible to the recipient, so do experiment with it: In any conversation, not necessarily at work, turn slightly towards the other person, look at his or her face, and stop talking. They will invariably start to speak after a pause of a second or two. For all cases, and particularly for less straightforward ones, you really want to move on to a dialogue stage between you and the examiner, so use every tool you have to stimulate this.

Diagnosis and differential diagnosis

If there is a single diagnosis (an 'Aunt Minnie' case, for example), then say so: 'The features indicate a diagnosis of...' or 'The features suggest...' (if you are less certain or generally more cautious).

If there is not a single obvious diagnosis then you must talk about differential diagnoses. The usual way of doing this is to list possibilities in descending order of likelihood. But below, we will suggest a different approach: A *conditional* differential diagnosis list. This will help you to be more confident in suggesting potential diagnoses when you are not certain of the definitive diagnosis.

Personal style plays a part here. Some candidates will naturally feel more willing to commit themselves to a diagnosis than others.

Suggested further investigation or management

Remember that you are sitting for a *clinical* radiology examination. Demonstrating your grasp of basic medical knowledge can go a long way towards persuading the examiners that you understand that each image you see corresponds to a real patient. What you say does not have to cover highly specialist ground: Good solid sensible suggestions are the order of the day, e.g. 'I would like to take this further by discussing the findings with the clinician and perhaps performing an ultrasound scan to confirm that these lesions are solid and not cystic'.

Subsequent steps should be *suggested* rather than described as being *required*. If there is a range of options, start the discussion with simple ones and escalate to more complex tests or interventions, if appropriate.

Discussion

There are relatively few spot diagnosis films or 'Aunt Minnies' in the senior radiology viva examinations. Candidates are sometimes surprised to find themselves engaged in discussions with the examiners, rather than just listing differential diagnoses. Do not be surprised if an examiner uses a case as a springboard to discuss anatomy, technical considerations as to how a study should be performed, what investigation would be the most appropriate in a particular circumstance or something else topical in modern day radiology.

Summary

Develop your own version of this standard structure for each case. Each film/case in your examination will be different, the history and the findings will be different, but if you always stick to your structured response pattern you will always know where you are in your responses because you will be using your own rehearsed turns of phrase, in an approach that you have developed to work for you.

Conditional differential diagnosis

The differential diagnosis is the stage at which a candidate who has picked up all the pertinent radiological signs can shine. Conversely, one way of losing momentum is to put all your mental energy into deciding which is the best order in which to list the differential diagnoses. So instead, consider using a *conditional differential diagnosis*: Speak about each of the diagnoses you think are likely, introducing each one with a suitable caveat.

For the real patient in the image, there is of course only one correct diagnosis, but senior radiology vivas are not all about giving the 'right' answer. They are about demonstrating that you have an understanding of how radiographic findings relate to real patients in real clinical scenarios. A 'conditional' approach to offering differential diagnoses allows you to show several possibilities and relevant clinical considerations. More than that, it allows you to score points for the wrong answers as well as the right ones.

Use the magic word 'If', for example, '*If* the patient is acutely unwell I would be wondering about...', 'On the other hand, *if* the presentation has been more insidious...', '*If* the patient is older...', and '*If* there is a past history of recent abdominal surgery...'.

Using this type of phrase before each suggested diagnosis shows that you are thinking about the patient not just the images. It is a 'considered' differential rather than just a list. Another bonus is that for each clinical scenario that you describe, the diagnosis that you are offering is correct, even if it is not the actual diagnosis for the patient whose image is being discussed.

This approach is far less stressful than having to decide which is the most likely diagnosis. It avoids having to commit to one diagnosis, and it can even include some of the most implausible options without over-committing, because you can preface them with an appropriate clinical scenario. This form of discussion can also act as a prompt for further clinical information in a much more elegant fashion than asking for it directly. It also acts as a prompt for dialogue, which may be more interesting for the examiner.

Many past candidates have described feeling as if they have 'changed up a gear' when they get used to presenting in this way. We strongly urge you to try it. It may feel unnatural at first, but once you have developed a few short phrases to link your imaginary clinical scenarios to your proposed different diagnoses you should feel relaxed and confident presenting your interpretations in this clinically-oriented fashion.

(Ultra) simplified surgical sieve

If your interpretation of the image(s) does not appear to add up to a specific diagnosis or even a broad class of disease, we suggest you use a form of 'surgical sieve' to structure your comments. This is not the list of more than a dozen options that you may recall from medical school, rather it is an effective and concise abbreviated list of categories:

- Congenital/acquired
- Trauma (including iatrogenic or postsurgical)
- Neoplastic – benign, malignant primary or secondary
- Inflammatory – infective, noninfective idiopathic, autoimmune or connective tissue disorder
- Cardiovascular – ischaemic, thromboembolic or haemorrhagic
- Endocrine – hormonally driven processes

In the viva setting, this helps you home in on the right disease 'territory'. If you have summarised your findings but are still not sure of the answer, then mentally working through this list can enable you to promptly exclude very unlikely options. For instance, you might say, 'I am not sure that I can tie all of the findings together neatly, but clearly the condition is an acquired one and is either inflammatory or neoplastic in nature'.

There are several ways of going forward from this point. Either the examiner will accept that it is time to open a dialogue or you can reach for the phrases we describe below in the section 'What to do if you get stuck' (p. 8).

Closing

For a few 'Aunt Minnie' cases you will be able to discuss your findings using an almost entirely rehearsed speech (e.g. rheumatoid hands), but for most you will not. For the majority, the non-'Aunt Minnie's, it is reassuring to progress with your own structured pattern, using many of your own rehearsed phrases. However, one thing that is common to both types of case is the importance of *closing* the film.

Closing is essential because it allows you to progress. If you do not close then you might be lucky and have examiners who help you out, but it is more likely you will end up either repeating yourself over and over again, or enduring an uncomfortable silence. Closing is easy but only you can do it, not the examiners. Practise it all the time so that it becomes natural for you before the viva itself.

As we have already described it is a good idea to use body language to animate the exchange with the examiner. When you want to close (and thereby start a dialogue), turn towards the examiner and talk to them as you would to a colleague at work, perhaps 10–15°, still predominantly facing the screen but also clearly engaging the examiner. As discussed earlier, this is a powerful everyday social cue that you have finished talking and that it is time for a dialogue (or perhaps the next image).

When you have come to the end of what you can say about a film you must stop yourself from talking (no one else will stop you). This simple turn-and-stop technique provides a mechanism to do this while simultaneously prompting the examiner that it is his or her turn to speak.

By doing this you will avoid repeating what you have already said and going around in circles and losing momentum, which will certainly not convince the examiners that you are about to 'crack' the case. It is very obvious to examiners when a candidate is failing to draw a case to a conclusion. It is far better to present what you have found, together with at least a stab at broad disease categories using your (ultra) simplified surgical sieve. You can even offer a way forward by following the suggestions in the 'What to do if you get stuck' section (p. 8), but whatever you do you must stop talking.

Requesting additional information

Sometimes you will think that you are stuck and there is no way forward without being able to compare the image with an earlier one or by knowing more about a specific aspect of the patient's clinical condition.

Different people will give different advice on this. Some will suggest that you should always ask for previous images or pre-contrast images if these would usually be available in clinical practice. However, we suggest that you consider why the examiner has selected a case for the viva. It may be an elegant example that does not require sight of a previous image (or pre-contrast images) to reach the diagnosis, for example, or a case that the examiners have found particularly interesting themselves.

We suggest that you should never ask for additional information or previous images. Examiners may not like knee-jerk requests like 'please may I see the pre-contrast images', in part because they may be proud that their films do not need any help to interpret, and in part because it just sounds so lame.

Instead, adopt an approach similar to the conditional differential diagnosis we described above, and receive credit for thinking of several ways of interpreting a film. It is easy to incorporate a request for further information into a conditional structure, again using the magic word '*if*': '*If* this is a new finding compared with previous films...; '*If* this is seen to be anterior on a lateral film.... On the other hand, *if* it is seen to be posterior...; and '*If* this is also evident on the pre-contrast images....'

By adopting this approach, you can resolve your indecision elegantly and in a way which, like a conditional differential diagnosis, allows you to score points for the 'wrong' answers as well as the 'right' ones.

What to do if you get stuck

You will get stuck on at least one case, maybe more, so it is vitally important that you anticipate this and practise a form of words that will help you to progress without losing momentum. No candidate will sail through all the cases without ever getting stuck. Examiners always have a supply of increasingly difficult cases in reserve, to stretch the most able candidates.

If you cannot think what to say then be prepared to say so, if not in so many words. There is no point in sitting in silence, becoming more uncomfortable. Keep talking and keep moving forwards.

Of course, in this situation what you really want to say is 'If I was stuck like this with a film at work I would discuss the case with the clinician and I would like to do that with you....' So why not say something like that? Develop your own form of words to indicate to the examiners that in the real-life world you would do whatever is necessary to work out the diagnosis and help the patient. This is exactly the sort of attribute that senior radiologists want to see in prospective colleagues: They want to see that you are prepared to admit when you cannot work something out, and that you will take whatever steps needed to help sort the patient out.

Other turns of phrase you might find useful are 'I am not comfortable that some of the findings I have described adequately explain the clinical picture...' or 'I am not comfortable that I have identified all of the pertinent radiographic findings on this image...; followed by a pause and then something like 'In ordinary clinical practice (or 'at work'), I would get in touch with the clinician and discuss the patient's presentation and past history to see if together we could get closer to understanding what we are seeing here and what is going on with this patient.'

If you say something along these lines then the examiner simply must step in, acting the part of the clinician and giving you at least some clinical information to guide you forwards. Once again, we suggest using the simple, powerful non-verbal cues that prompt a dialogue: A slight twist of the body, a glance at their face (or look directly at the camera if not face-to-face).

Getting stuck is stressful: It is important that the turns of phrase you use are so well-rehearsed, automatic and embedded that you can use them even when you feel things are going wrong.

'Bad' cases

It is normal to have one or more 'bad' cases. It would be quite extraordinary if you emerged from your viva feeling that there had been no tough cases. Everyone will tell you to forget a 'bad' case, and they are right. Prepare for this by accepting, ahead of the viva, that there are going to be some bad cases in your viva.

When a bad case comes along it is just part of the process. Just accept it and use the tools and tricks which we have described to get as far with it as you can: Use the techniques you have developed for those times that you get stuck or need to request further information. A dialogue will ensue and no matter how that goes the film will come down. And as soon as it is down, move on.

Complex cases

In the examination, just as in real life, you will occasionally see extremely complex cases with so much going on that it is almost impossible to know where to start. Outside the context of a viva, these might take a long time to report and necessitate detailed discussions with radiological or clinical colleagues. In the viva, time is of the essence and you have nobody to ask for a second opinion. The examiners know this: They are not necessarily looking for definitive answers, just a considered response that proves you know how to handle the situation.

Do not be deterred when facing images with multiple findings: Start as you would with any case and go on to describe the abnormalities, keeping to the system you normally use.

Talk about the really important elements first

In clinical practice, if you identified an immediately life-threatening finding then you would not keep it to yourself for 10 minutes while you painstakingly reviewed every additional finding. You would ensure that it was dealt immediately before moving on to identify less relevant features. Do the same in a viva. For example, for a CT scan of a polytrauma patient you might conclude 'There is an active extravasation of intravenous contrast from the thoracic aorta. I would immediately explain this to the trauma team leader making sure they appreciate this patient may require immediate cardiothoracic surgery or endovascular intervention.'

Be systematic

Develop your own systematic approach to describe other findings, and stick to it. If there are lines and tubes, list them and state whether they are appropriately positioned (if they are not, mention what you would do about this). And remember, misplaced lines and tubes are *far* more common in viva films than they are in real life, so be particularly vigilant about these. Then describe the other findings according to your system.

For a chest radiograph, this might be to look at the heart and mediastinum, lungs, upper abdomen, bones, and soft tissues, in that order, revisiting your review areas at the end. In an abdominal CT scan, you might review all solid viscera before looking at bowel, lymph nodes, peritoneal surfaces, bones, muscles, lung bases, and subcutaneous tissues.

Multiple similar findings

With complex cases, it is particularly tempting to spend time counting or listing things. This is not necessary. There might be enlarged left inguinal iliac, right common iliac, para-aortic, aortocaval and portocaval lymph nodes, or multiple rib fractures in trauma, but it is not worth spending time identifying every enlarged node or fractured rib. Instead say something like 'There is widespread abdominal and pelvic lymphadenopathy' or 'There are multiple bilateral rib fractures, of which the most significant are displaced fractures involving the right first and second ribs.'

Remember to highlight any particularly pertinent findings, for instance, 'There are multiple thoracolumbar vertebral fractures, of which the most significant is a burst fracture of T12 with retropulsion of a large fragment of bone into the spinal canal.'

Summarising

In a straightforward case, it may not be necessary to summarise the findings when closing, because this risks repeating almost everything you have just said. In complex cases, however, summarising may help by refreshing own memory of the findings and by giving you extra time to pull together the pieces of the puzzle.

Diagnosis or differential diagnosis?

Now you need to draw your conclusions based on the findings. If you are not sure of the exact diagnosis then proceed by offering a conditional differential diagnosis, as described above. However, if you feel confident, state the diagnosis, e.g.: 'In summary, there is a mass in the stomach which is likely to represent gastric carcinoma accompanied by ascites and features in keeping with nodal, hepatic and sclerotic bone metastases. Bilateral ovarian masses are also evident. These may be unrelated to the other findings but I am suspicious that they represent Krukenberg tumours....'

What about a syndrome you do not recognise?

You might be fairly sure that various findings can be tied together as part of a syndrome but you cannot remember what the syndrome is. Do not worry. It would be reasonable to say something along the lines of: 'In summary, this infant has multiple abnormalities including cerebellar hypoplasia, grey matter heterotopia, absence of the corpus callosum and microphthalmos. These findings are almost certainly part of a complex congenital disorder although I am unsure which syndrome or condition they represent. In my usual practice, I would consult a textbook or clinical or radiological colleagues to help to make the diagnosis.'

If you cannot put it all together

The case could have a range of findings or you may be unable to decide whether the findings are linked. In either instance just say so. If you have clearly described the clinically relevant findings and have stated what you would do next, then it is likely that you are doing alright. Consulting textbooks and colleagues is something that everyone does in real life at work, including the examiners, and saying so is an indication that you are safe to practise rather than an admission of weakness.

A few specifics and exceptions

Mention lines and tubes first

If you do not do this first then you may forget. Mentioning them demonstrates that you are thinking about the clinical status of the patient, which will help to guide you into the right clinical zone for interpreting the film. Keep in mind that misplaced lines and tubes are far more common in vivas and teaching collections than they are in real life, so be particularly vigilant for this.

Lumps and masses

Anywhere in the body, on any modality, your primary task is to determine whether the lesion is benign/nonaggressive or malignant/aggressive. Once you have done this, it will be easier for you to talk through a differential diagnosis.

Changing your mind

As you progress through a case you may wish to revise an initial observation. That is fine, we all do it all the time at work. Simply say 'on reflection…' and move on.

Terminology

Radiographic images are 'radiographs' not 'X-rays', though they can still be called 'films' (see p. 1).

Use the correct terminology for each modality: Density for plain films, attenuation for CT, reflectivity (rather than echogenicity) for ultrasound, signal intensity for MRI, tracer uptake for radioisotope studies.

Consider using 'high' or 'low' rather than 'hyper' and 'hypo', particularly if you have a strong accent or tend to speak quickly, because they are less easily misheard and harder for you to confuse.

Radioisotope examinations

You may not see these studies every day at work. It is worth spending a couple of hours reminding yourself how the basic radioisotope studies are performed. In the viva, a good way of working out what is going on in a radioisotope image is to talk through the actual methodology of how the test is performed as you describe the image. It sounds good, helps to prompt you in the right direction and buys you thinking time.

Trauma

Trauma is a very common topic in senior radiology viva examinations, and is widely regarded as an excellent discriminator between good and bad candidates. Whenever you have practice sessions with your seniors ask them to show you the trauma cases in their collections. You cannot see too many examples of trauma before your examination. Make the rules of trauma reporting second nature, mention what might be seen on the orthogonal view (rather than ask for it), and always mention the soft tissues.

Trauma to the cervical spine is a common examination film, and it is the only one where you should be seen to count the vertebrae to ensure that coverage is adequate. Otherwise, do not count ribs and vertebrae: It is time consuming and implies that you think that getting the number right is as important as giving an appropriate opinion on the pathology.

Chest radiographs

There is a limited number of lung spaces for diseases to occupy so restrict yourself to the terms 'airspace', 'interstitial' and 'pleural' and use the more elaborate terms 'reticulo-nodular', 'ground glass', etc. only when you are confident that they are right for the film. Sticking with the plain anatomical terms will also help to guide you through your differential, especially if you have had the foresight to think about what would be on your conditional differential diagnosis lists for disease in each of the three anatomical spaces.

Arthropathies

Avoid drawing too many conclusions from a film of a single joint: You need to know the distribution between joints. For a severely damaged joint, it may be very difficult or impossible to work out what has caused the damage or there may be a secondary condition involved. Also look carefully at some of the less severely affected joints, where more classic (and diagnostic) features may still be visible.

Mammograms

Ensure that you are familiar with the way in which mammograms are displayed and reported. This may be less of an issue in a digital examination but a sure-fire way of making a bad impression is to display the images in the wrong order. Also make sure you use the right terms to localise abnormalities (using quadrants or a clock face). Make sure you know how to use the magnification function on the DICOM viewer, if needed.

Emergency management

For a variety of diagnoses, it is appropriate that you indicate that you recognise the urgent need to communicate the findings to the clinical team. You should develop a form of words which shows that you would not rely on anyone but yourself and the referring clinician to recognise the gravity of the situation, e.g. 'The diagnosis is emphysematous cholecystitis. This is a surgical emergency. At work, I would pick up the phone and ask switchboard for the bleep number of the senior surgeon on call and speak to them myself immediately.'

You might worry about what you will say if you see a tension pneumothorax. We have spoken to a lot of radiologists in a lot of countries and have not found anyone who has seen a tension pneumothorax film in a senior radiology viva examination. But in case you do, remember that you should say you would immediately insert a wide-bore cannula in the second intercostal space in the midclavicular line on the affected side and then insert a formal chest drain.

And finally…

- If there is any written information on the images then mention it: Erect, pre-contrast, 30 minutes, etc.
- A brief appropriate silence is better than a 'er…' or 'um…'
- The viva is not the place to air your opinion on any deficiencies in your training scheme so do not offer an excuse like 'I have not seen many radionuclide studies.' It will not elicit leniency from your examiners and it may make them work harder to seek weaknesses in your experience and knowledge.
- If an image is diagnostic then say so. If not, you should be closing with a plan, using your rehearsed structure.

- For 'classic' cases you absolutely must learn the terms and phrases that earn all the points. This includes diffuse interstitial lung disease, rheumatoid arthritis, aggressive bone lesion, etc. You will not use your whole rehearsed response but the rehearsed phrases will be invaluable.

Personal appearance

Most examination rooms for in-person examinations are too small and too hot. Have a good shower in the morning and brush your teeth.

Whether in person or online, the examiners are judging your radiology knowledge, nothing more, but your clothing should be appropriate for a senior radiologist at work. If you would not be comfortable wearing your outfit to speak to patients or their relatives then do not wear it in the viva. For men, we suggest that you are either clean shaven or have a proper beard (avoid in between). Wear a suit with a tie, and do up the top shirt button. For women, wear a suit or similarly smart outfit: Avoid low-cut tops or tight-fitting clothes.

If your first language is not the language of the examination, or you have a strong regional accent

Senior radiology examinations do not often contain language tests per se. However, they are intended to determine whether you can function safely in the local radiology departments, where an appropriate level of fluency and clarity of local language is required.

When examiners are trying to decide if you should pass the examination, they can only presume that your ability to communicate with them is the same as it would be with your colleagues. If they cannot understand you or you cannot understand them, they will come to the conclusion that you would not be safe simply because you cannot communicate effectively.

Most people find it harder to communicate in a second language when they are under stress. They may respond in several ways. They may speak more quickly, their accent may become stronger, or they may become very hesitant. Similarly, people with strong regional accents may find their accents becoming stronger when under pressure.

Take time to talk to close friends and colleagues who are not from the same region as you, or who do not share the same first language. Ask them to tell you how you behave under stress and particularly what happens to your speech, especially in terms of speed and accent. Listen carefully to their feedback and act on it. If they say your speech speeds up and/or your accent becomes thicker and more difficult to understand, then you must rehearse minimising these effects in your practice sessions.

Handling films

This book is written with the digital workstation examination format in mind, in keeping with contemporaneous radiology practice. If your examination still uses traditional films–or indeed if you attend teaching sessions or courses with radiologists who still make use of their film collections–then you should be familiar with how to handle them. Never touch a film without asking the examiner first (no-one wants to see their precious cases covered in fingerprints) and use a pen or similar for pointing to the relevant abnormalities. Be aware of how to read cross-sectional studies. You may need, or suggest to the examiner, a magnifying glass, particularly for mammograms.

Homework

Arrange as many practice viva sessions with as many different qualified radiologists as you can. Colleagues who have recently passed the same examination are often particularly helpful. Use the relevant workstation and DICOM viewer software, if and when you can. Do not underestimate the value of practising with colleagues who are sitting the examination at the same time as you. Taking turns at playing the 'examiner' gives you an interesting insight into what comes across well (and what does not). You can work out good turns of phrase together and refine them for the 'classic' images.

Rehearse your own structure until it flows without any need to think about what comes next: Silence → description → summary → differential → suggestions. In particular, you must ensure that you close every film by stopping talking.

Practise using the magic word 'If' for a conditional approach to differential diagnosis and when you think you would ask for an extra image or additional clinical information.

Work out your own reliable routines for cases where you get 'stuck' and for 'bad cases,' and rehearse them until you are comfortable using them. And expect to use them. Do not be knocked sideways by bad cases–they are just part of the viva.

You do not need to be lucky. Be prepared instead.

Case 1

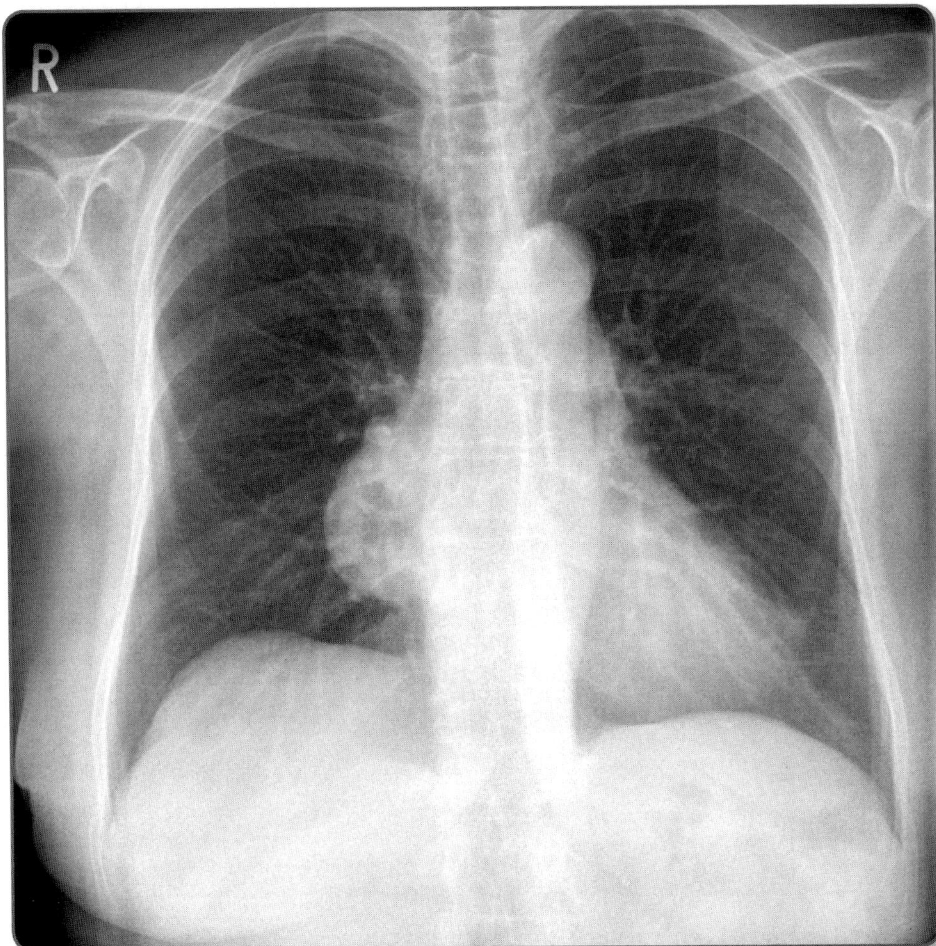

Suggested response

This is a frontal chest radiograph of a skeletally mature female patient. A homogeneous soft tissue density is projected medially in the right mid and lower zones. It is rounded and well-defined laterally but the medial aspect is not visualised separately from the mediastinum. It forms obtuse angles with the lung, implying a mediastinal rather than a pulmonary mass. The right hilum is clearly visualised through the mass. The right heart border at this level is not visualised, although it is evident inferior to the mass. These features suggest that the mass is localised to the anterior mediastinum.

The lungs are clear and there are no abnormalities of the thoracic cage. Both breast shadows are present.

Review of any available and relevant previous imaging would be useful to assess for change, together with consideration of the patient's current symptoms. If this is the first presentation, further investigation will be necessary, probably with a CT scan in the first instance. At this location, the differential diagnosis should include pericardial cysts and cardiac aneurysms as well as lymphoma and germ cell tumours.

Diagnosis

Right-sided pericardial cyst in an adult female.

Tips: Mediastinal mass on a chest radiograph

This is a very common case, so it is important to recap the differential diagnoses relating to the anterior, middle and posterior mediastinum.

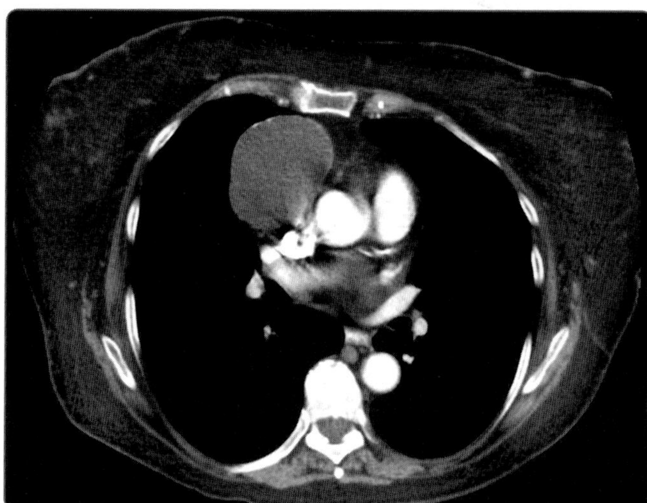

Figure 1 Post-contrast CT image from this case, demonstrating the homogeneous, well-defined pericardial cyst.

Key points

Consider whether the mass is mediastinal or pulmonary in origin. In general, pulmonary masses form acute angles with the mediastinum and mediastinal masses form obtuse angles.

On a frontal view, the visualisation of the hilar vessels through a mass (*hilum overlay sign*) localises the mass to the anterior or posterior mediastinum (more commonly the anterior mediastinum). Paraspinal line deviation indicates a posterior mediastinal mass, and any mass located above the superior aspect of the clavicle is either posterior mediastinal or cervical in origin.

On the lateral view, the retrosternal space may be obliterated by anterior mediastinal masses. However, this space may be filled by fat in people who are obese.

Posterior mediastinal masses cause loss of the normal increasing transradiancy (in a craniocaudal direction) down the vertebral column.

Pericardial cyst

Pericardial cysts are rare (prevalence around 1 in 100,000) and are typically incidental findings. They may present with symptoms such as dyspnoea and atypical chest pain if sufficiently large due to pressure effects. They are usually right-sided and are most commonly located at the cardiophrenic angle. (Note that the differential diagnoses for abnormalities at this location should include Morgagni hernia and bronchopulmonary sequestration, rather than the typical mediastinal mass differential diagnoses). However, they may be found in any of the anterior, middle or posterior mediastinal compartments. A CT scan of a pericardial cyst typically demonstrates a thin-walled, well-defined, rounded mass which is homogeneous nonenhancing and slightly hyperattenuating relative to water (30–40 HU).

Case 2

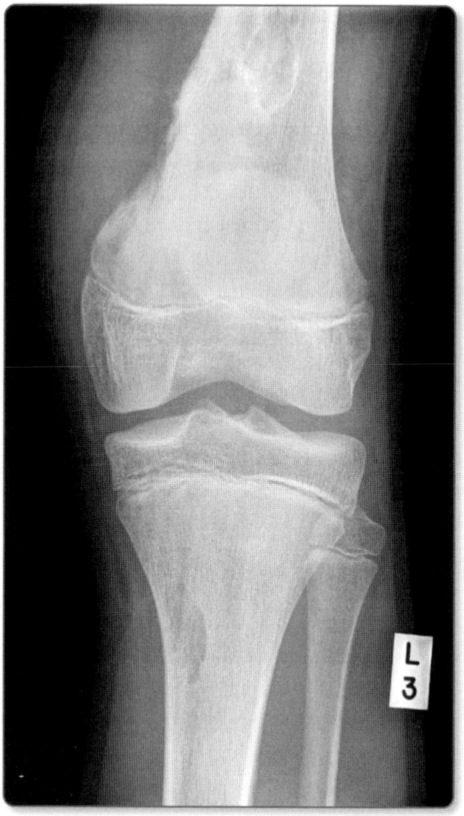

Suggested response

This is an anteroposterior radiograph of the knee of a skeletally immature patient.

There are two abnormalities on this radiograph. There are lesions in both the femur and tibia with very different characteristics.

In the femur, there is a lesion of mixed sclerotic and lucent density with destruction of the lateral cortex of the distal diaphysis and metaphysis and a small Codman's triangle at the inferior margin of this area. The lesion extends proximally beyond the margin of this radiograph but does not appear to involve the physis or cross into the epiphysis. The joint appears normal. There is the impression of a soft tissue mass but no soft tissue calcification. Appearances are consistent with an aggressive lesion. The age of the patient would be relevant; the osseous development in this radiograph suggests an early adolescent, in which case the lesion is most in keeping with an osteosarcoma.

In the lateral aspect of the proximal tibial metaphysis, there is a well-defined, lucent lesion. The margins are clearly defined but not sclerotic, with a narrow zone of transition. It does not appear expansile and there is no visible matrix calcification within the lesion. There is no periosteal reaction, soft tissue mass or other aggressive feature. The most likely aetiology is a nonossifying fibroma.

This patient would be best managed in a specialist bone tumour centre. I would routinely review an orthogonal view and, if these findings are not previously known, then I would urgently discuss the findings with the referring clinician and suggest appropriate referral. The patient will require further imaging with MRI of the entire femur for local staging and assessment for skip metastases, in the first instance. This imaging would also confirm that the apparently nonaggressive tibial lesion is not a metastasis. This patient is likely to need further staging of the tumour, as per local protocol, with at least a CT scan of the chest. Imaging of the other bones with bone scan or whole-body MRI should also be considered, depending on local protocols. A biopsy should only be considered in consultation with the regional specialist tumour centre and is usually avoided until local staging has been completed and surgical planning has been discussed.

Diagnosis

Osteosarcoma of the distal femur in a 13-year-old patient. Small nonossifying fibroma (NOF) in proximal tibia.

Tips: Aggressive bone lesions

Use the terms *aggressive* and *nonaggressive* or *indolent* instead of *malignant* and *benign* when describing bone lesions as they are broader and encompass non-neoplastic pathologies such as infection.

Key points: Focal bone lesion description

Location is important: Which bone and where in the bone? Central or eccentric? Diaphysis, metaphysis or epiphysis? Has it been completely imaged?

Describe lesion features: Is the lesion expansile? Does it cross the physis or involve any visible joint? Is there cortical destruction? Is there a soft tissue mass? Is there calcification within the lesion? If so, is the matrix chondroid or osteoid? Is the zone of transition narrow or wide, well-defined or ill-defined (wide and ill-defined zones of transition are an aggressive feature)?

Mention periosteal reaction: Rapidly growing lesions may have a hair-on-end or sunburst periosteal reaction. However, the most aggressive lesions grow too quickly for periosteal reaction to form. Codman's triangle refers to ossification of periosteum which is raised at the margins of the lesion (with the remainder of the lesion too aggressive for periosteal reaction to form).

Differential diagnosis

It is important to revise the differential diagnoses of focal bone lesions as this is a very common case. The likelihood of a diagnosis depends primarily on the patient's age and site of the lesion (both in terms of the skeleton and in the bone itself), especially for less aggressive lucent bone lesions. In the over-40s, metastasis is the most likely diagnosis when there is a known malignancy, and still very probable even if there is not. Typically, lucent metastases arise from bronchogenic, renal cell and thyroid cancers and melanoma (compare with sclerotic lesions from breast and prostate cancer). Always consider infection.

Osteosarcoma

Osteosarcoma is the most common malignant primary bone tumour and may occur anywhere in the body, but tends to occur in long bones (most frequently the femur). It typically involves the metaphysis and most commonly presents with pain. There is usually at least some sclerotic component and very frequently an aggressive periosteal reaction.

Nonossifying fibroma

NOF were previously referred to as fibrous cortical defects. They are classically eccentric, slightly expansile and have a sclerotic margin, but these findings are not constant. They are extremely common, asymptomatic and are frequently incidental findings. They generally disappear as a child grows and may be metabolically active. There should not be an associated periosteal reaction or internal matrix.

These lesions may be complicated by fracture. The management of large NOFs (which may be at risk of fracture) is controversial.

Case 3

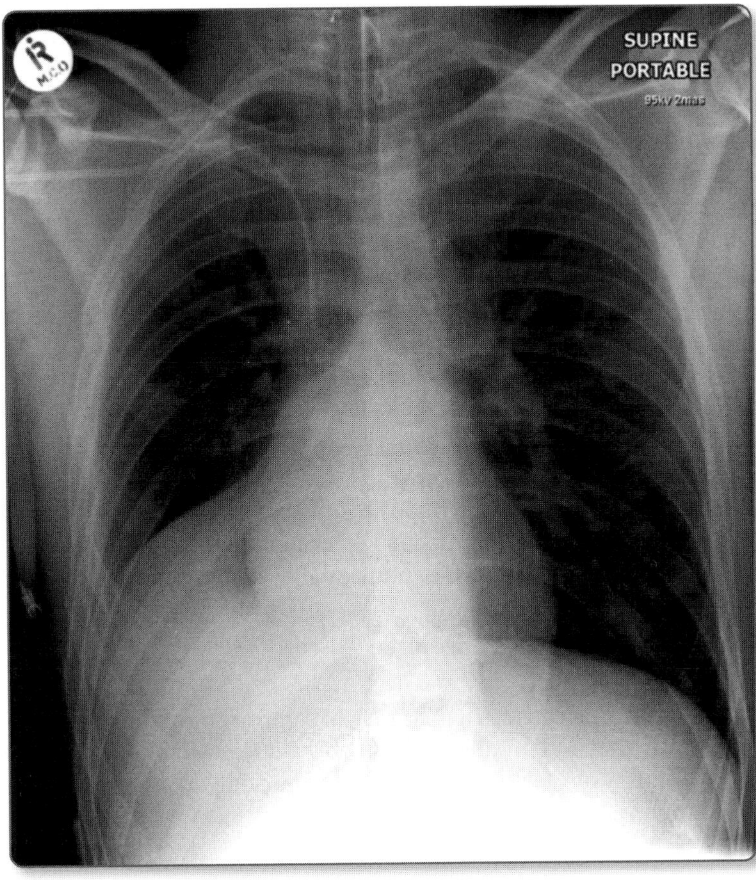

Suggested response

This is a supine chest radiograph of an adult patient.

There is an endotracheal tube (ETT) in an apparently satisfactory position and a right-sided central venous catheter, presumably a subclavian line, which also appears appropriately sited with the tip projected over the superior vena cava (SVC). The patient is also wearing a collar for immobilisation of the cervical spine.

There is volume loss in the right hemithorax with mediastinal shift to the right. The right heart border remains visible but the right hemidiaphragm is obscured by a uniform soft tissue opacity with a linear superior boundary. A very dense triangular opacity is projected over the right side of the mediastinum in the region of the right lower lobe bronchus. The right lower lobe pulmonary artery is not clearly visualised. The remainder of the right lung and the whole of the left lung are clear, but there are several right-sided rib fractures laterally.

The appearance is that of right lower lobe collapse and the cervical immobilisation and rib fractures suggest that the patient may have suffered recent trauma. The very dense opacity could represent a tooth which has been displaced and aspirated.

I would discuss this case urgently with the referring clinician to confirm the history and convey these findings. Assuming that the patient has aspirated a tooth following trauma I would consider a CT and suggest retrieval with bronchoscopy.

Diagnosis

Right lower lobe collapse secondary to aspiration of a tooth following trauma.

Tips: Lobar collapse on chest radiographs

Key points

The 'silhouette' sign occurs when the collapsed lobe obscures the clarity of the edge of the mediastinum or diaphragm which it usually abuts.

Volume loss is indicated by a raised hemidiaphragm, tracheal or mediastinal shift to the side of the collapse, increased transradiancy of the hyperexpanded lung on the side of the collapse, herniation of the opposite lung across midline and hilar elevation/depression (the right hilum should not be higher than the left; middle lobe collapse does not affect hilar position). A mass or effusion may compensate for volume loss.

An underlying cause of the collapse may be visible. For instance, a misplaced ETT (a common example in vivas), neoplastic disease (primary or metastatic), or a radio-opaque foreign body.

When considering the cause of a collapse, take into account the patient's age. The most common cause beyond middle age is an obstructing carcinoma. In children, consider the possibility of a foreign body. Mucous plugging may occur at any age and is common in asthma.

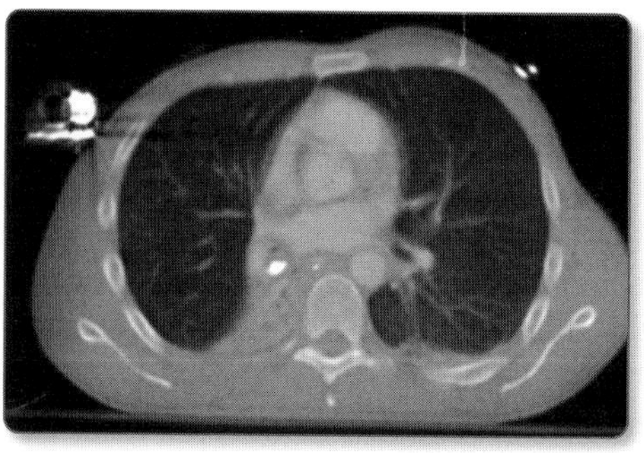

Figure 1 CT through the right lower lobe bronchus, showing a tooth impacted in the bronchus, with associated right lower lobe collapse.

Lobar collapse

Lobar collapse is common in both radiological examinations and everyday radiological practice. It can be subtle, particularly in complete collapse, so ensure that you can recognise the relevant signs and the underlying cause, if possible. Remember that by sitting further away from the radiograph you are more likely to spot any major asymmetry of the volumes of the hemithoraces than if you are very close to the screen. A recommended approach for reviewing chest radiographs is to start well back from the image to gather an overall picture and then close in. Handling a lobar collapse radiograph well is a good opportunity to demonstrate sound knowledge to an examiner.

If a cause is not apparent, then give a conditional differential diagnosis and suggest appropriate further investigations. Be ready to stage a lung carcinoma accurately using a CT scan, or approximately using a plain radiograph, as this is a common cause of lobar collapse.

Case 4

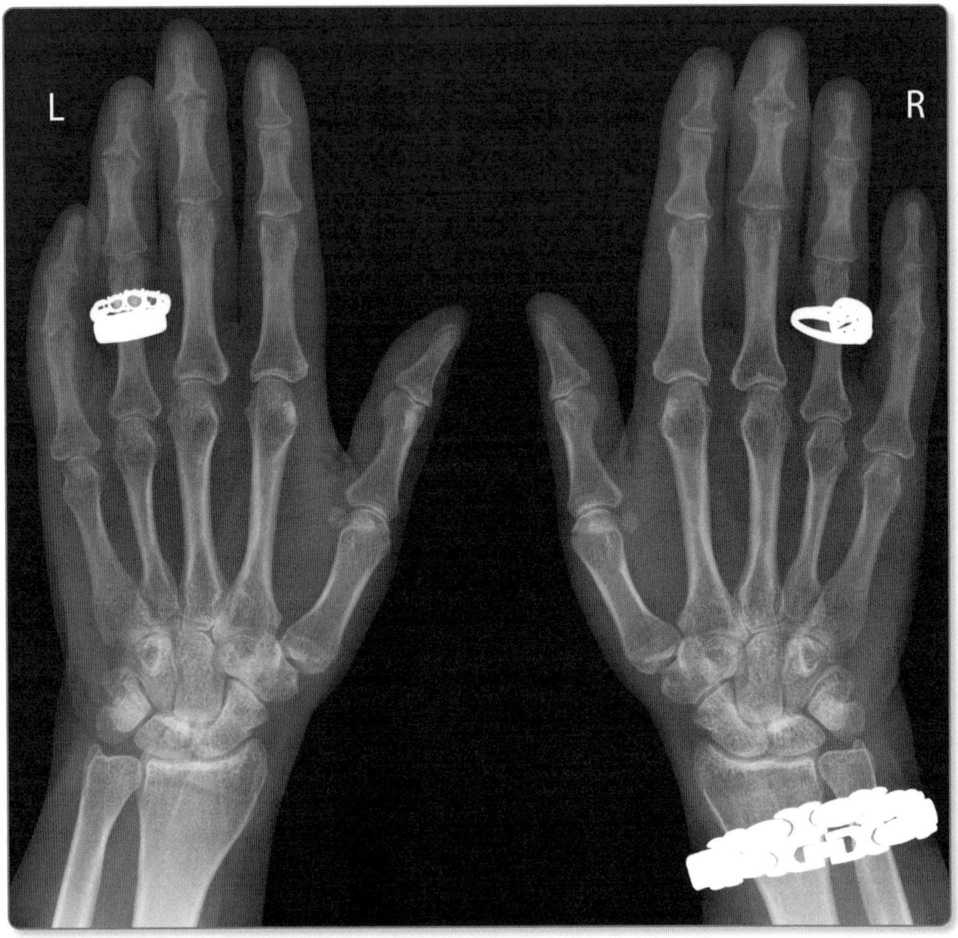

Suggested response

These are dorsipalmar (DP) views of both hands. There is ankylosis of the right little finger proximal interphalangeal (PIP) joint and asymmetrical, erosive polyarthritis involving the whole of the articular surfaces in many other joints. This affects the middle finger distal interphalangeal (DIP) joint in both hands and multiple other joints in the left hand – the DIP joints of the middle, ring and little fingers as well as the left little finger PIP joint.

The metacarpophalangeal (MCP) joints and wrist joints appear normal and the bone density is normal. I cannot see any resorption of the terminal tufts of the phalanges or any soft tissue calcification.

There is marked soft tissue swelling around the right middle finger of DIP joint. The patient has not removed their jewellery and it is possible that pain and swelling prevented them from doing so.

I would like to correlate the findings with those of any other joints which have been imaged now or previously and also the clinical history. However, overall I think the most likely diagnosis is psoriatic arthropathy, although an atypical form of another erosive arthritis could also give this appearance.

Diagnosis

Psoriatic arthropathy.

Tips: Erosive arthropathy (hands)

When reviewing a radiograph of a patient with arthropathy using a systematic approach, it is essential to start with general observations. As you progress through your review you may wish to revise an initial observation; say, 'on reflection...', and move on. If available, refer to other radiographs, e.g. other hand, feet and other joints.

Key points

Comment on deformity and bone density (e.g. periarticular osteopaenia in rheumatoid arthritis).

Consider the distribution and symmetry of disease. Rheumatoid arthritis tends to be symmetrical and spares the DIP joints, erosive osteoarthritis may or may not be symmetrical and tends to spare the MCP joints, while psoriatic arthropathy tends to be asymmetrical but can affect all joints.

Consider the site and appearance of any erosions. Erosions are asymmetrical and 'overhanging' in gout, but marginal in rheumatoid arthritis.

Finish your description by commenting on any soft tissue swelling or calcifications, any ankylosis (which is unusual in rheumatoid arthritis) and any bone resorption (terminal tufts or subperiosteal).

Psoriatic arthropathy

Appearances of erosive arthropathies can overlap considerably, but particular features make a diagnosis of psoriatic arthropathy highly likely. Look for the characteristic 'pencil-in-cup' appearance, which reflects ill-defined erosions with adjacent periosteal new bone formation. Examination of the soft tissues often reveals a 'sausage digit' due to diffuse swelling. If faced with a foot radiograph, then destruction of the great toe interphalangeal joint with a florid periosteal reaction and bony proliferation at the base of the distal phalanx is classic. Ankylosis may be seen but it is not specific to psoriatic arthropathy; it is also a feature of erosive osteoarthritis and ankylosing spondylitis.

Case 5

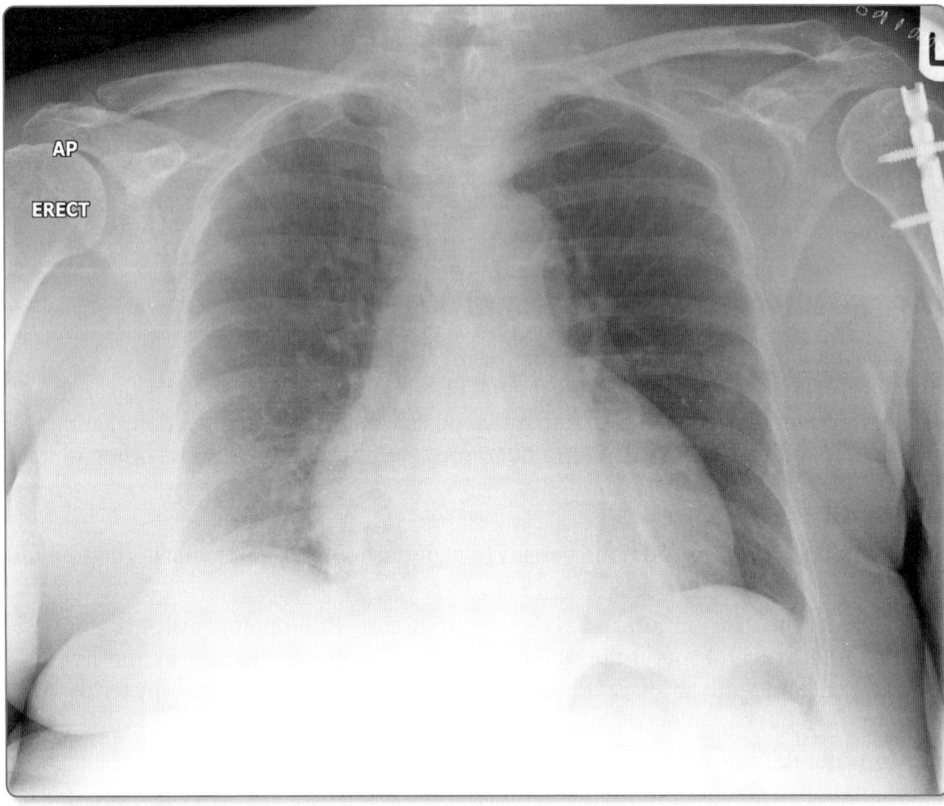

Suggested response

This is an anteroposterior erect chest radiograph of an adult female patient. There are several findings of note. Firstly, at the right base the appearance is suggestive of free subdiaphragmatic gas.

There is also a rounded mass, measuring approximately 3 cm, projected over the right heart border. There has been a left mastectomy.

Skin staples are projected over the left shoulder and there has been internal fixation of the left humerus with an intramedullary nail, presumably recently.

The lungs are otherwise clear. Allowing for the projection, I cannot see any mediastinal lymphadenopathy and no other fractures or bone destruction are visible.

In conclusion, I suspect that this patient has pneumoperitoneum and also metastatic breast carcinoma, with a lung metastasis and a recent pathological fracture of her left humerus secondary to a bone metastasis. Understandably, knowledge of the clinical presentation will be relevant in this case and it would be useful to review any available relevant previous imaging. Nevertheless, I suspect an intra-abdominal surgical emergency and, in the first instance, I would urgently discuss the case with the referring clinicians or, if I cannot get hold of them, the on-call surgical team. Once acute problems have been appropriately managed, the need for further investigation of the other findings will depend on the overall clinical picture, so discussion of the case between the members of the breast cancer multidisciplinary team may be appropriate.

Diagnosis

Pneumoperitoneum and metastatic breast cancer with right lung metastasis, previous left mastectomy and recent internal fixation of a pathological humeral fracture.

Tips: Breast cancer

Key points: Chest radiograph

In females, consider previous breast surgery on all chest radiographs, including bilateral mastectomy if other findings suggest disseminated breast cancer. Look for evidence of a mastectomy, asymmetry of the breast contours, surgical clips from an axillary clearance, implants and evidence of breast reconstruction. Review for evidence of lymphangitis, radiotherapy changes, lymphadenopathy, effusions and lung and bone metastases (which are often sclerotic, but may be lytic or mixed). Other findings might represent a complication of treatment, e.g. heart failure due to chemotherapy.

Key points: Mammograms

Assess for the presence of a mass, any architectural distortion, asymmetrical density, microcalcifications (you may need to magnify the image), skin changes (e.g. thickening, peau d'orange) and axillary nodes.

Key points: Ultrasound

Lesion appearances depend on the tumour type, but look for any ill-defined, hypoechoic mass (typically 'taller than it is wide') and comment on any acoustic shadowing or enhancement.

Breast cancer

Breast cancer is very common in the general population and has many manifestations. Consequently, it features very commonly in radiological examinations where radiographs depicting mastectomy and metastatic disease are classical cases. Mammograms may not be a common viva case but they can still crop up [as can breast ultrasounds and MRI, so ensure that you can interpret (and correctly view) them]. Lack of exposure to these modalities in your training cannot be used as an excuse for an inability to interpret them in an examination if they are within the curriculum.

Case 6

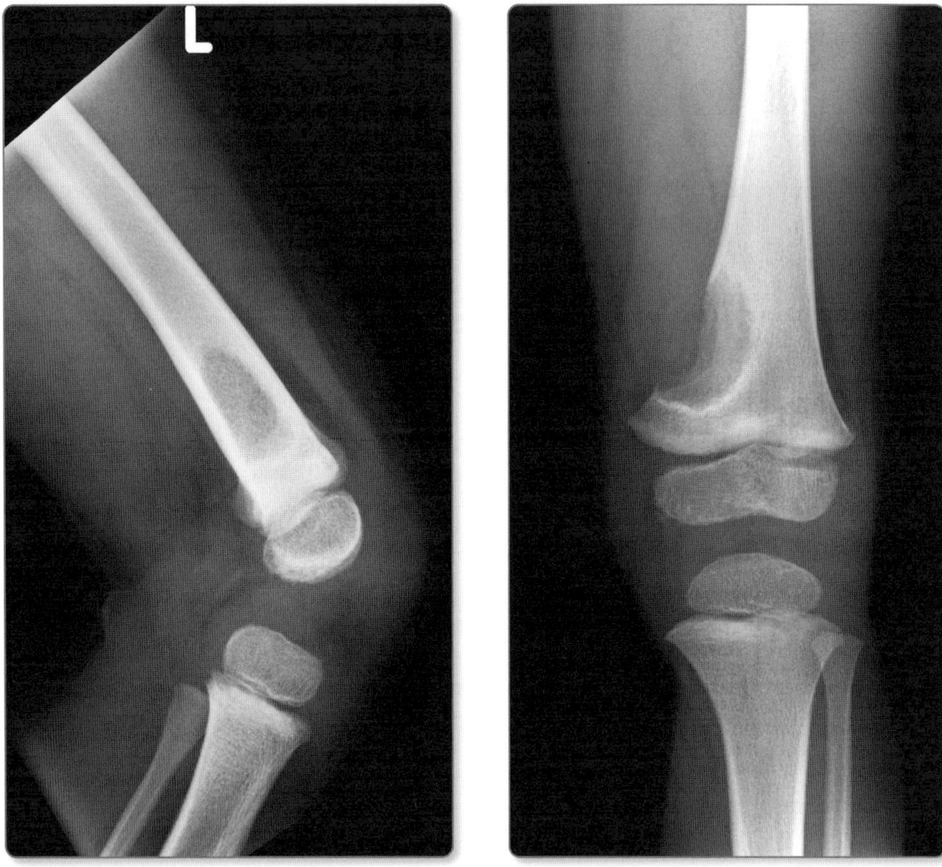

Suggested response

These are anteroposterior and lateral views of the left knee of a skeletally immature patient, likely a very young child given the stage of osseous development. There is a longitudinally oriented ovoid lucency located eccentrically in the medial aspect of the distal metaphysis of the left femur. This is well-defined and measures several centimetres in long axis. The medial cortex is absent and there is a small extra-osseous component. The zone of transition is narrow and fairly well-defined, especially laterally and inferiorly where there is a sclerotic rim. At the inferior margin, the cortex is undercut by the lesion, but there is no discernible periosteal reaction. This lesion appears solitary and does not extend to the physis. The bones are otherwise normal.

The features are mostly nonaggressive, but the lesion could still represent an aggressive process. I think the appearance is not typical for infection. In a patient of this age, a primary bone tumour would be more likely. An osteosarcoma or Ewing's sarcoma could have these appearances and my differential would lie between these lesions and less aggressive lesions such as eosinophilic granulomas and possibly nonossifying fibromas or chondromyxoid fibromas.

I would seek specialist advice and discuss the case with the referring clinician to correlate my findings with the clinical history. An MRI of the femur and referral to the regional bone tumour centre, without local biopsy, are likely to be appropriate.

Diagnosis

Eosinophilic granuloma in the distal femur of a 2-year-old child.

Tips: Indolent lucent bone lesions

Refer to 'Key points: Focal bone lesion description' in Case 2.

Key points: Nonaggressive (or indolent) bone lesions

These lesions usually exhibit a central location in bone (especially simple or aneurysmal bone cyst, fibrous dysplasia, enchondroma), a narrow zone of transition and thick or dense periosteal reaction, implying slow growth. Several indolent lesions only cause periosteal reaction in association with a fracture (e.g. enchondroma, simple bone cyst, nonossifying fibroma and fibrous dysplasia).

Consider the age of the patient. Although a narrow zone of transition usually suggests an indolent diagnosis, it may be seen in plasmacytoma or metastases in older patients.

Unless all features point to an indolent diagnosis, you should not discard possible aggressive causes for lucent bone lesions; equivocal lesions with mixed features are difficult to deal with and you should say so.

Eosinophilic granuloma

This is uncommon and represents the localised form of Langerhans cell histiocytosis. It predominantly affects children and young adults and may be unifocal or multifocal. Typically it affects the skull, ribs or diaphyses of long bones. Imaging appearances are variable and these lesions may show aggressive features. Consequently, it is a difficult diagnosis to confidently make on a single plain radiograph, but features frequently on differential lists.

Case 7

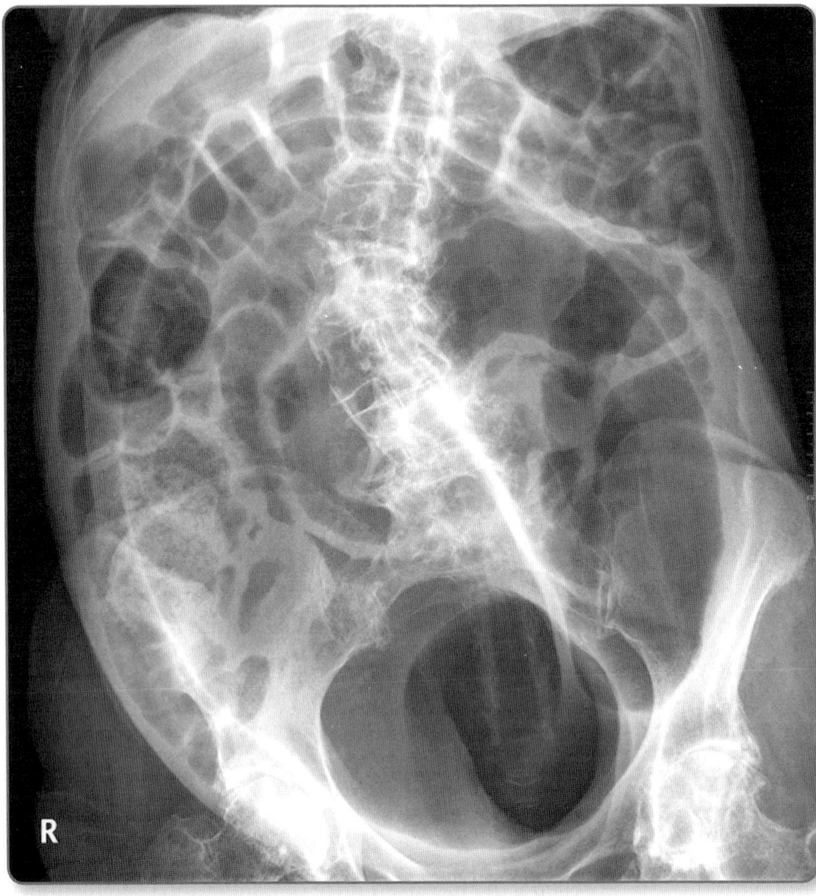

Suggested response

This is an abdominal radiograph of an adult patient.

There is massive dilatation of a gas-filled loop of large bowel which extends superiorly from the pelvis and has a 'coffee bean' configuration. The remainder of the large bowel is gas-filled and mildly dilated. Faeces is visible in the caecum and there are also nondilated loops of small bowel in the central abdomen.

I also note severe osteoarthritis of the hips, much more so on the left, and a scoliosis convex to the right which is centred on L2/L3. Depending on the clinical findings, these are likely to be long-standing and unrelated to the patient's current presentation.

The appearance suggests sigmoid volvulus. There is no Rigler's sign or other feature of free gas. However, if this is a clinical concern, I would suggest confirming this with an erect chest radiograph.

I would urgently contact the referring clinicians and suggest that decompression of the bowel with a flatus tube may be appropriate.

Diagnosis

Large bowel obstruction, secondary to a sigmoid volvulus, without perforation.

Tips: Large bowel obstruction

Key points

Remember that fluid-filled loops of bowel are generally not visible radiographically, only gas-filled loops are visible. Try to recognise which segment of the bowel is obstructed by tracing to it from any segment you can confidently identify. Alternately, try to trace the bowel proximally from the rectum or distally from the caecum.

There are a number of ways to help to distinguish between large and small bowel.

Location: Large bowel is generally peripheral, whereas small bowel is more central.

Number of loops and radius of curvature: Small bowel tends to have multiple loops with frequent tight turns, whereas large bowel tends to have fewer, longer and less-curved loops.

Size: Small bowel is rarely as large as normal large bowel, even when there is severe obstruction.

Bowel markings: Haustra and valvulae conniventes are distinguishing features, but do not conflate incomplete visualisation of valvulae conniventes with the presence of haustra and therefore large bowel, especially when all other features point to a segment being small bowel, and vice versa.

Other signs: Also look for intramural and portal venous gas. Look specifically for perforation and state your findings out loud.

Differential diagnosis

This is contingent on the age of the patient, but includes carcinoma, hernia and volvulus for large bowel obstruction and adhesions (presuming previous surgery), hernia, Crohn's disease and intussusception for small bowel obstruction.

Sigmoid volvulus

While caecal volvulus tends to occur in younger adults, sigmoid volvulus is predominantly seen in elderly patients. The 'coffee bean sign' seen here is a classical finding on a supine plain radiograph, with the midline crease corresponding to the root of the sigmoid mesentery. Erect radiographs may demonstrate fluid-fluid levels within the distended loop.

Cases such as this can form the basis of patient management-centric discussions in a viva. Urgent discussion with the on-call surgical team is necessary. Further imaging (single contrast enema or CT scan) may be necessary in some instances to help to confirm the diagnosis in the event of uncertainty, aid operative planning, or determine whether conservative management is possible.

Case 8

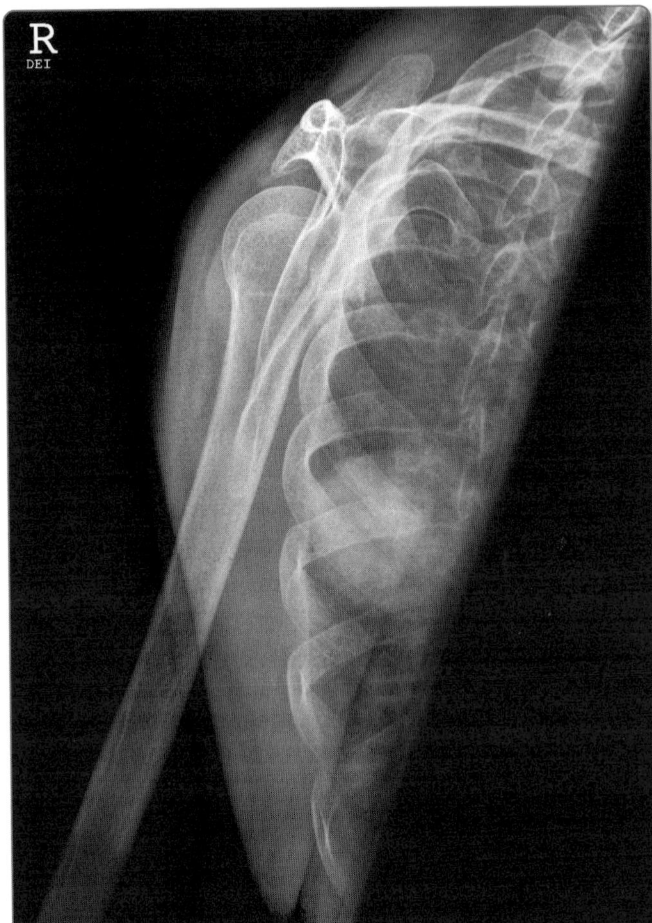

Suggested response

This is a 'Y' view of the right shoulder of a skeletally mature patient. There is a posterior glenohumeral dislocation. I also suspect that there is a fracture of the humeral head, although this is not well-visualised. In my usual practice, I would review a second view of the shoulder, or request one if not available. There is a further significant finding on this radiograph – a large rounded soft tissue mass projected in the right lung. In the first instance, I would review any available relevant previous imaging to establish whether this is a new finding. If not previously reported, I would discuss it with the referring clinicians and advise a frontal chest radiograph.

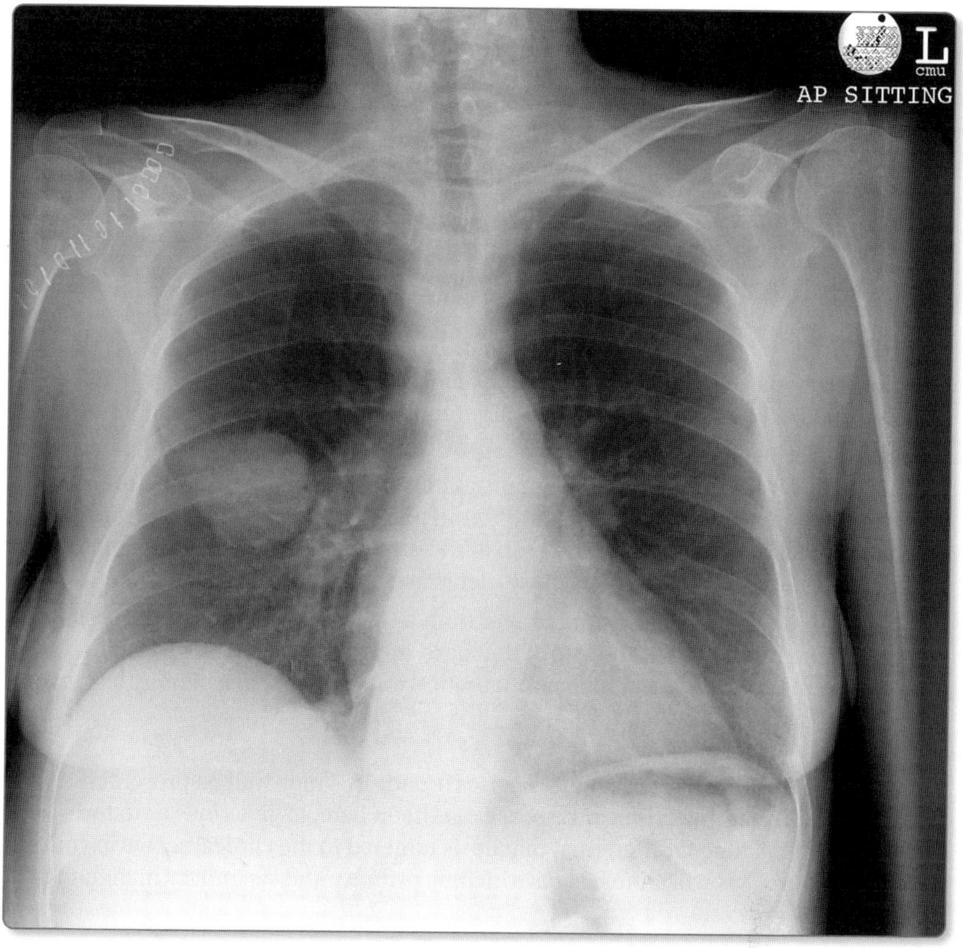

Suggested response

This is an anteroposterior sitting chest radiograph in an adult female patient. There are skin staples projected over the right shoulder and the dislocation appears to have been reduced on this view.

The chest radiograph confirms the finding of a large solitary mass which is projected in the right lung. The lungs are otherwise clear. Assessment of the mediastinum and heart size is limited by the projection, but I suspect that the superior pole of the right hilum is bulky.

The thoracic wall, including the breast shadows, appears normal.

I cannot see any definite metastatic disease and the lung lesion may have been detected incidentally following investigation of trauma.

The differentials for a solitary lung mass are broad. In an adult patient, by far the most likely diagnosis is primary or secondary malignancy. If this is a new diagnosis, then I would suggest a respiratory referral and a staging CT scan. Discussion at a multidisciplinary team meeting is usually appropriate and I would facilitate this.

Diagnosis

Metastatic carcinoma with pulmonary metastasis. Fracture/posterior dislocation of the right shoulder caused by a fit secondary to a cerebral metastasis.

Tips: A solitary lung mass

Key points

Determine whether the lesion is a nodule or a mass. Nodules measure <3 cm and are usually visualised on radiographs when larger than 8 mm (visualised smaller nodules suggest internal calcification). In contrast, masses are ≥3 cm in diameter.

The patient's age is relevant: Malignant solitary pulmonary masses are rare in children (consider congenital causes and round pneumonia, particularly in early childhood). Solitary pulmonary masses in adults should convey high suspicion for primary pulmonary malignancy (solitary metastases are uncommon).

Ensure that you can stage a lung cancer from a CT scan and approximately stage one on a radiograph. Look at the size of the mass, any further pulmonary lesions, the proximity to the mediastinum, hilar configuration and the presence of bony lesions.

Differential diagnosis

Acknowledge that the differential diagnosis is broad. This may well be presented as part of a more complex clinical case, as it has been here, to give clues as to the diagnosis. Offer a limited differential diagnosis targeted to the clinical scenario you have been given. This will almost always include primary and secondary malignancy and infection.

Solitary pulmonary mass

When faced with a solitary pulmonary mass, a review of previous imaging is essential: very rapid (days) or very slow (years) doubling times favour benign aetiologies. Various patterns of calcification (popcorn, laminated, central or diffuse) are also more suggestive of a benign aetiology. Although often not possible, primary and secondary malignancies can sometimes be differentiated on thoracic imaging. Calcification is seen in up to 10% of primary bronchogenic carcinomas, but it is very rare in metastases. A metastasis is usually sharply demarcated and lobulated, whereas a primary bronchogenic carcinoma tends to have ill-defined margins.

Case 9

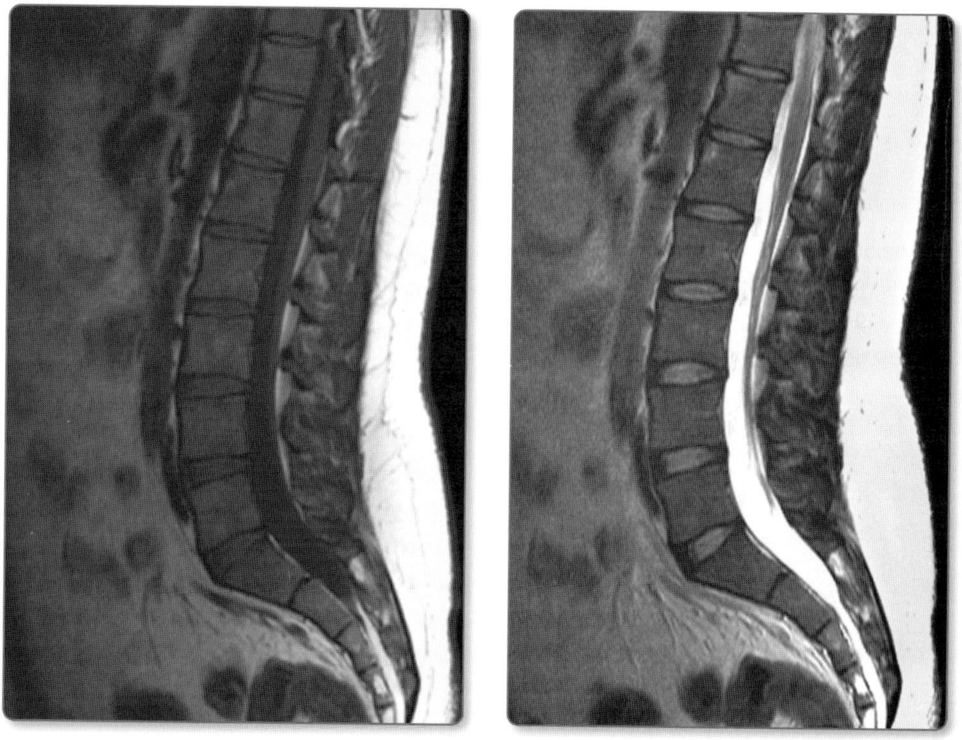

Suggested response

These are selected sagittal T1 and T2 MRI images of the lumbar spine.

There is normal alignment. I cannot see any abnormality of the distal cord, conus or cauda equina and the central canal is widely patent. The intervertebral discs are well-preserved.

There are small focal abnormalities of the marrow signal at the anterior superior corners of the vertebral bodies. These are oedematous at L1 and fatty at T11 and T12.

The marrow signal elsewhere is normal and there are no visible soft tissue masses.

The finding of changes in the marrow at the anterior superior margins of the vertebrae at the thoracolumbar junction gives the appearance of 'shiny corners' and raises the possibility of spondyloarthropathy.

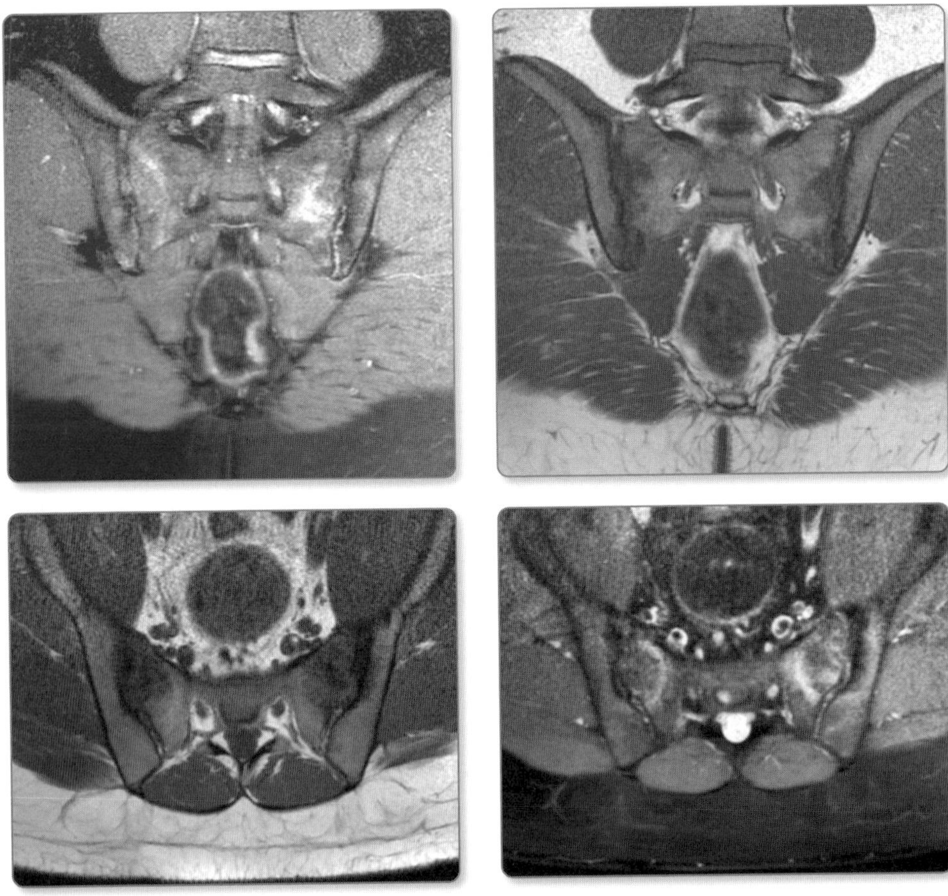

Suggested response

These are selected images from an MRI scan of the sacroiliac joints.

There are florid symmetrical changes with multiple erosions and widespread surrounding oedema.

I cannot see any ankylosis on these images, but in my usual practice I would review the whole of the examination.

The findings support the diagnosis of spondyloarthropathy and, as there is symmetrical involvement of the sacroiliac joints, the most likely diagnoses are either ankylosing spondylitis or an arthropathy associated with inflammatory bowel disease.

Diagnosis

Ankylosing spondylitis.

Tips: Spondyloarthropathy

Key points and differential diagnosis

Syndesmophytes and osteophytes can be distinguished as follows. Syndesmophytes are paravertebral ossifications that run vertically between the margins of adjacent vertebral bodies, whereas osteophytes run more horizontally and originate a few millimetres from the edge of the vertebral body. Large osteophytes and syndesmophytes can appear identical, in which case say so and look at other levels for smaller areas of ossification that may give a clue.

On MRI, the earliest sign of change in the spine is oedema, which is visible on fluid-sensitive sequences in the corner of the vertebra (most commonly anterosuperior – 'shiny corners'). With more chronic inflammation these changes may become fatty. This is the MRI counterpart or precursor to the plain radiograph 'Romanus lesion'.

Look for sacroiliitis, which is common in all seronegative spondyloarthropathies. It is usually reasonably symmetrical in ankylosing spondylitis and arthritis associated with inflammatory bowel disease, but is usually asymmetrical or unilateral in psoriatic arthropathy and reactive arthritis (Reiter's syndrome).

Ankylosing spondylitis

Ankylosing spondylitis usually presents in young adults (under the age of 35 years). The majority of patients are HLA-B27 positive. The spinal and sacroiliac abnormalities in ankylosing spondylitis are well-known, but remember that the disease can manifest in a variety of ways, including erosive arthropathy of the hands, pulmonary fibrosis (upper zone predominance) and aortic valve insufficiency. While you may encounter changes of advanced spondyloarthropathy on radiographs in a viva, there has been a shift in day-to-day practice towards earlier investigation of suspected inflammatory spondyloarthropathy with MRI and it is much more likely in clinical practice that the diagnosis will be made on MRI.

Case 10

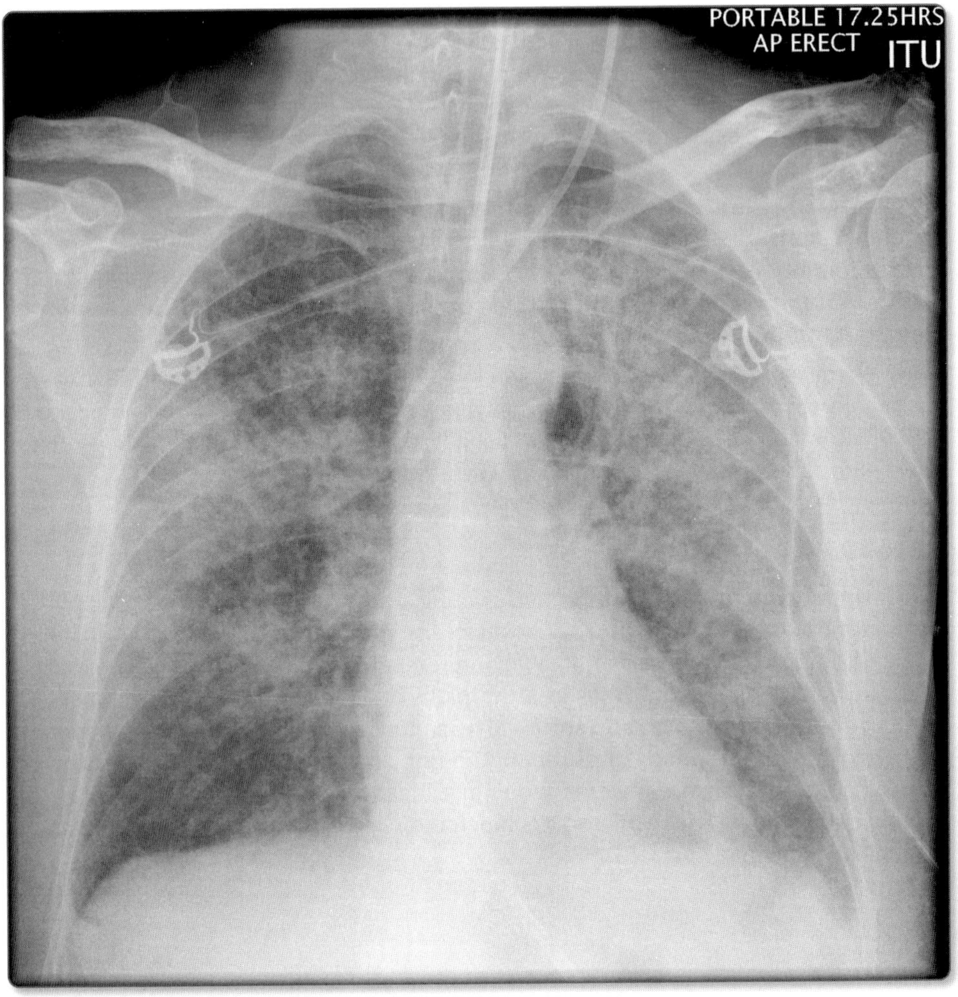

Suggested response

This is a portable anteroposterior erect chest radiograph of an adult patient taken in ITU. There are features that suggest this patient is very unwell. There are ECG monitoring leads and also a number of lines. An endotracheal tube and left internal jugular venous catheter appear to be appropriately positioned. A nasogastric tube is evident, the tip of which is not visualised although it passes below the diaphragm.

There is widespread shadowing throughout both lungs, predominantly in the right mid and left mid and upper zones. In the right lung, there is the impression of a peripheral predominance while in the left lung the changes are more widespread.

There are some interstitial features but overall this has the appearance of airspace opacification.

This is an anteroposterior radiograph, but allowing for this the mediastinal contour is normal and the heart does not appear to be enlarged. There are no pleural effusions or pneumothoraces.

In summary, there is widespread bilateral airspace opacification with a normal heart size and no effusions. The differential is broad, but the most likely aetiologies are oedema (particularly noncardiogenic causes), acute respiratory distress syndrome (ARDS) and extensive infection. Knowledge of the overall clinical picture and, in particular, whether the patient exhibits features of sepsis, would help to clarify the diagnosis. Review of any available relevant previous imaging may also help to refine the interpretation.

Diagnosis

Bilateral pulmonary oedema with normal heart size and no effusions, secondary to fat embolism.

Tips: Bilateral airspace shadowing

This is a common scenario in both everyday practice and the examination. Describe the findings, recognise that there is bilateral airspace opacification and begin by saying that there is a wide differential. Do not list every cause you can remember; if you do, you will finish with long pauses between suggestions and your final suggestion will be the diagnosis about which you know the least. Instead, stick to a 'top three' and make it clear that you are aware that it is the clinical picture which is the most important factor in refining the radiograph interpretation (consider presenting your options in a 'conditional differential diagnosis' format; e.g. if the patient has presented with central crushing chest pain this may represent pulmonary oedema; if the patient has been on ITU for several weeks it could be ARDS; or if the patient has features of systemic sepsis it could be widespread pneumonia).

Key points and differential diagnosis

Most cases of bilateral airspace shadowing will be due to oedema or infection. For oedema, cardiac causes are by far the most common, either due to cardiac failure or induced by fluid overload. Do not forget noncardiac causes such as raised intracranial pressure, aspiration injury and re-expansion. It can be very difficult to distinguish pneumonia from oedema and ARDS and they may co-exist. **Table 10.1** highlights the differences between these entities.

Note that the terms 'airspace shadowing/opacification,' 'consolidation' and 'alveolar shadowing' can be used interchangeably.

Fat embolism

Fat embolism can be seen after skeletal trauma (particularly pelvic or long bone fractures) or orthopaedic surgery. It harbours a significant mortality rate, in the order of 10–20%, and often presents 24–72 hours after the traumatic event. Chest radiographs are often normal initially, but subsequently show diffuse bilateral airspace opacification. ARDS may subsequently develop. Fat embolism may not be suspected clinically due to multiple confounding factors or other possible causes for radiographic appearances. The presentation may also be subclinical. Therefore, always keep the diagnosis in mind when reporting imaging of polytrauma patients or those who have recently undergone orthopaedic procedures.

Table 10.1 Tips for distinguishing pneumonia, oedema and acute respiratory distress syndrome (ARDS)

Characteristic	Pneumonia	Oedema	ARDS
Type of shadowing	Airspace	Interstitial and airspace	Initially interstitial, rapid progression to diffuse airspace
Proximal vessels	Unaffected unless adjacent to airspace shadowing	Hazy	Well-defined
Distribution	Usually focal, at least initially	Predominantly basal and central	All zones (symmetrical)
Heart size	Normal	Large	Normal
Pleural effusion	Common	Very common	Uncommon
Timing of changes	Chest radiograph changes delayed	Changes when symptomatic, quick resolution	Delayed appearance, may persist even with clinical improvement

Case 11

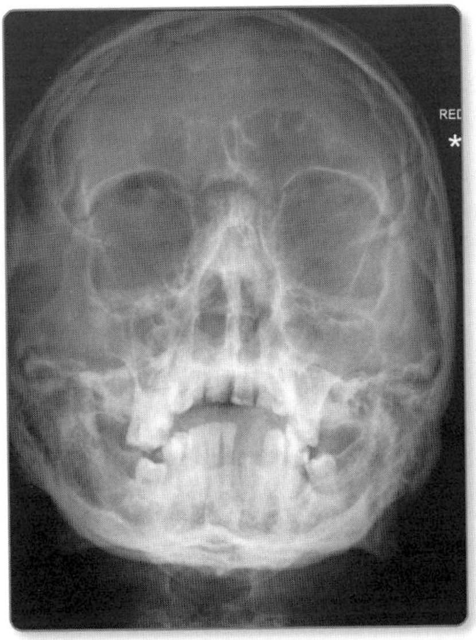
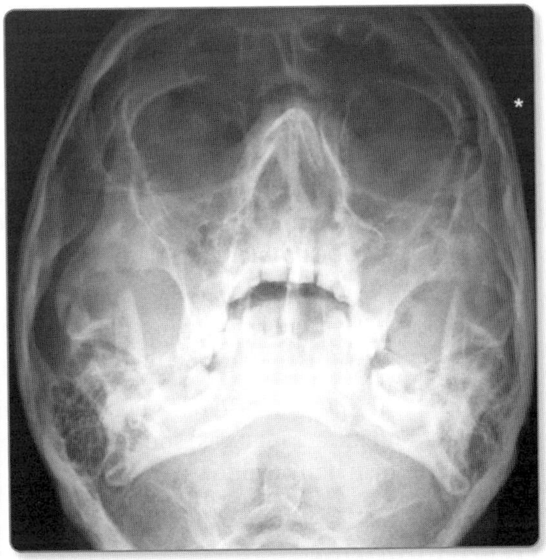

Suggested response

This is a 'facial views' series of a skeletally mature patient. Multiple fractures are evident. The most significant injury extends from one frontozygomatic suture to the other (with diastasis of both sutures), involving both medial and lateral walls of both orbits. A further fracture is evident through the body of the left hemimandible with loss of at least one lower left tooth. Appearances are suspicious for another fracture through the inferior margin of the left orbital floor. There are clearly extensive facial fractures which warrant CT scanning to more accurately delineate their extent and assess for intracranial injury.

The most significant injury, however, is craniofacial dysjunction in keeping with a Le Fort type III fracture. I would convey these findings to the referring clinicians immediately since the patient is at a high risk of airway obstruction.

Diagnosis

Le Fort type III fracture in an adult male.

Tips: Craniofacial trauma

Key points

Facial views: Remember McGregor's three lines. Disruption of the lines is seen with tripod fractures, orbital floor fractures [in blow-out fractures look for maxillary antrum 'teardrop' (may be seen even if fracture is not apparent) and 'black eyebrow' sign due to air within the orbit], isolated zygomatic arch fractures and Le Fort fractures.

Orthopantomogram: It is far more common to see two fractures of the mandible or a fracture and a dislocation at the TMJ rather than a single fracture in isolation, so beware of satisfaction of search and scrutinise the TMJ alignment bilaterally. The symphysis menti is a problem area: fractures here can be obscured due to technical factors and a mandibular view would usually provide clarity if required.

Skull views: Linear calvarial fractures and vascular grooves have similar appearances but can be distinguished from one another: a fracture line is dark and well-defined, whereas a vascular groove is grey with marginal sclerosis and branching. Differentiation from sutures may be problematic, particularly in children, hence knowledge of sutural positions is vital.

Look for an air-fluid level in the sphenoid sinus in particular (it is also a good practice to review this area on lateral trauma C-spine radiographs).

CT of the head: Any manifestations of potential intracranial trauma (e.g. haemorrhage, contusions and intracranial gas) should stimulate careful assessment of the skull base and calvarium on bony windows.

Le Fort injuries

Le Fort fractures are typically the result of significant impact to the face such as in road traffic accidents. All fractures involve the pterygoid process. Le Fort type I fractures consist of a transverse fracture through the maxilla to produce a floating palate. Le Fort type II fractures extend up through the maxillae and inferior and medial walls of the orbit (no involvement of the zygoma) to produce a floating maxilla. Le Fort type III fractures are the most clinically significant due to the high risk of airway compromise. As in this case, a fracture passes in a more or less transverse direction through the medial and lateral walls of the orbit (again without involvement of the zygoma) and causes complete craniofacial dysjunction, i.e. a 'floating face'.

Case 12

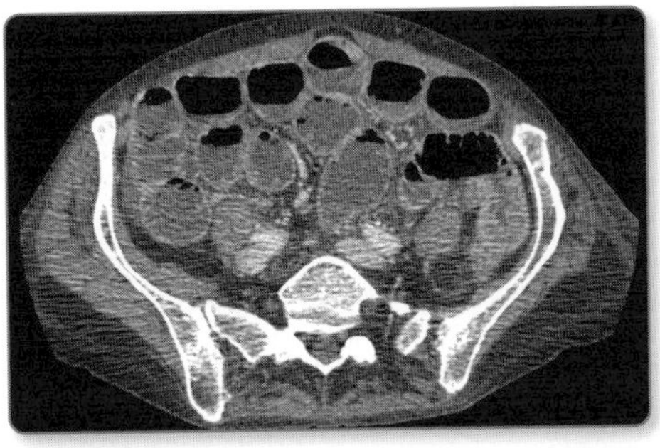

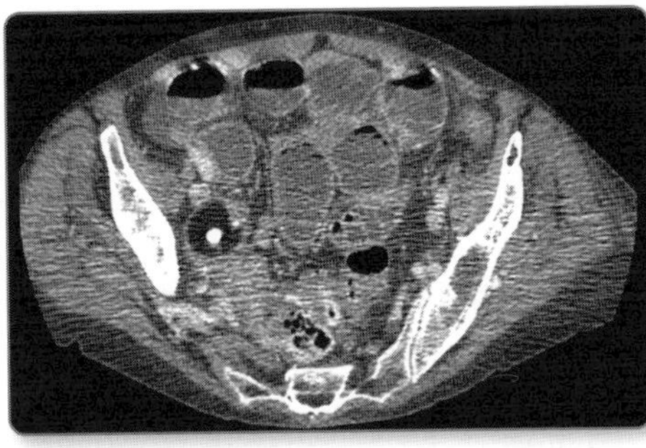

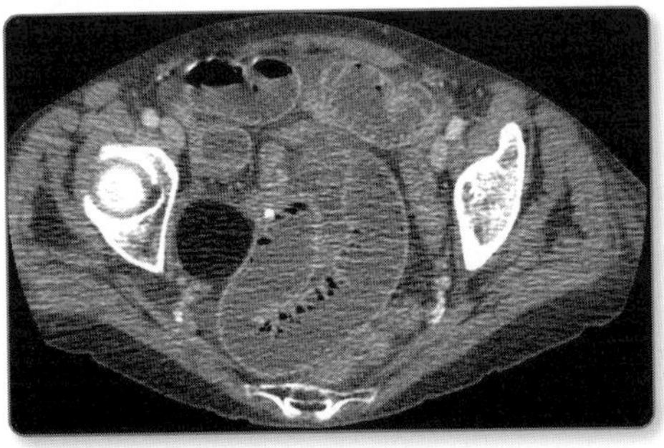

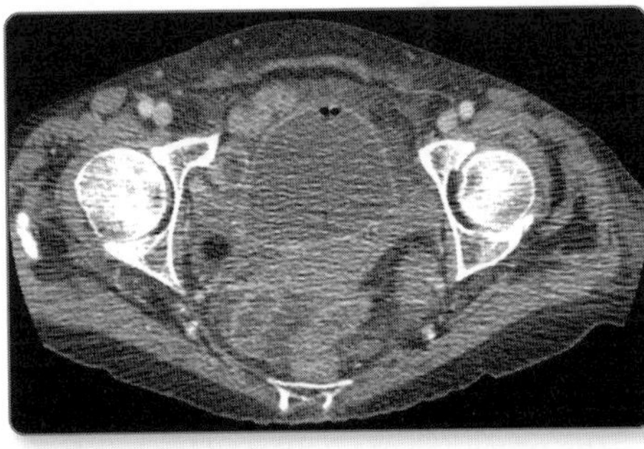

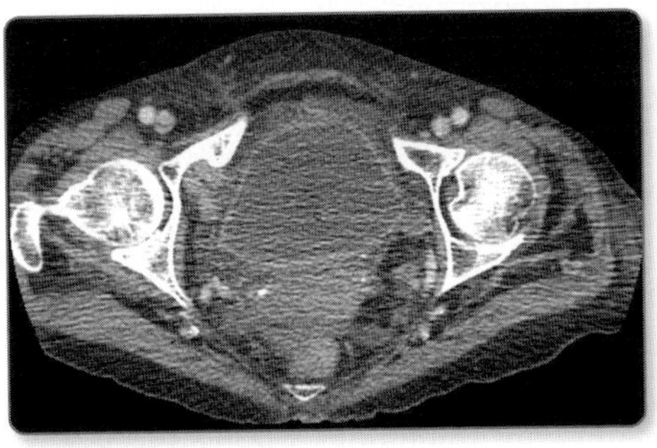

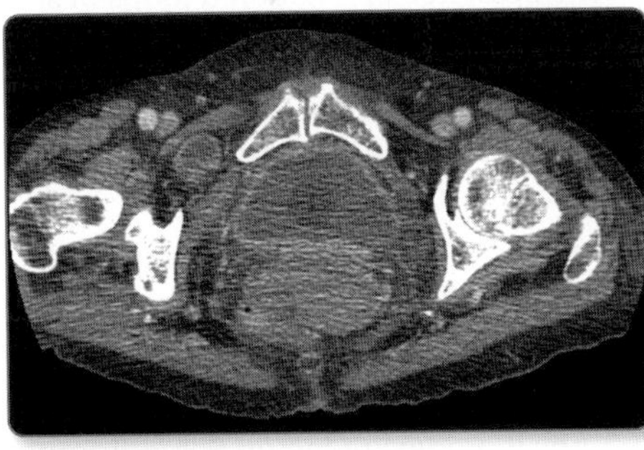

Suggested response

These are selected axial images from a post-contrast CT scan of the pelvis in a skeletally mature female patient. There are multiple dilated loops of fluid-filled small bowel. One loop of bowel is seen to pass through the right obturator foramen, where it exhibits a narrow neck, into the extra-pelvic fat. The findings are consistent with small bowel obstruction secondary to a right obturator hernia.

The small bowel folds do not appear thickened. A small volume of ascites is evident in the pelvis. No free intraperitoneal gas is identified on these images, although in my usual practice I would review all images on lung windows to more accurately assess for the presence of free gas.

A second abnormality is evident on these images. Lying medial to the right acetabulum is a rounded mass of fatty density measuring several centimetres in diameter, with a calcific density at its superior aspect. The appearance is almost certainly that of a right ovarian dermoid tumour. While this is unlikely to be relevant to the current presentation, the lesion is at risk of torsion, rupture and malignant transformation. Consequently, these findings should also be conveyed to the referring clinicians when discussing the more immediately life-threatening diagnosis of small bowel obstruction.

Diagnosis

Obturator hernia causing small bowel obstruction in a 59-year-old female. Incidental right ovarian dermoid.

Tips: Small bowel dilatation

Key points and differential diagnosis

There are a number of specific features that should be sought and described:

- Hernial orifices are a critical area for review on a CT scan or radiograph. Look for gas projected over the upper thigh on a radiograph. Mention that you would want to review images of the hernial orifices if they are not included in the imaging available in a viva.
- The presence of angulated loops of small bowel suggests adhesions.
- Thickened walls ± hyperenhancement are seen in Crohn's disease and ischaemia.
- Assess for gas in the bowel wall. It is usually easier to be confident of the finding when it is in the dependent portion of the bowel. Also consider whether or not there is free intraperitoneal gas.
- Review the small bowel folds to see if they are normal or thickened. Normal folds are seen in mechanical obstruction, ileus and malabsorption, e.g. coeliac disease. Thickened folds are a feature of ischaemia, Crohn's disease, lymphoma and radiotherapy.

Age is a relevant factor. For children, remember the mnemonic, 'AIM': adhesions, appendicitis, intussusception, incarcerated hernia, malrotation and Meckel's diverticulum. In adults, consider adhesions (most common), hernia and tumour.

Obturator hernia

Obturator herniae are rare, but are considerably more frequent in women (usually elderly), in part as a consequence of the larger diameter of the obturator canal. It is often unsuspected clinically because, unlike with femoral and inguinal herniae, there is often no externally palpable lump. Delays in the diagnosis of incarcerated obturator herniae incur a high mortality rate (up to 70%) relative to other incarcerated herniae, which highlight the role of the radiologist in making the diagnosis and guiding management. It presents with small bowel obstruction in around 90% of cases, but can also present with neurological symptoms due to compression of the obturator nerve.

Case 13

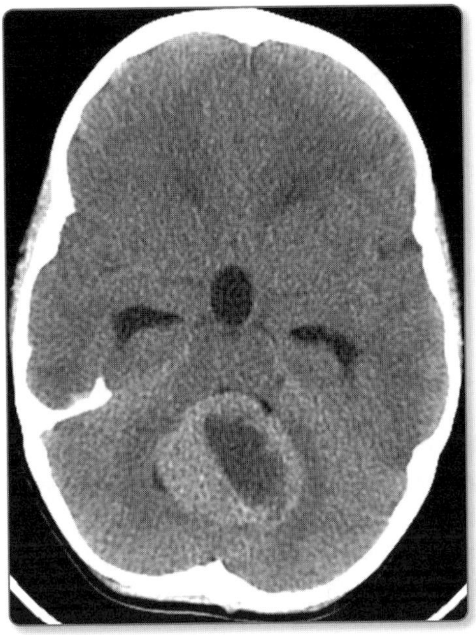

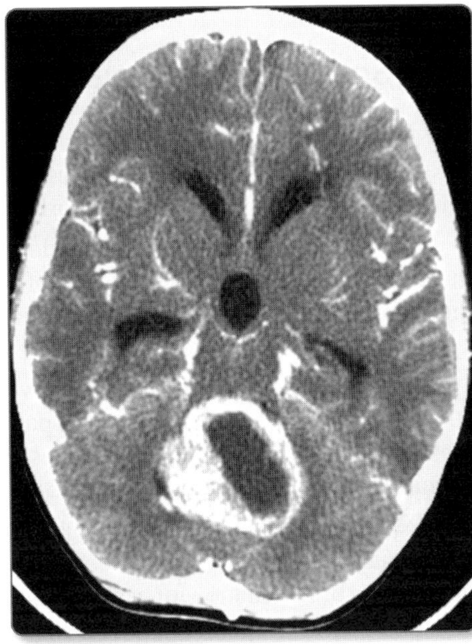

Suggested response

These are selected axial slices from a cranial CT study, one image being before and one after injection of intravenous contrast.

There is a large, vividly enhancing mass with a central cystic area in the region of the fourth ventricle, which appears to be expanded by the lesion. There is associated hydrocephalus with dilation of the visible components of the upstream ventricular system, namely the third ventricle and the temporal horns of the lateral ventricles.

No other masses are visible on these slices, although I would routinely review the whole of the study and also consider the clinical history. Knowledge of the age of the patient would be relevant, but appearances suggest that these images are of a young child. If this is correct, in light of the location of this mass, i.e. close to the vermis, and this being a paediatric patient, the most likely diagnosis is a medulloblastoma. Cystic change is not classical but can occur.

Cystic change is typical for a cerebellar astrocytoma, but with that lesion I would have expected the rim of the lesion to be thinner. An ependymoma is also a possibility, but is much less likely. In view of the presence of a mass causing hydrocephalus, I would immediately discuss the case with the referring clinicians or, if they could not be contacted, directly with the neurosurgical team.

Diagnosis

Obstructive hydrocephalus in a 6-year-old child, secondary to medulloblastoma (previous classification primitive neuroectodermal tumour).

Tips: Solitary intracranial mass lesions

Key points

Firstly, consider the location of the lesion. Determine whether it is intra-axial or extra-axial and supratentorial or infratentorial.

The next discriminating factor in determining the type of tumour is the age of the patient. In children under the age of approximately 4 supratentorial tumours are more common, with infratentorial tumours usually presenting between the ages of approximately 4 and 11 years.

It can be difficult to distinguish between a primary lesion and a metastasis. About 90% of solitary intracranial masses in patients with known primary malignancies are metastases and one-third of metastases will be solitary. Gliomas are the most common primary brain tumour in adulthood. Gliomas are usually less well-defined and cause less extensive vasogenic oedema than metastases.

Some primary tumours are seen as part of a syndrome that also affects other parts of the brain, so look for associated findings. Commonly encountered tumours are: giant cell astrocytomas in tuberous sclerosis; optic tract glioma in type 1 neurofibromatosis; and haemangioblastoma in Von Hippel–Lindau syndrome.

Medulloblastoma

The most common paediatric infratentorial tumour, medulloblastomas tend to occur in 5–9-year-old children and are seen more frequently in boys. They usually arise from the vermis and there is typically hydrocephalus at the time of presentation. They are generally quite aggressive and commonly spread through the subarachnoid space by seeding.

Case 14

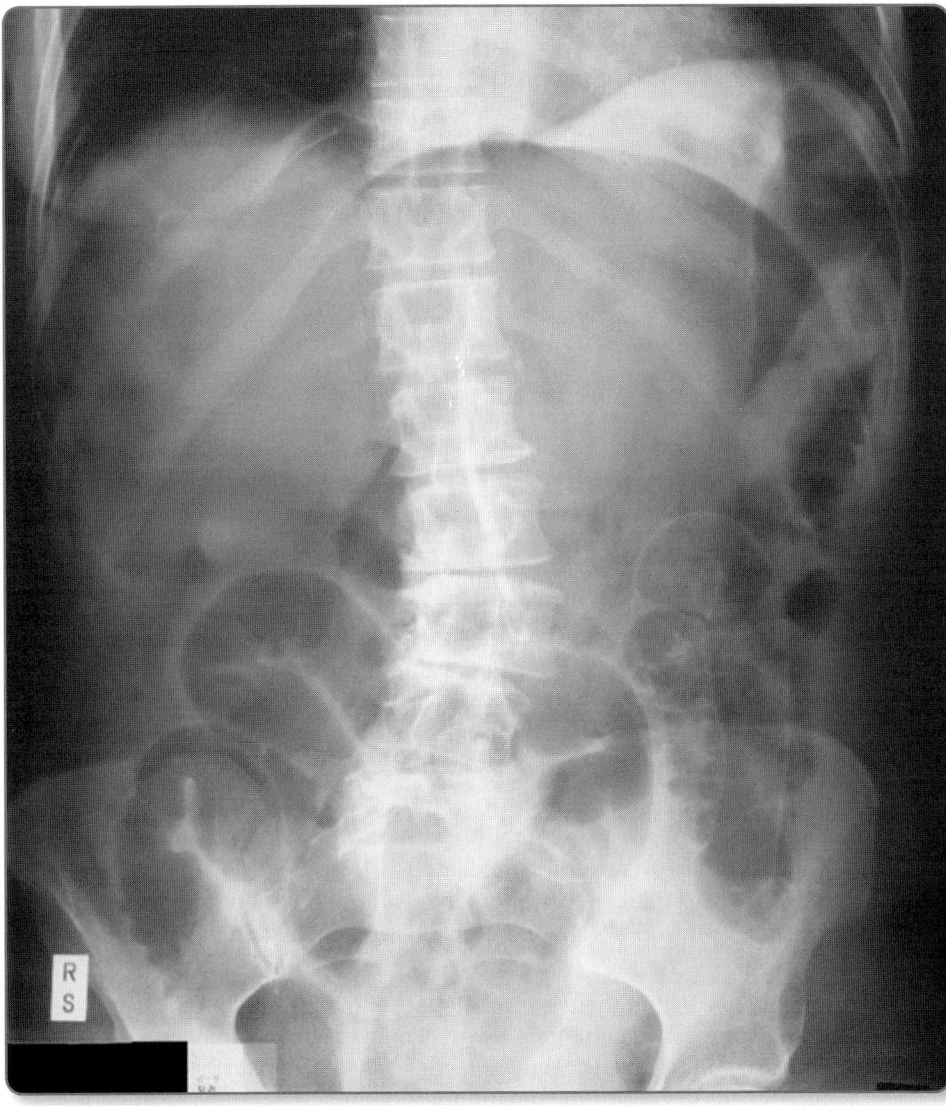

Suggested response

This is an abdominal radiograph of an adult patient. There is a very large area of relative lucency in the upper abdomen and multiple gas-filled, distended loops of small bowel in the central abdomen and pelvis. On the left side of the abdomen, there is a clear Rigler's sign with both sides of the bowel wall clearly visible, indicating perforation. There is some gas and faeces in what is presumably the splenic flexure and descending colon, which are of normal calibre, but the remainder of the large bowel cannot be positively identified.

A background of some degenerative changes in the lower lumbar spine is also noted with a mild scoliosis that is convex to the right and centred on L3/L4.

In summary, there is evidence of small bowel obstruction with a large volume of free gas secondary to bowel perforation. If the patient has had previous surgery, the most likely cause for the obstruction is adhesions. An obstructed hernia is the next most likely cause although the hernia orifices are not visualised on this radiograph.

Regardless of the cause this is a surgical emergency and I would immediately telephone the on-call surgical team to discuss the findings.

Diagnosis

Massive pneumoperitoneum with small bowel obstruction (in this case, secondary to inflammation and obstruction at the terminal ileum, although this is not apparent from the radiograph).

Tips: Pneumoperitoneum

All of the signs can be very subtle on an abdominal radiograph. It is therefore worth specifically considering pneumoperitoneum whenever you are presented with one, even if it is part of another study, such as an intravenous urogram.

Findings vary depending on the volume of free gas. With a large amount of free gas Rigler's sign may be visible; with very large amounts of gas the entire abdomen may be outlined by gas (the 'Football' sign). Triangular pockets of gas may be visible between bowel loops. The anterior abdominal wall ligaments may be outlined by gas with an inverted 'V' sign outlining the lateral umbilical ligaments or the 'urachus' sign outlining the median umbilical ligament.

Smaller collections of gas are generally best seen when they are in the right upper quadrant. Gas here may outline the falciform ligament or ligamentum teres, cause an area of increased lucency over the liver, outline the right or posteroinferior edges of liver or be visible as a triangular pocket of gas in the pouch of Rutherford–Morison.

If you are unsure whether there is pneumoperitoneum, it is generally better to say so and state your recommendations, as you would in clinical practice. Usually, an erect chest radiograph will answer the question (if it adds no further delay) as it offers a quick means of confirming pneumoperitoneum. It may also be helpful to evaluate the lungs preoperatively. Some authorities favour an erect lateral chest radiograph centred on the diaphragm. You may also encounter a lateral 'shoot through' abdominal radiograph, which was historically the preferred option in neonates and young children. Make sure that you can interpret these investigations, particularly if you recommend one. In clinical practice, the use of CT in the evaluation of cases of suspected pneumoperitoneum is now very common. A review of images on lung windows is useful when looking for abnormal gas patterns.

Pneumoperitoneum

Most commonly caused by perforation of a hollow viscus, pneumoperitoneum can also be caused by transperitoneal instrumentation and extension from abnormal intrathoracic gas collections (e.g. pneumomediastinum). However, beware of false positives, including the 'pseudo-wall' sign (in which closely applied adjacent loops of distended bowel mimic Rigler's sign), colonic interposition and retroperitoneal gas (which may also feature in a viva; look for gas outlining the kidneys, adrenal glands and psoas major muscles – it is usually secondary to duodenal perforation).

Case 15

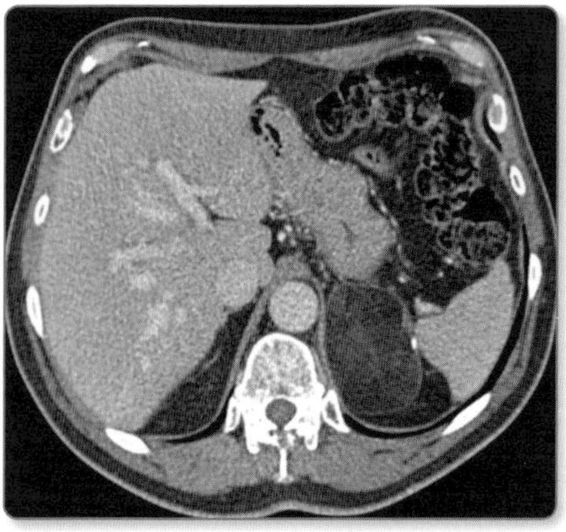
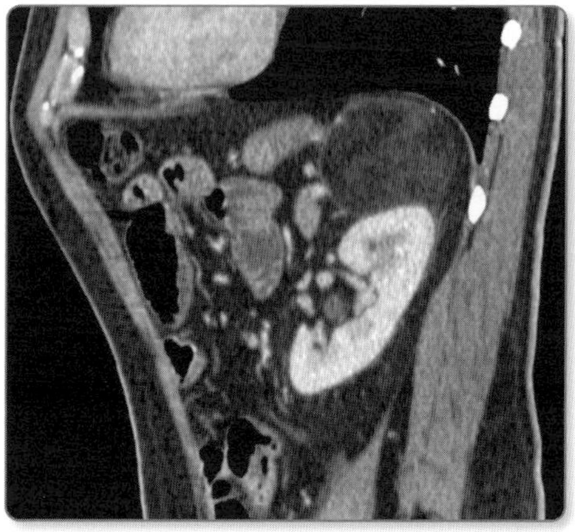
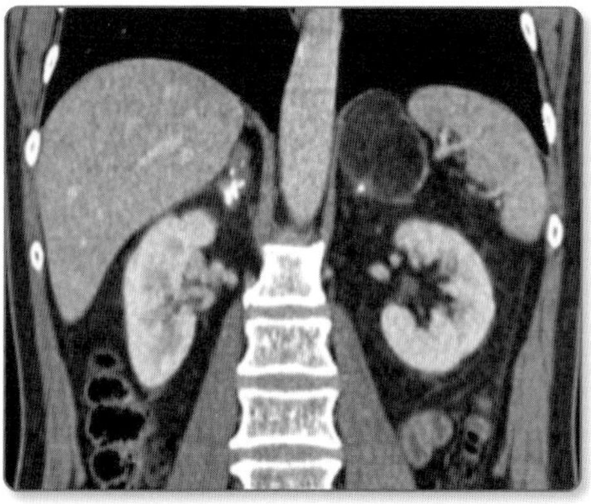

Suggested response

These are selected images from a contrast-enhanced CT scan of the upper abdomen.

There is an encapsulated retroperitoneal mass which is predominantly of fat density. The mass measures several centimetres in diameter and lies superior to the left kidney. On these images, the mass appears to arise from the adrenal gland (which is not visualised separately) and abuts, but appears to be separate from, the kidney. It contains wisps of soft tissue attenuation material and there is some calcification within the wall. There is also right adrenal calcification.

In my usual practice, I would review the remainder of the scan, but I do not see any further definite abnormalities on these images.

The most likely diagnosis is a myelolipoma and, unless the patient is symptomatic, no further investigation is required and treatment is unlikely to be necessary.

Diagnosis

Myelolipoma (an incidental finding in a study performed to evaluate lung disease which is not visible on these images).

Tips: A retroperitoneal mass

Key points

A good understanding of anatomy is the key to reaching a differential diagnosis. Most retroperitoneal masses arise in the perirenal space. The kidney and adrenal gland lie laterally in the perirenal space and the inferior vena cava and aorta lie in the midline in the perirenal space.

Differential diagnoses

Distinguishing between retroperitoneal fibrosis and lymphoma is an easy topic to examine in a viva setting. Retroperitoneal fibrosis causes medial deviation of the ureter, whereas lymphoma causes lateral deviation and also tends to displace the aorta anteriorly.

Age is a useful factor in reaching a differential diagnosis as retroperitoneal malignancies such as neuroblastoma and Wilms' tumour are comparatively common in the first 5 years of life.

Cases incorporating a syndrome occur frequently in viva scenarios. Tuberous sclerosis is associated with multiple renal angiomyolipomas (which lead to a well-described risk of haemorrhage), renal cysts and also a risk of renal cell carcinoma. Possible manifestations of Von Hippel–Lindau syndrome include solid organ cysts, phaeochromocytoma and renal cell carcinoma.

Myelolipoma

This is an uncommon benign retroperitoneal mass which usually arises from the adrenal gland and often comes to light as an incidental finding, as in this case. There is no risk of malignant change; its origin from the adrenal gland and well-defined nature distinguish it from the main differential of retroperitoneal liposarcoma. Areas of calcification are present in around 20% of cases. The appearance of this pathology on ultrasound and MRI varies with the relative proportions of myeloid and adipose tissue. Extra-adrenal myelolipomas may occur but are exceedingly rare.

Case 16

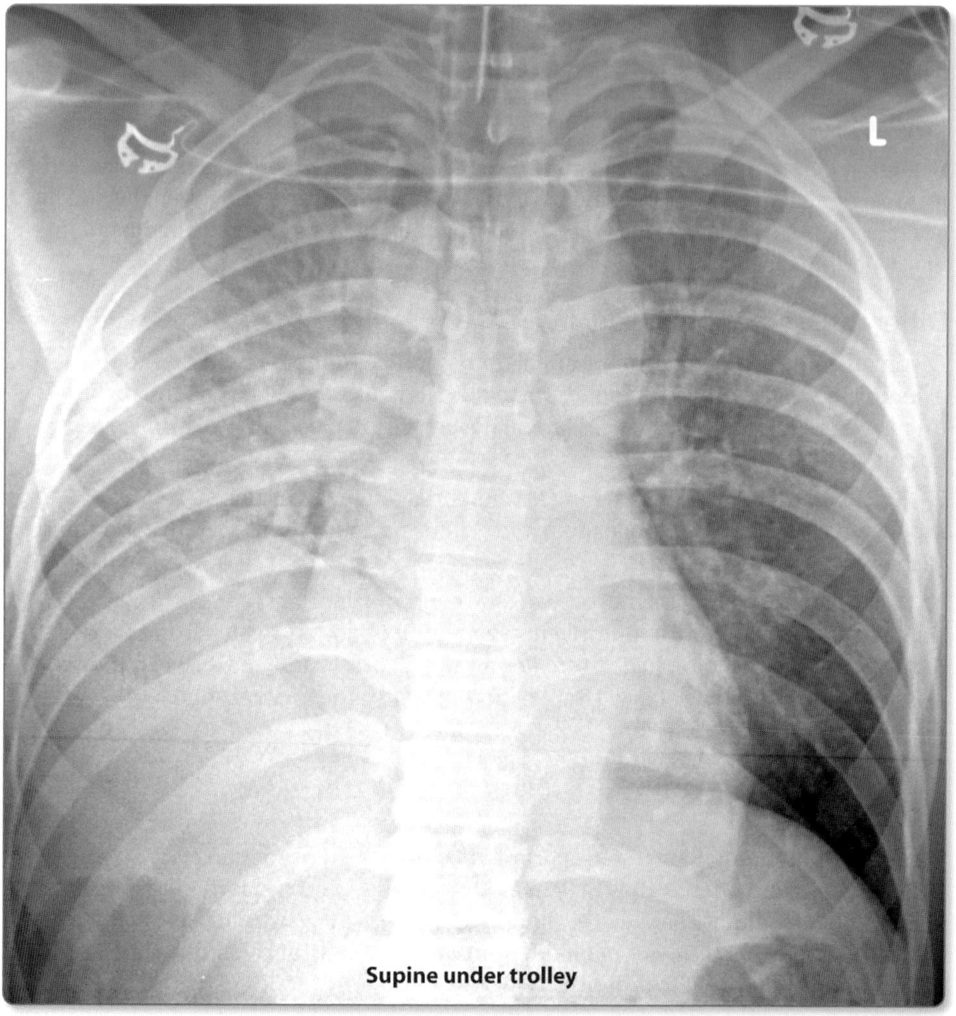

Suggested response

This is a supine chest radiograph with several significant findings.

An endotracheal tube is present, the tip of which is projected slightly high in the trachea at the level of T1/T2 and may benefit from being advanced further; this should be discussed with the referring clinicians. Cardiac monitoring leads are also noted. These findings suggest a very unwell patient.

Even allowing for the supine projection, there is widening of the upper mediastinum, with the aortic knuckle not clearly visualised and with 'apical capping' bilaterally. No obvious vertebral fractures or other bony injuries are identified, but if there is a history of blunt trauma this appearance raises suspicions for an aortic injury.

There is also a discrepancy in translucency between the two hemithoraces, with increased opacity on the right. Increased opacity of the right hemithorax in this nonrotated supine radiograph could be due to consolidation (including contusion), haemothorax or effusion. No pneumothorax is identified.

Furthermore, the right hemidiaphragm is indistinct and sits higher than the left. If there is a history of trauma, this raises suspicions for diaphragmatic rupture, although review of any available previous imaging would clarify whether diaphragmatic elevation is a new feature.

In summary, there are multiple potentially life-threatening features on this radiograph including strong suspicion of aortic rupture. I would convey these findings to the referring clinicians immediately with a view to discussing urgent CT scanning.

Diagnosis

Adult male pedestrian hit by car causing contained aortic rupture. Getting to the full diagnosis may not be possible from this radiograph but it should be possible to identify many abnormalities and be able to talk around them, trying to reach a unifying diagnosis.

Tips: Trauma chest radiographs

A systematic approach is vital in reviewing these radiographs. These studies can be very 'busy', so use a logical system that is suited to you. It does not matter particularly whether you look at lines and tubes or mediastinal contours first (although the authors prefer the former), providing that everything relevant and important is covered.

Key points

Misplaced lines and tubes are far more frequent in examinations than in real life, so consider each one carefully, particularly when presented with a radiograph from an emergency situation in which rapid placement may have been necessary. Clues such as cardiac monitoring leads, defibrillator paddles, a spinal board or neck support may help to clarify the clinical status of the patient.

Remember that trauma radiographs are often acquired in the supine projection which reduces their sensitivity with respect to examination of the lungs. A supine projection may make pneumothoraces and pneumoperitoneum less visible, but will exaggerate the cardiac and mediastinal contours. In the context of trauma, true mediastinal widening may be due to vertebral fractures, aortic injury, haemorrhage secondary to damage to small mediastinal vessels, or other incidental findings such as vascular tortuosity.

Look for abnormal gas patterns that may indicate pneumomediastinum, pneumoperitoneum or pneumothorax. Do not forget that the signs of a pneumothorax on a supine radiograph differ from those on an erect radiograph and may include the 'deep sulcus' sign and increased lucency over the upper abdomen.

As well as scrutinising all the bones for fractures, it is important to be alert for certain specific patterns of injury. Fractures of the first to third ribs imply significant force and are often associated with neurovascular damage or bronchial rupture. Fractures of the 11th and 12th ribs increase the likelihood of abdominal visceral injury. If there is a sternal injury, it is important to look specifically for a mid-thoracic vertebral fracture and vice versa. With either of these findings, look for a great vessel injury.

Traumatic injury to the aorta

Aortic ruptures are typically caused by rapid deceleration injuries (as seen in road traffic collisions). Most patients with an aortic rupture do not survive sufficiently long to undergo imaging in hospital. A normal appearance on an erect chest radiograph makes traumatic aortic injury highly unlikely. In traumatic injury, the usual finding on a radiograph is mediastinal widening, but this is a very nonspecific finding (mediastinal haematoma is more likely to be caused by damage to smaller vessels). The presence of ancillary signs such as apical capping (representing extrapleural extension of a haematoma along aortic arch vessels), left main bronchus depression and upper rib fractures increase the likelihood that the patient has sustained significant vascular damage. Great vessel injury is not something that can be diagnosed on radiographs; CT scanning is effectively mandatory in patients who sustain the kind of traumatic force that would be sufficient to cause aortic injury. On arterial phase imaging – or biphasic, single-acquisition CT which is now common in the assessment of trauma – look out for intraluminal filling defects, pseudoaneurysm formation or intramural haematoma.

Case 17

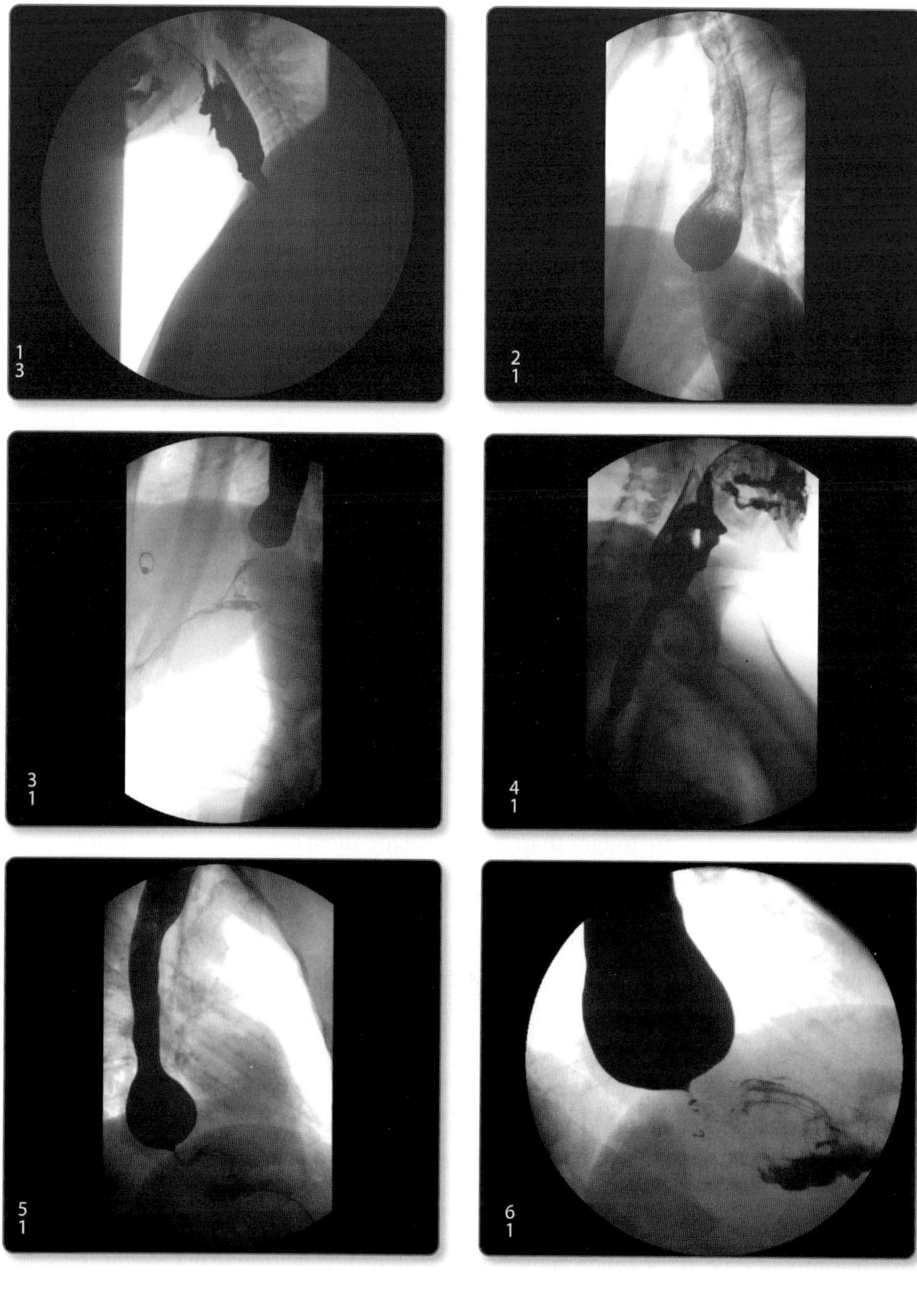

Suggested response

These are selected images from a contrast examination of the oesophagus in an adult patient.

The contrast passes into the oesophagus without visible aspiration, but the oesophagus, which is predominantly visualised in single contrast only, is markedly abnormal. The lower half in particular is widely dilated and contains what appears to be food residue. Just below the level of the diaphragm there is smooth, rapid tapering of the lumen which becomes very narrow over a short segment. A small amount of contrast has passed beyond this and what is visible of the stomach appears normal.

Further clinical details may sway the emphasis in the differential diagnosis, but there is a tight, smooth-looking stricture in the distal oesophagus, hence the main differential lies between achalasia, malignancy and an inflammatory stricture. The margins are smooth and there is no appreciable mass, so I would favour achalasia. I would discuss this case with the referring clinician and suggest endoscopy to exclude a carcinoma. A diagnosis of achalasia can be confirmed with oesophageal manometry.

Diagnosis

Achalasia

Tips: Focal oesophageal narrowing

Key points

Look at the (craniocaudal) length of the lesion to decide if it is a web, ring or stricture. Webs and rings are the most common oesophageal structural abnormalities.

A web is <3 mm long and most commonly occurs in the cervical oesophagus. Webs usually arise anteriorly, are typically post-inflammatory and may undergo malignant transformation.

Oesophageal rings are longer than 3 mm and are most common in the distal oesophagus. They are due to concentric extension of normal oesophageal tissue. Note that a Schatzki or 'B' 'ring' is actually a web.

Strictures are longer than 10 mm and can be short or long (paradoxically very long strictures may not be malignant). Crohn's disease can cause strictures of a variable length. Long strictures can be caused by conditions which increase exposure to acid such as causes of reflux, nasogastric tubes and Zollinger–Ellison syndrome. Strictures secondary to ingestion of corrosives may develop years after the initial insult.

Differential diagnoses

The vast majority of irregular strictures are malignant and inflammatory strictures are more likely to be smooth. Classically, achalasia gives a smooth 'rat's tail' or 'bird's beak' appearance.

The appearance of the mucosa may help to identify infection (e.g. *Candida*), ulceration or ectopic gastric mucosa (Barrett's oesophagus).

Do not forget that extrinsic compression, for instance from a mediastinal mass, may also be a possibility and remember that some normal anatomical structures cause impressions on the oesophagus (cricopharyngeus, aortic arch and the left main bronchus).

Primary achalasia

This is a motility disorder which is usually idiopathic but may be caused by Chagas' disease. It is characterised by a lack of peristalsis and failure of relaxation of the lower oesophageal sphincter. In the examination setting and real life, it may initially present as a 'posterior mediastinal mass' (containing gas and food residue) on a chest radiograph. Look also for an absence of gas in the gastric fundus.

In a viva, if a chest radiograph has a truly bizarre appearance and you have no idea where to start, then consider the oesophagus as the offending organ. The so-called 'neo-oesophagus' (after oesophagectomy) and grossly dilated examples of achalasia can produce extraordinary appearances.

Case 18

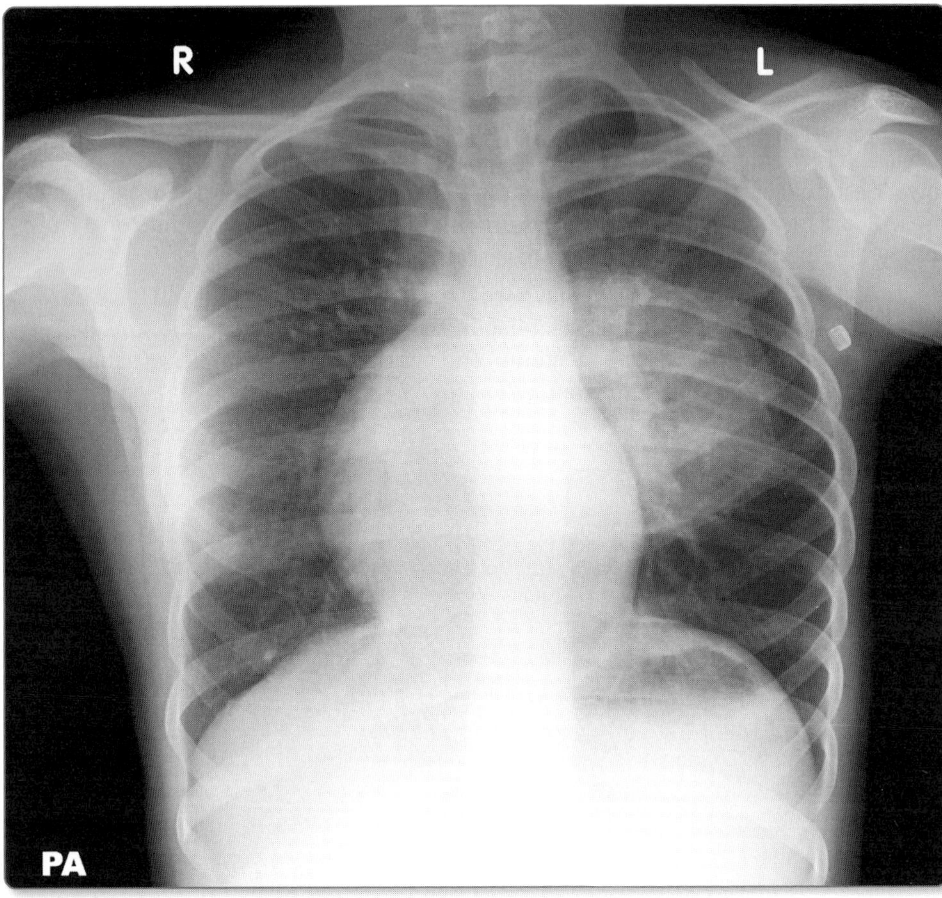

Suggested response

This is a posteroanterior chest radiograph of a skeletally immature patient. A large rounded opacity of soft tissue, measuring approximately 10 cm in diameter, is projected over the left mid and lower zones. This is well-defined laterally, but the medial border is not clearly visualised. All intrathoracic structures on the left side of the mediastinum are present and are clearly defined, although the mediastinum is shifted to the right. Otherwise the lungs are clear, although I note that there is increased transradiancy of the left lung field compared to the right.

A metallic density is present in the left axilla and the pectoral girdle appears asymmetric, being deficient on the left. The left second to fifth ribs are slender in comparison with the corresponding right ribs. The lungs, mediastinum and thoracic skeleton appear otherwise normal.

The difference in transradiancy cannot be explained by patient rotation since the patient is slightly rotated to the right side. The fact that the borders of the mediastinal structures remain clearly visible suggests that the large density is not in contact with these structures and, accordingly, may not be intrathoracic. The chest wall anomalies are likely to explain the mediastinal shift, although it is possible that the large density contributes anteriorly.

The combination of left-sided chest wall deformity, metallic density in the left axilla and a large left-sided opacity suggest that this is a surgical implant (most likely pectoral) with an underlying diagnosis of Poland's syndrome. Review of any available relevant previous imaging would be useful to clarify and assess for change, and it would be useful to confirm whether there is a past history of surgery.

Diagnosis

A 14-year-old girl with Poland's syndrome and left-sided pectoral implant.

Tips: Unilateral increased transradiancy

Check that the side contralateral to the increased transradiancy is not abnormally dense (pneumonia or pleural effusion).

Differential diagnoses

Consider if the findings could be explained by technical factors such as the anode heel effect (rarely) or patient rotation (most common). In a rotated patient, the more lucent lung is usually seen on the side to which the patient is rotated (i.e. the side on which the medial aspect of the clavicle is furthest away from the spinous process). On a rotated radiograph, increased transradiancy which does not obey this rule cannot have been caused by the rotation.

If technical factors do not offer an explanation, then consider chest wall, pleural and parenchymal causes. Unilateral mastectomy, Poland's syndrome or previous poliomyelitis may give a reduced amount of soft tissue on one side of the chest. A pneumothorax is the most common cause in the pleural cavity. Within the parenchyma, there may be too much gas (as in emphysema or congenital lobar emphysema with air trapping, compensatory expansion following collapse or resection of a lobe, or air trapping behind an inhaled foreign body); restricted arterial flow, as is seen with pulmonary artery hypoplasia (alone or as part of Swyer–James syndrome); or a lesion constricting the pulmonary artery.

Poland's syndrome

More commonly affecting males, Poland's syndrome is a rare congenital disorder. It is characterised by unilateral hypoplasia of the chest wall (including breast, pectoral muscles, ribs and costal cartilage) as well as unilateral hand deformities. Surgical correction depends on the degree of deformity; surgical options include pectoral implant and breast augmentation or implants, but these are often not performed until after puberty.

Hand involvement may take the form of syndactyly (short middle phalanges with cutaneous webbing) or even complete absence of the hand.

Case 19

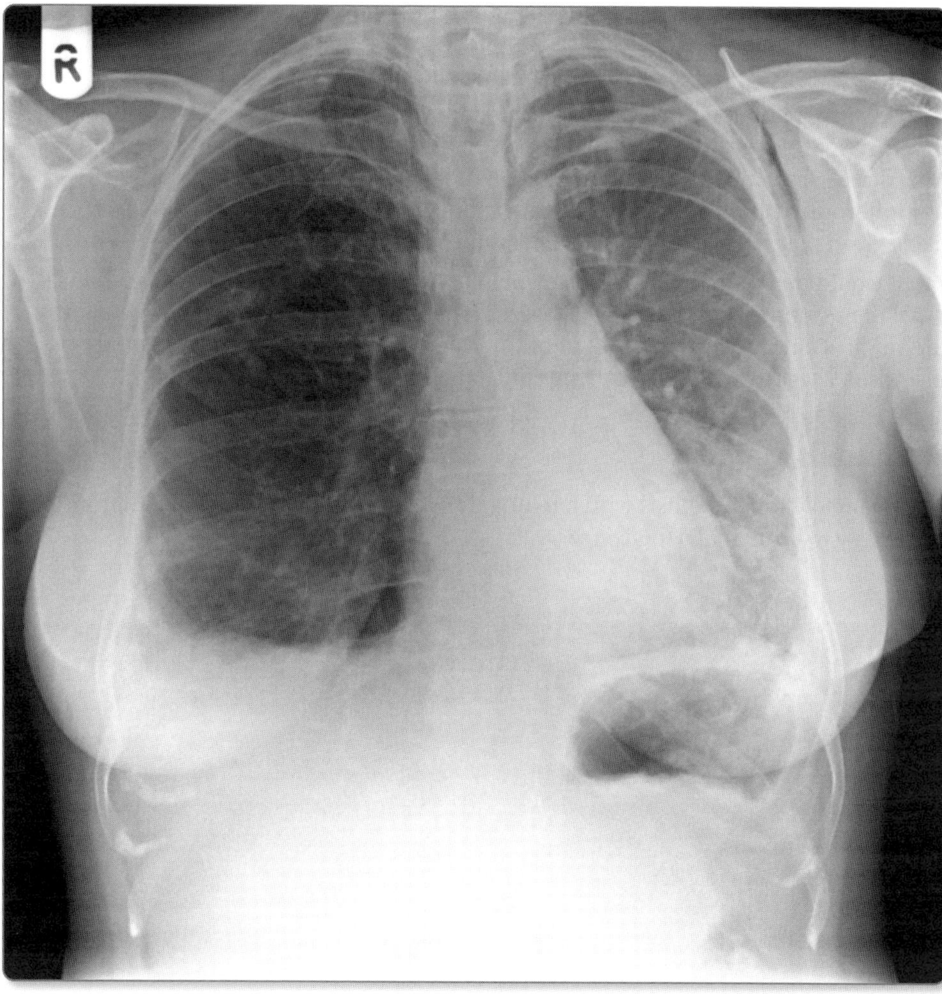

Suggested response

This is a frontal chest radiograph of a skeletally mature female. Several abnormalities are evident. Although the radiograph is fairly well-centred, the right hemithorax is more lucent than the left. The right lung is of greater volume with coarse interstitial shadowing and the impression of cystic change involving all zones.

There is subcutaneous emphysema, most conspicuous lateral to the left upper ribs. A linear opacity running between and parallel to the right third and fourth ribs posteriorly could represent the lung edge with a small apical pneumothorax. A line of gas running parallel to the left side of the mediastinum could feasibly represent pneumomediastinum although appearances are inconclusive and there are no ancillary signs such as the 'continuous diaphragm' sign. No left-sided pneumothorax is identified.

There is pleural reaction at both costophrenic angles. The left hemidiaphragm and left heart border are clearly visualised and increased density in the left mid and lower zones is more in keeping with effusion than collapse or consolidation.

One explanation for the marked discrepancy in the appearances in the lungs is that there has been a lung transplantation on the left. Differentials for the underlying lung disease include lymphangioleiomyomatosis (LAM), tuberous sclerosis (TS), neurofibromatosis and Langerhans' cell histiocytosis (LCH), the latter two being less likely given that cystic change is evident at the right base.

It would be useful to review any available previous imaging to assess for change, but if the assumption that there has been a left lung transplantation is correct and the surgical emphysema and pneumothorax are new findings, this case should be discussed urgently with the referring clinician.

Diagnosis

Lymphangioleiomyomatosis with left lung transplant and pneumomediastinum secondary to bronchial dehiscence.

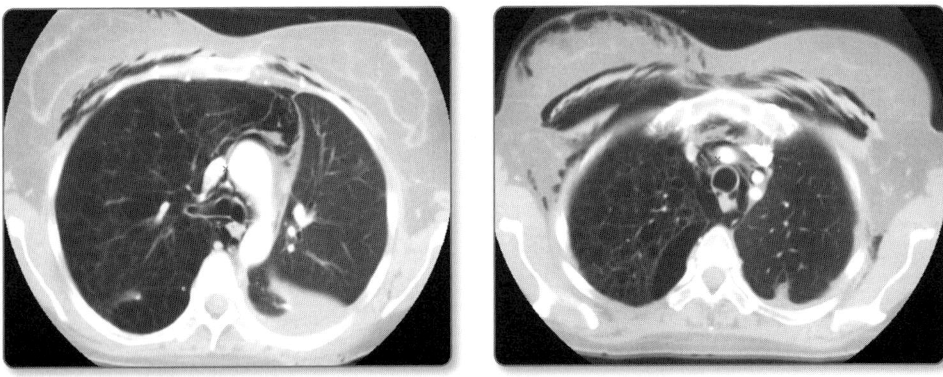

Figure 1 Axial CT images (lung windows) showing lymphangioleiomyomatosis of the right lung and post-transplant appearances of the left lung with pneumomediastinum, small right apical pneumothorax and left pleural effusion.

Tips: Cystic lung disease

Key points

Consider the zonal distribution of the disease. LCH tends to spare the lower zones, whereas neurofibromatosis is predominantly apical. In contrast, LAM and TS have no zonal predominance.

Consider the size and shape of cysts. LCH nodules evolve into thick- and then thin-walled cysts of varied size and shape (characteristically 'bizarre'), whereas the cysts in LAM and TS are more uniform.

Ancillary findings may provide clues that aid diagnosis. The fact that a patient is male effectively excludes LAM as a diagnosis. LAM or TS should be suspected if there are renal cysts or angiomyolipomas, and LCH and neurofibromatosis may be associated with bony abnormalities.

Lymphangioleiomyomatosis

Lymphangioleiomyomatosis is rare in real life (it has a prevalence of around one in a million) but is far more common in examinations. It affects only females, typically those of child-bearing age. Abnormal smooth muscle proliferation in the walls of small airways results in postobstructive cyst formation throughout the lungs, the cysts being randomly distributed (with normal intervening lung). These cysts typically exhibit more uniformity of size than the irregular cysts seen in LCH. TS and LAM involve, in essence, the same pathological process, hence they exhibit identical features on thoracic imaging. Pneumothorax is a common presentation and chylothorax (a consequence of smooth muscle proliferation in the lymphatics) is also commonly seen. Chylothorax can be differentiated from a 'simple' effusion on CT scanning by its fatty attenuation. Lung transplant may be considered for end-stage LAM although recurrence in the transplanted lung has been reported.

Case 20

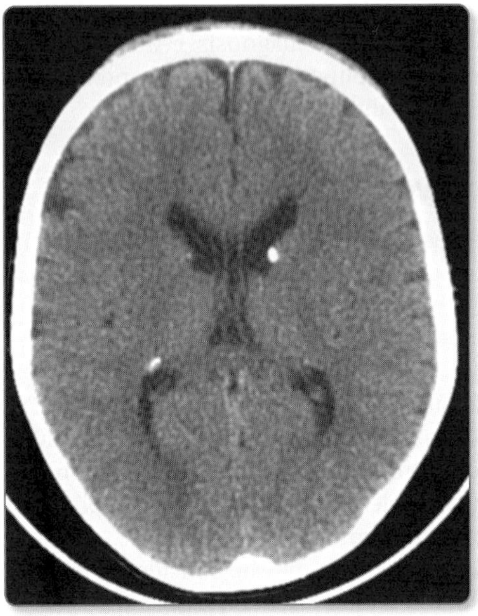

Suggested response

This is an axial image through the level of the thalami and head of the caudate nuclei from an unenhanced CT study of the head. There are multiple subependymal foci of calcification. No other abnormality is visible on this slice.

The appearance is nonspecific and could be due to old infection (such as cytomegalovirus or toxoplasmosis) or secondary to a condition such as tuberous sclerosis, although there is a wider differential of rarer conditions that could also give this appearance.

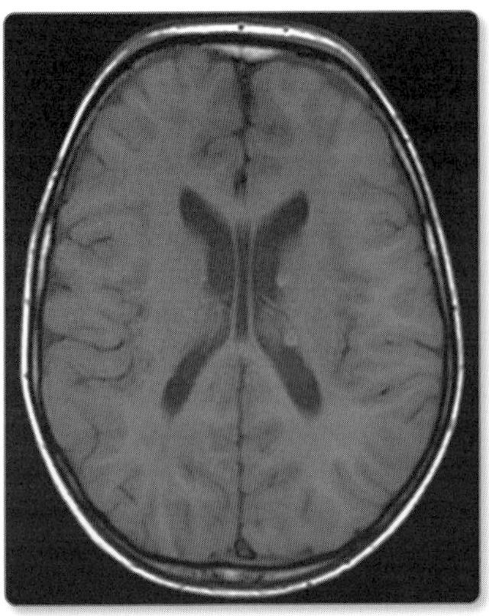

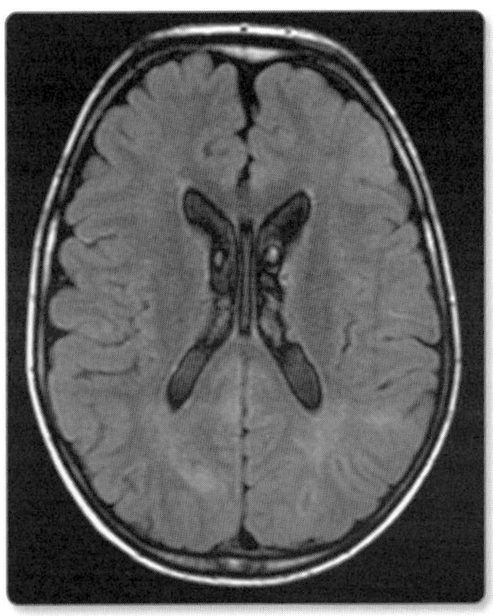

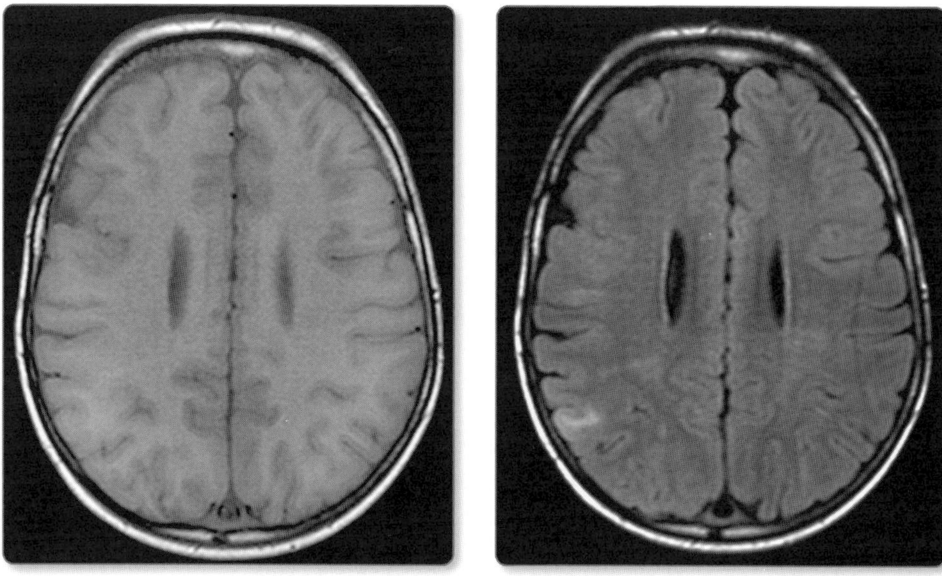

Suggested response

These are selected axial images from an MRI study of the brain.

There are multiple small subependymal nodules. On the fluid-attenuated inversion recovery (FLAIR) images, several cortical and subcortical foci of high signal are evident. These are likely to represent cortical tubers.

I note a septum cavum pellucidum which is a common incidental finding, but I am not aware of any association with the likely diagnosis of tuberous sclerosis. I cannot see any complication of TS such as a subependymal astrocytoma on these images, but would of course review the whole study.

Diagnosis

Tuberous sclerosis without identifiable complication.

Tips: Intracranial calcification

Key points

Intracranial calcifications are usually pathological in children but are more often physiological with increasing age. Calcification of the pineal gland may be seen in the under 20s and is increasingly common with age, as is calcification of the dural reflections, arachnoid granulations, choroid plexus and dentate nucleus of the cerebellum. Calcification of the basal ganglia is a common incidental finding, usually of no clinical significance, but may raise the possibility of Fahr's disease.

Differential diagnosis

The differential diagnosis is extensive but may be ordered with a simplified surgical sieve.

Congenital causes include tuberous sclerosis with subependymal and/or cortical hamartomas, and Sturge–Weber syndrome with gyriform lesions.

Acquired causes include dystrophic calcifications associated with trauma from injury or previous surgery, ischaemic insults and previous radiotherapy.

Inflammatory causes include sarcoidosis with leptomeningeal, periventricular, pituitary or pontine calcifications, and systemic lupus erythematosus with calcifications in the basal ganglia or cerebellum. Infective inflammatory causes may be congenital such as toxoplasmosis, rubella cytomegalovirus, herpes simplex and human immunodeficiency virus (HIV) (TORCH) infections, with periventricular and/or subependymal calcifications (which may resolve with treatment in the case of toxoplasmosis), or congenital HIV, with periventricular frontal or cerebellar calcifications. Acquired infective causes include cysticercosis (associated with calcified cysts in ventricles, basal cisterns and at the grey–white matter junction), tuberculosis, *Cryptococcus* infection (associated with parenchymal or meningeal calcifications) and HIV (associated with calcifications in the basal ganglia).

Neoplastic causes are those tumours which commonly calcify. Intra-axial lesions include oligodendrogliomas (up to 90% calcify) and low-grade astrocytomas, while extra-axial lesions include meningiomas and pineal gland tumours.

Cardiovascular and metabolic causes include calcifications associated with atherosclerosis and vascular malformations. Hyperparathyroidism is associated with calcification in the basal ganglia and subcortical regions, whereas in Fahr's disease calcifications are seen in basal ganglia, cerebral white matter and the cerebellum, although idiopathic calcification of the basal ganglia in older patients is not uncommon.

Tuberous sclerosis

The incidence of spontaneously occurring tuberous sclerosis is similar to that of inherited (autosomal dominant) tuberous sclerosis. The classic triad of findings is adenoma sebaceum, mental retardation and seizures. However, only one-third of cases exhibit all three findings, and multiple other features may be identified, including subependymal nodules, cortical and/or subcortical tubers, cardiac rhabdomyoma, angiomyolipomas, ungual fibromas, retinal hamartomas and subependymal giant cell astrocytoma.

Case 21

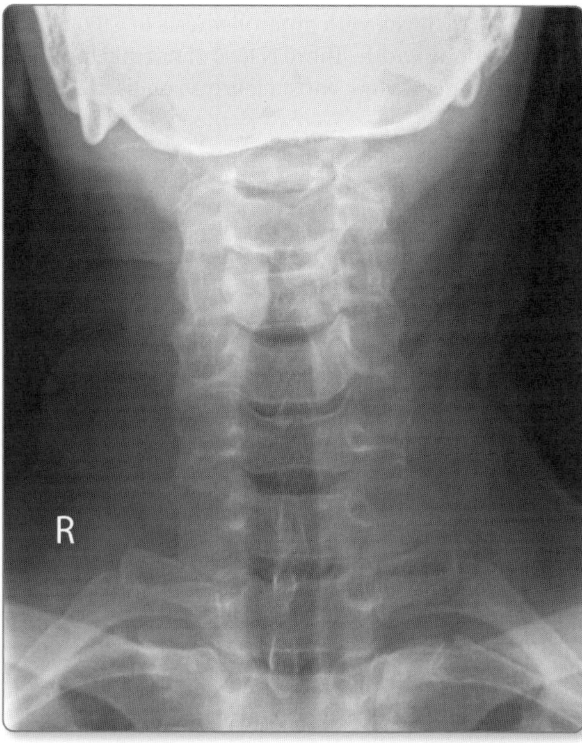

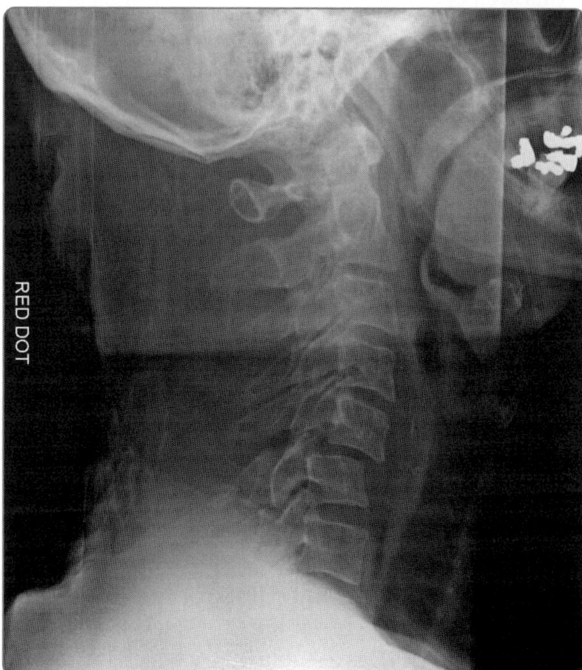

Suggested response

These are anteroposterior and lateral views of the cervical spine. A spinal board is evident, suggesting that this is a trauma case. There is loss of normal alignment of all three spinal lines at the C5/C6 level, with anterolisthesis of C5 on C6 of approximately one-quarter of a vertebral body width. There is loss of normal facet joint alignment with a 'bow tie' sign on the lateral view, most clearly visualised at C5. No convincing fracture is identified.

Findings are most in keeping with unilateral facet joint dislocation. Although this is typically a stable injury, the patient has suffered a very significant injury and I would not consider these views sufficient evaluation of their cervical spine. I would contact the referring clinician immediately to highlight this injury with a view to an urgent CT scan of the cervical spine to further characterise this injury and look for other injuries, ensuring that spinal support is maintained in the meantime.

Diagnosis

Unilateral facet joint dislocation in an adult patient following a 1.5 m (5 feet) fall onto a hyperflexed neck.

Tips: Cervical spine trauma diagnosis

Key points

You must be seen to ensure that the whole cervical spine is adequately visualised by counting out the vertebral levels from the base of skull to T1. If the cervicothoracic junction is not clearly identified, then say so and state that in ordinary practice you would ensure that this area is visualised. A 'swimmer's view' is one possibility, but it is increasingly common to proceed directly to CT depending on other findings and the clinical situation. Remember that Jefferson's fractures may be subtle on standard anteroposterior and lateral views, hence 'peg views' should be scrutinised for alignment of the lateral masses.

You must assess the three lines on the lateral view – anterior to vertebral bodies, posterior to vertebral bodies and anterior to spinous processes – and ensure that all facet joints are normally aligned. Beware of pseudosubluxation which may be seen in paediatric patients.

Comment on the prevertebral soft tissues using the 'rule of 4s': On the lateral view, soft tissue should measure up to 4 mm down to the level of C4 and up to the anteroposterior diameter of C4 inferior to this.

Remember to review key areas such as Harris' ring (composite shadow at the base of the odontoid peg) and also the calvaria and skull base for injuries. Do not forget to inspect the sphenoid sinus for a possible fluid level.

Unilateral facet joint dislocation

Dislocation or lock of a unilateral facet joint (UFJD) occurs as a result of a flexion-rotation injury. It most commonly occurs at the C5/C6 level, as in this case. Unlike bilateral facet joint dislocation, UFJD is a stable injury which is most readily appreciated on oblique radiographs of the cervical spine. It can be recognised by a 'bow tie' sign of vertebrae above the level of the dislocation as a result of viewing four rotated facets, with anterolisthesis of less than one-quarter of a vertebral body width. Spinous processes can be seen to be rotated on anteroposterior views (subtle in this case). Findings can be confirmed on CT: locked facets will be seen on sagittal reformats (see **Figure 1**) and loss of normal facet joint alignment will be apparent on axial imaging (see **Figure 2**). Normally, facet joint alignment is seen on axial CT as a 'Hamburger' sign. Loss of this sign should be sought carefully as it indicates facet joint dislocation.

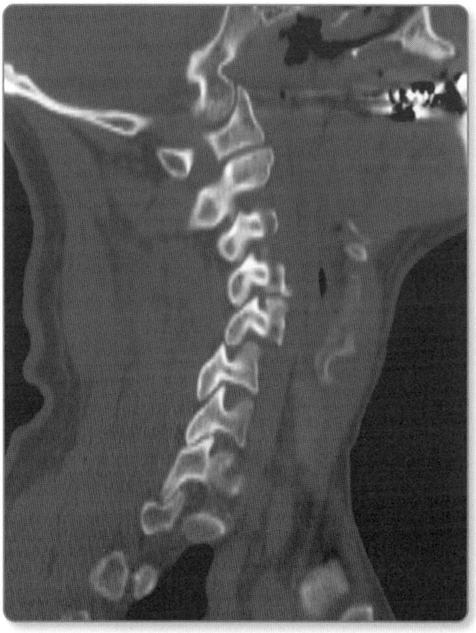

Figure 1 Sagittal reformat demonstrating locked facets.

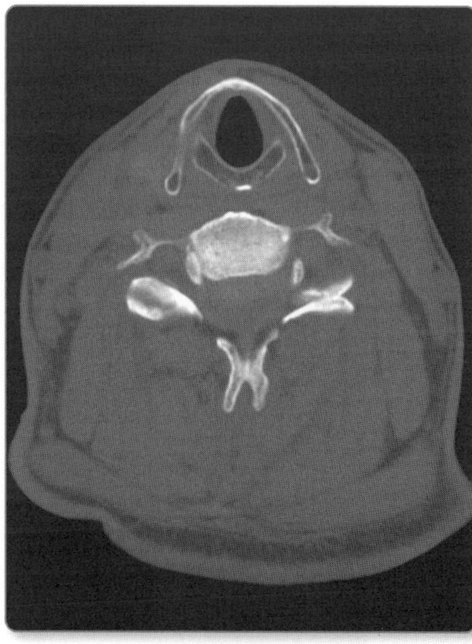

Figure 2 Axial CT showing loss of the normal left facet joint alignment (loss of the 'Hamburger' sign).

Case 22

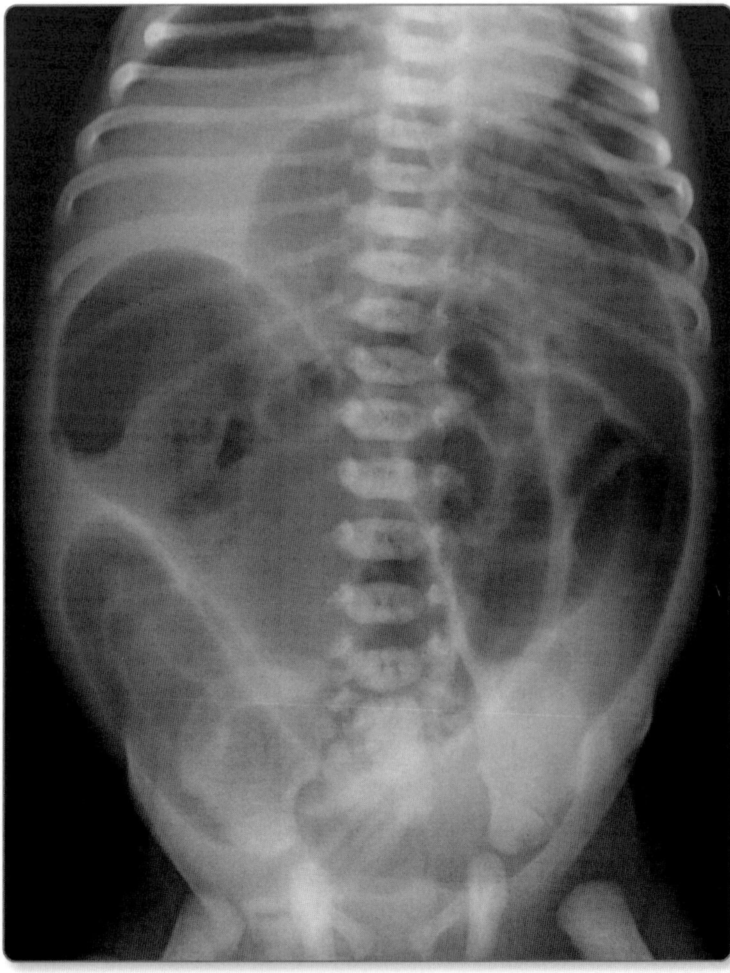

Suggested response

This is an abdominopelvic radiograph of a neonate. A nasogastric tube is present and appears to be in an appropriate position. There are multiple grossly dilated bowel loops without any visible gas–fluid levels. Loops of nondistended bowel are evident centrally. The main differential diagnosis here is meconium ileus with other possibilities including ileal atresia, Hirschsprung's disease and imperforate anus. If this neonate has not yet passed meconium, I would favour meconium ileus.

I would discuss this case with the referring clinicians with a view to excluding imperforate anus clinically, and to consider a contrast enema for further evaluation.

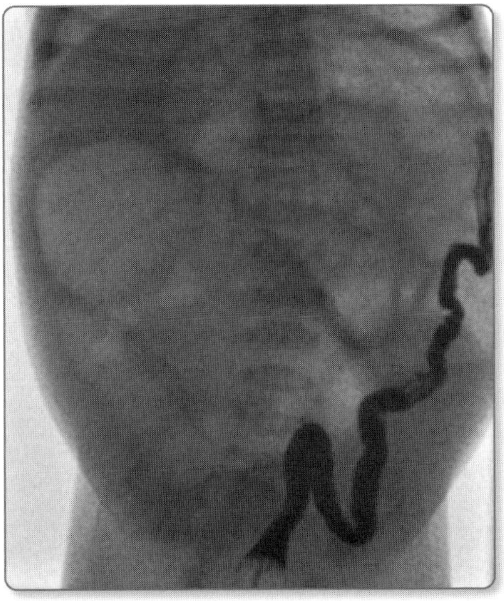

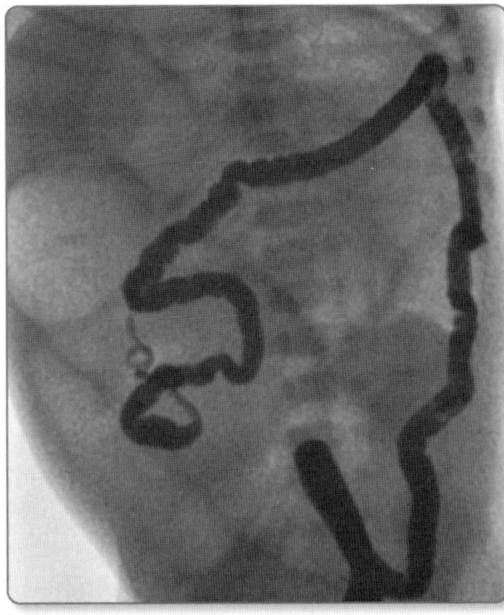

Suggested response

These two spot images from a contrast enema show a very narrowed colon, consistent with microcolon, with a few filling defects evident in the colon. Multiple dilated loops of small bowel are again visible. Although both meconium ileus and ileal atresia can cause microcolon, the lack of air-fluid levels makes meconium ileus the most likely cause. I would recommend that the neonate should be tested for cystic fibrosis.

Diagnosis

Meconium ileus in a 2-day-old neonate with cystic fibrosis (CF).

Tips: Neonatal low bowel obstruction

Key points

Differentiate between high and low bowel obstruction. In the neonate, distinguishing between small and large bowel is extremely challenging. However, high bowel obstruction (up to the jejunum, e.g. jejunal/duodenal/pyloric atresia) tends to present with vomiting, whereas low bowel obstruction (distal to the jejunum, e.g. ileal/colonic atresia, meconium ileus) tends to present with failure to pass meconium.

Consider the size of the colon. Microcolon may be evident in cases of meconium ileus and ileal atresia, whereas a distended right and transverse colon with small left colon may be seen in meconium plug syndrome (related to CF) and small left colon syndrome (not related to CF). Proximal distension of the colon with normal distal colon may be seen in Hirschsprung's disease, whereas proximal distension of the colon with a small distal colon may be seen in colonic atresia and anorectal malformations (usually with no gas in rectum).

Consider and mention any air-fluid levels in the bowel. These are typically absent in meconium ileus but prominent in ileal atresia. Check the hernial orifices for evidence of an inguinal hernia and mention the need to look for imperforate anus on clinical examination while assessing for manifestations of VACTERL association (gas in the bladder suggesting fistula, sacral agenesis). Peritoneal calcifications may be seen in cases of meconium ileus as a consequence of in utero perforation.

Meconium ileus

Meconium ileus is often the initial manifestation of CF and proven meconium ileus is almost always associated with CF. Meconium is a normal finding in the neonatal intestine but pancreatic insufficiency secondary to CF makes it more viscous than normal, such that the meconium impacts in the distal small bowel. The associated microcolon is not specific to meconium ileus but is seen in any case of underused bowel in a neonate, including ileal atresia. The water-soluble contrast enema has a dual role, being both diagnostic and therapeutic. Although a nonspecific finding, a characteristic 'soap bubble' appearance is strongly suggestive of meconium ileus and is a result of gas being mixed with the viscous meconium. Although not seen in this case, reflux of contrast into the terminal ileum often demonstrates pellets of meconium in the distended distal small bowel.

Case 23

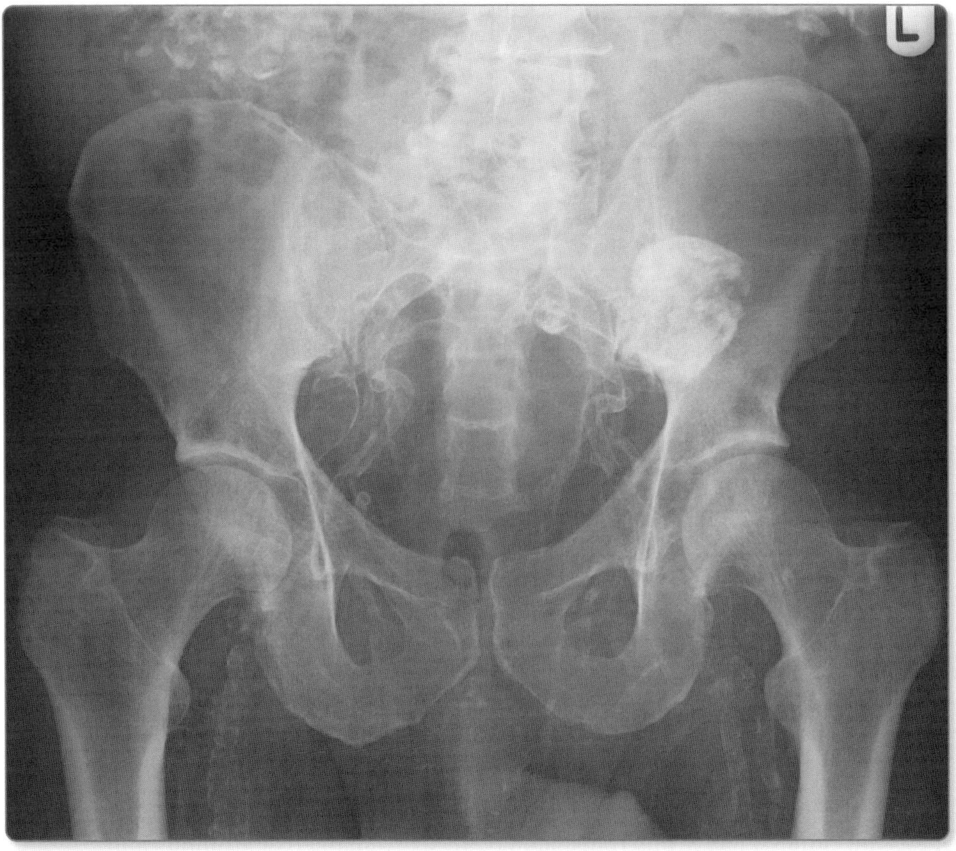

Suggested response

This is a pelvic radiograph of a skeletally mature male. Several abnormalities are evident. Firstly, there is a well-defined area of dense calcification projected over the left ilium, measuring at least 5 cm in diameter. Secondly, clusters of predominantly curvilinear calcification are projected in both flanks above the iliac crests. The upper extents of these areas of calcification are not visualised on the current radiograph. Thirdly, there is florid vascular calcification. The age of the patient would be relevant but while vascular calcification may be a normal ageing process, the extent of calcification here suggests an underlying disease process such as chronic renal failure. The area of dense calcification in the left iliac fossa is in a typical location for a renal transplant and, particularly given its morphology, could represent transplant autonephrectomy.

Correlation with clinical history and review of any available and relevant previous imaging would be valuable to assess for change and to establish whether or not the clusters of abdominal calcifications have been visualised in their entirety. Based on appearances of the current radiograph, however, the calcifications in the flanks could represent enlarged, polycystic kidneys, with a subsequent failed renal transplant.

Diagnosis

Renal transplant autonephrectomy with calcified native polycystic kidneys.

Tips: Renal transplant

Patients with renal transplants often have multisystem disorders with multiple imaging findings. These may be due to the underlying condition, the transplant or its complications. The relative frequency of the many potential complications of renal transplantation varies over time.

Key points: Ultrasound

You must be able to identify features of transplant rejection and other complications. Look specifically at renal size, parenchymal reflectivity and the collecting system for features of obstruction. Also look for perinephric collections and any evidence of renal vein thrombosis. An elevated resistive index (RI) > 0.9 is strongly predictive of renal dysfunction but is not specific to rejection because it is elevated above the normal value in all cases of renal dysfunction. It is calculated as follows:

$$RI = \frac{\text{(Peak systolic velocity – lowest diastolic velocity)}}{\text{Peak systolic velocity}}$$

Key points: Radiographs and fluoroscopic images

Assess all kidneys, native and transplanted, for size (enlarged or atrophic) and calcifications (parenchymal, collecting system and vascular). Scrutinise the bones for features of hyperparathyroidism. Look for evidence of a nephrostomy, a perinephric drain or a ureteric stent. If possible, look for evidence of vascular complications including renal artery stenosis/thrombosis, pseudoaneurysm and arteriovenous fistula.

Renal transplant imaging

Patients with renal transplants are encountered not infrequently in everyday radiological practice, often for assessment of complications. These occur in around one-tenth of transplant patients, so evaluate available imaging for both evidence of complications and of the underlying pathology necessitating transplant in the first place (this may also recur in the transplanted kidney and is responsible for up to 4% of allograft failures). Transplant-related immunosuppression significantly increases the risk of a range of malignancies (typically non-Hodgkin's lymphoma, but also lung, colorectal and bladder cancer).

Case 24

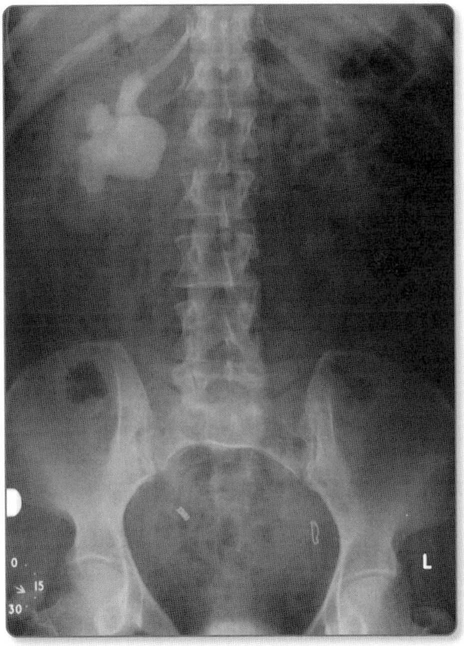

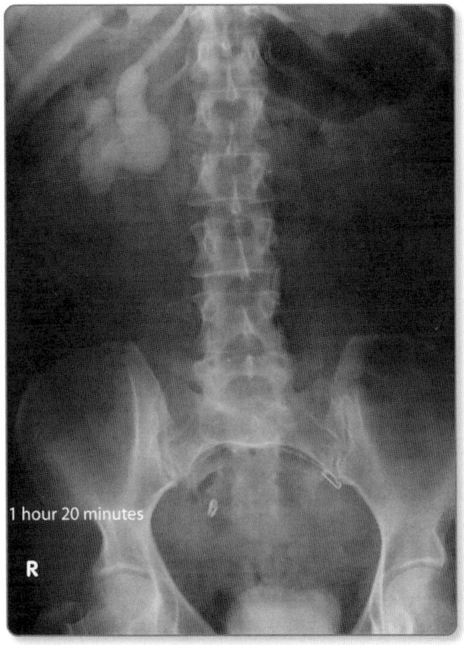

Suggested response

These are two radiographs taken from an intravenous urogram (IVU) series in a skeletally mature female patient, the first acquired at 20 minutes and the second at 80 minutes. There is an abnormality in the right kidney. The pelvicalyceal system is dilated, with calyceal clubbing which may obscure any calcification that could have been present on the control radiograph. In my usual practice, I would always review this in conjunction with the control radiograph. The right renal outline is dense on both radiographs, consistent with a persistent dense nephrogram. No contrast is evident in the right ureter on the 20-minute radiograph although contrast is seen in the proximal and mid ureter, which is of normal calibre, on the later radiograph.

The left renal outline is largely obscured, although contrast is faintly seen in the pelvicalyceal system and proximal ureter on the 20-minute radiograph. If there is clinical concern regarding the left kidney, it may be appropriate to acquire conventional tomographic views for more accurate assessment. Contrast is seen in the incompletely visualised bladder from 20 minutes.

Clips projected in the pelvis are most likely to represent sterilisation clips. Tubing projected over the right side of the abdomen is of uncertain origin, but presumably lies outside the body.

In summary, there is persisting dilatation of the right pelvicalyceal system with no evidence of ureteric dilatation. This is most in keeping with pelviureteric junction obstruction; however, no convincing cause is demonstrated. Urological referral is warranted if this is a new diagnosis and further imaging may be appropriate, for example, if there is suspicion of an obstructing calculus at the pelviureteric junction.

Diagnosis

Adult female patient with right pelviureteric junction obstruction.

Tips: Intravenous urography

Key points on the control radiograph

Calcifications in the renal area are most commonly assessed with CT although tomography or oblique radiographs were historically common and may potentially feature in the examination setting. Similarly, these techniques may help to distinguish between a calculus or phleboliths projected over the distal ureter. Urethral calculi may be projected behind the symphysis pubis. Remember to review the radiograph as you would for any abdominal radiograph (bowel gas, free gas, bones and joints, etc.).

Differential diagnosis for nephrographic patterns

A persistent or increasingly dense nephrogram may be seen in hypotension, renal vein thrombosis or with renal parenchymal damage. A striated nephrogram may reflect acute obstruction, renal vein thrombosis, medullary sponge kidney or acute pyelonephritis. A diminished nephrogram, reflecting reduced clearance, is seen in chronic obstruction. A striking rim nephrogram may be seen in severe chronic obstruction or with acute arterial occlusion.

Differential diagnosis for calyceal clubbing

The term calyceal clubbing applies when the sharp forniceal angle is obliterated. It is characteristic of urinary tract obstruction, but is also seen in pyelonephritis and papillary necrosis.

Pelviureteric junction obstruction

Intravenous urography has been largely superseded by CT urography in clinical practice. CT datasets are large and take time to digest so it should not come as too much of a surprise to see other types of imaging in a viva. You should familiarise yourself with the various nephrographic patterns and a few important differential diagnoses for each. Renal tract obstruction can cause a number of nephrographic patterns, as highlighted above. Pelviureteric junction obstruction is the most common cause of neonatal hydronephrosis, but more frequently affects adult patients. It may be primary (arising due to functional problems, anatomical variants or other extrinsic causes) or secondary (to infection or calculi, for instance). The frequency of the latter is one of the important reasons for scrutinising the control radiograph. If faced with a postcontrast IVU radiograph in a viva, ensure that the examiners are made aware that you would always review the control radiograph.

Case 25

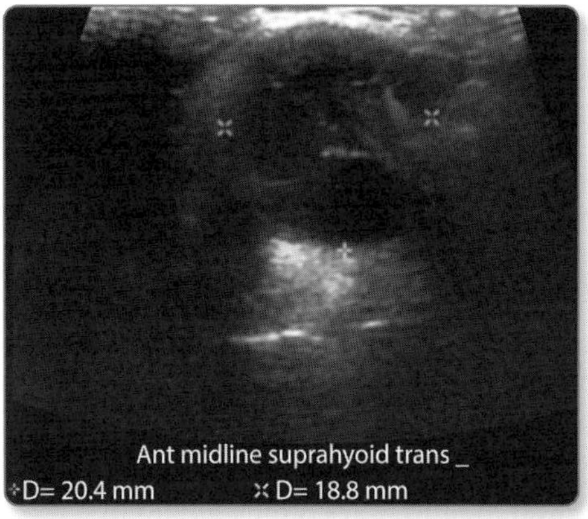

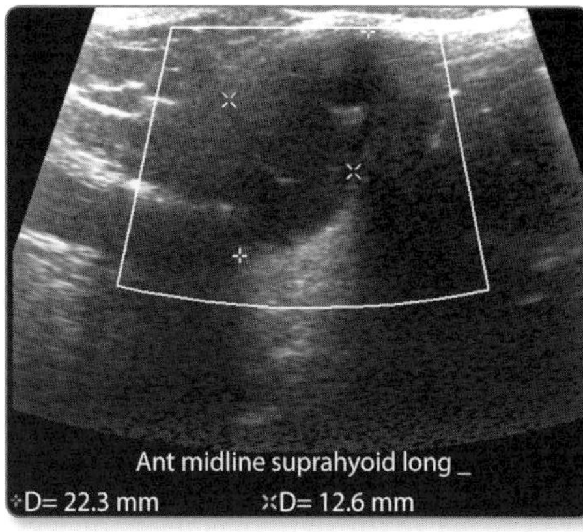

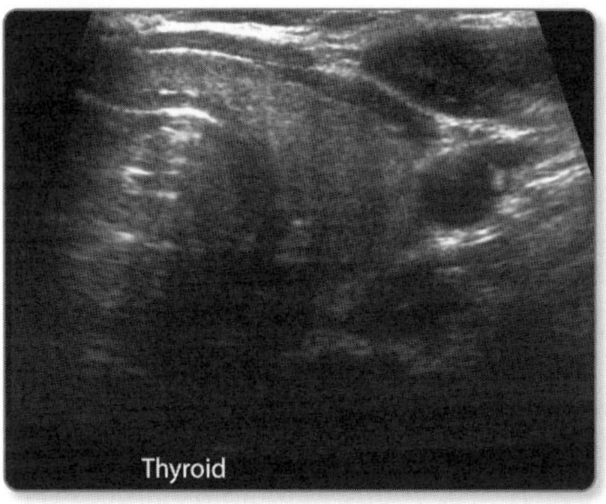

Suggested response

These are selected views from an ultrasound scan of the neck. There is an abnormality centred in the anterior midline in the suprahyoid region. The abnormality is a complex ovoid mass which is predominantly of low reflectivity, with posterior acoustic enhancement and which measures up to 22 mm in diameter. No internal flow is demonstrated on the Doppler images. The area of the thyroid visible on this image, in particular the isthmus, appears normal. Findings are consistent with a midline cystic lesion in the suprahyoid neck. The most common cause of a midline cystic mass in this region is a thyroglossal duct cyst. In this case the internal complexity raises the possibility of infection. I would discuss this case with the referring clinicians. If this diagnosis does not correspond with the clinical presentation, or if there is clinical concern regarding malignant transformation, MRI may be appropriate for further evaluation.

Diagnosis

Thyroglossal duct cyst in an adult female.

Tips: A lump in the neck

Key points and differential diagnosis

Consider whether the mass is midline or lateral. Thyroglossal duct cysts lie in the midline, whereas most other cystic structures (e.g. branchial cleft cyst, laryngocele) are laterally placed. Ectopic or accessory thyroid tissue may also occur in the midline, so ensure that the thyroid is in a normal position.

Consider whether the mass is solid or cystic. Solid masses are more likely to be neoplastic (necrotic small cell carcinoma being an exception which manifests as a thick-walled cystic structure). Cystic masses are more likely to be congenital (e.g. branchial cleft cysts, thyroglossal duct cyst, cystic lymphangioma).

The age of the patient is relevant. Cystic lymphangiomas are often evident in neonates. Branchial cleft cysts and thyroglossal duct cysts present in children and young adults. In older patients the development of a neck lump is very suspicious for neoplastic disease.

Thyroglossal duct cyst

Embryologically the thyroid descends to its normal position in the neck along the line of the thyroglossal duct, which extends inferiorly from the base of the tongue. Cysts may form along the course of this duct. Ectopic thyroid tissue is one of the main differential diagnoses for a midline neck mass and can be seen in addition to, or even inside, thyroglossal duct cysts. This can be detected using thyroid scintigraphy.

A thyroglossal duct cyst usually presents in a child or young adult as a painless midline or paramedian mass. Unlike in the example above, it is more common in the infrahyoid neck and elevates when the tongue is protruded. Cysts are typically around 2 cm in size, as in this case, and can become infected or undergo malignant transformation.

Case 26

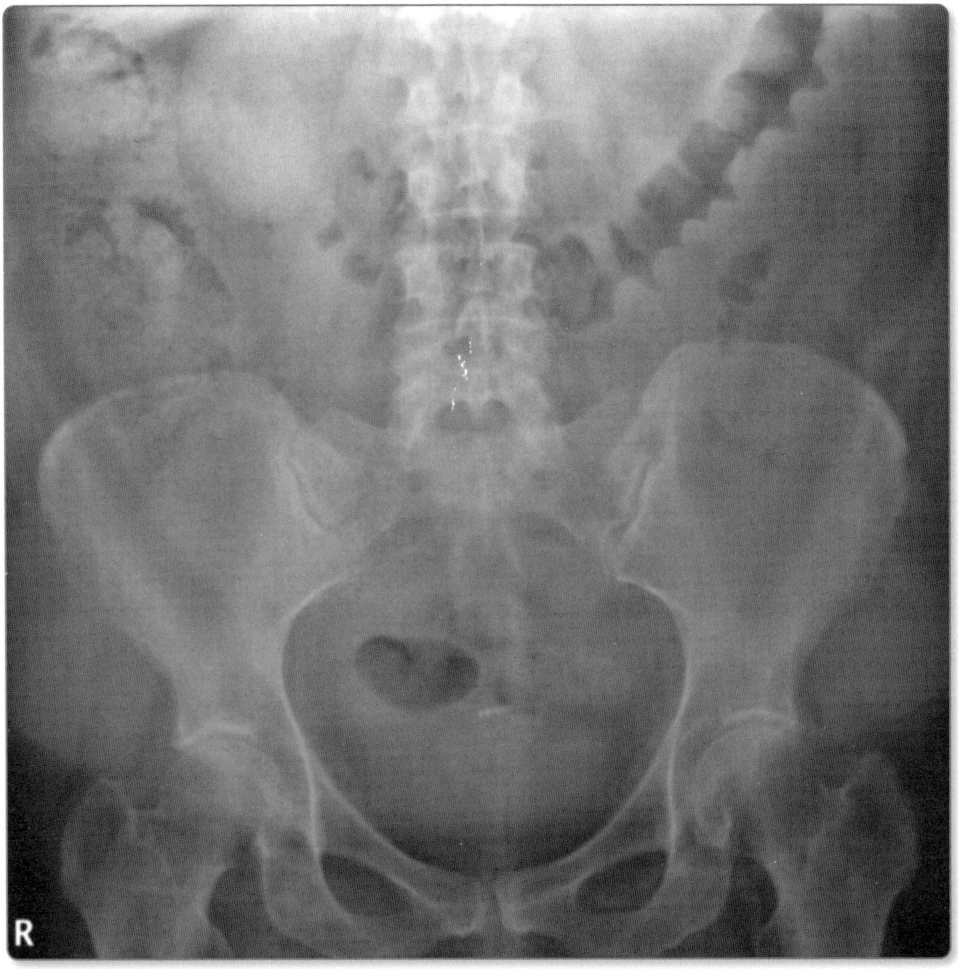

Suggested response

This is a plain radiograph of the abdomen and pelvis in an adult patient.

There is thickening of the colon wall with thumbprinting from the mid-portion of the transverse colon distally. The caecum and ascending colon appear to be normal and contain faeces, but no faeces is visible elsewhere in the colon.

There are no features to suggest bowel perforation, but I would routinely confirm this with an erect chest radiograph if it were a clinical concern.

The appearances indicate colitis and the distribution from mid-transverse colon distally, without any normal bowel being visible, suggests a diagnosis of ulcerative colitis. I cannot see any associated features such as sacroiliitis. If the patient has been on broad-spectrum antibiotics and has recently developed diarrhoea, then pseudomembranous colitis is another possibility. Other possibilities include ischaemic colitis and Crohn's disease and knowledge of the overall clinical picture will be necessary to clarify the diagnosis. I would discuss this case with the referring clinician to refine the diagnosis and to determine what further investigations might be helpful.

Diagnosis

Ulcerative colitis (UC) with mucosal thickening and an impression of 'thumbprinting'.

Tips: Bowel wall thickening on abdominal radiographs

Bowel wall thickening on a plain radiograph can be subtle or not visible at all, so only comment if you are reasonably confident of the finding and cannot see more dramatic pathology (or if you are led to it by the examiner). Be careful not to overinterpret collapsed segments of bowel as demonstrating mucosal thickening.

Key points and differential diagnosis

Look at the distribution of the thickening and determine whether it involves the large and/or small bowel. If it involves the large bowel, consider whether it is in a watershed area for ischaemia (splenic flexure). Assess whether the thickening is continuous from the rectum (suggestive of UC) or multifocal (suggestive of Crohn's disease).

Assess for intramural and free intraperitoneal gas.

If presented with CT images, also consider the enhancement pattern and specifically look for inflammatory changes and filling defects in the vessels. Assess to see whether there is any free fluid or a collection.

Various ancillary findings can help to narrow the differential diagnosis. Prominent vascular calcification raises suspicions of ischaemic colitis. Bone and joint changes (e.g. sacroiliitis, osteoporosis in a younger patient, osteomalacia, spondylitis, peripheral/rheumatoid arthritis) are features of UC and Crohn's disease, as is hepatobiliary disease (e.g. fatty liver and primary sclerosing cholangitis).

Ulcerative colitis

Ulcerative colitis is relatively common and different manifestations of the disease could appear in the viva. Although features do overlap significantly, you should be aware of the various features that enable differentiation between Crohn's disease and ulcerative colitis on imaging (including barium studies which are now a problem-solving tool rather than common clinical practice in most settings).

Case 27

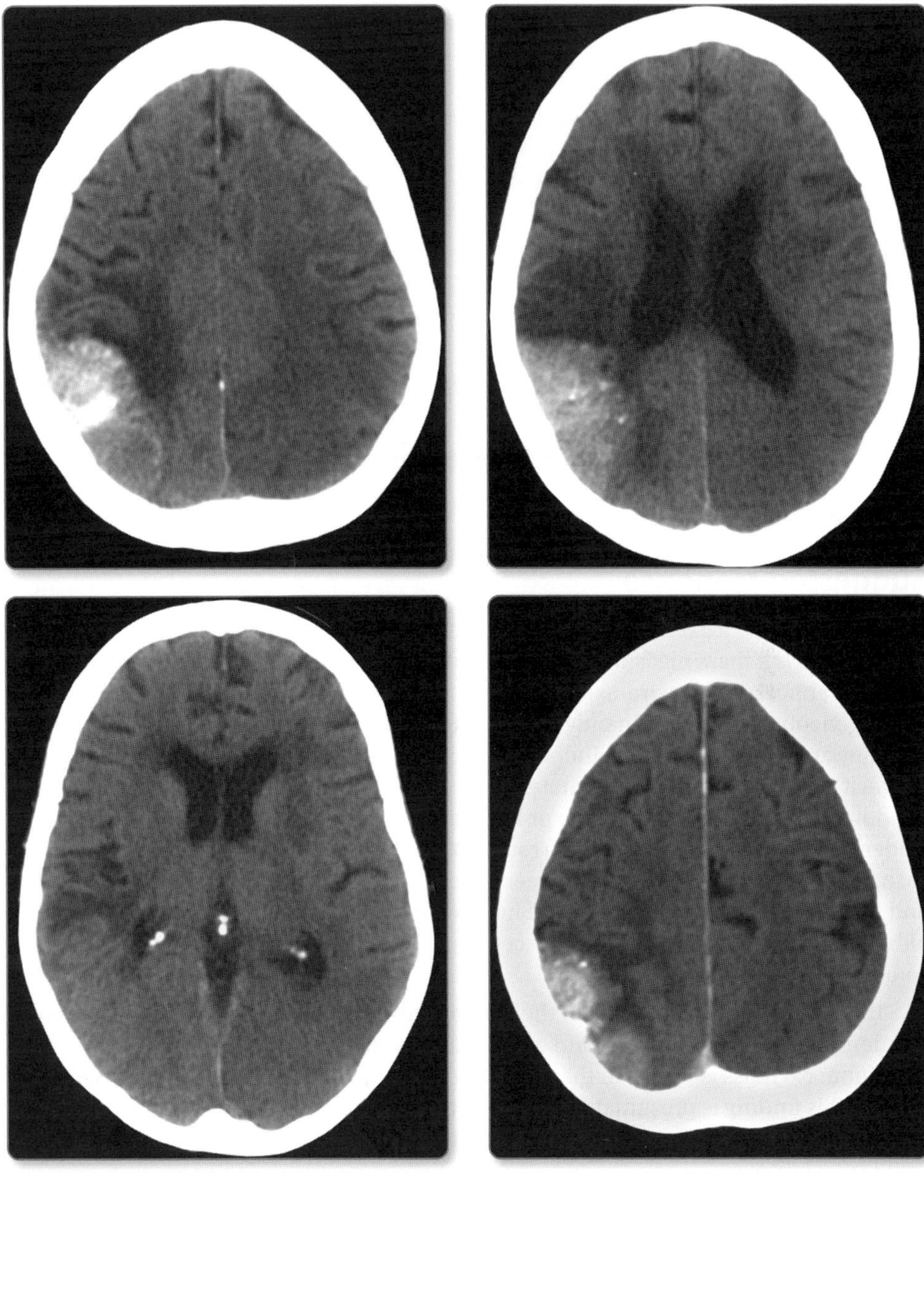

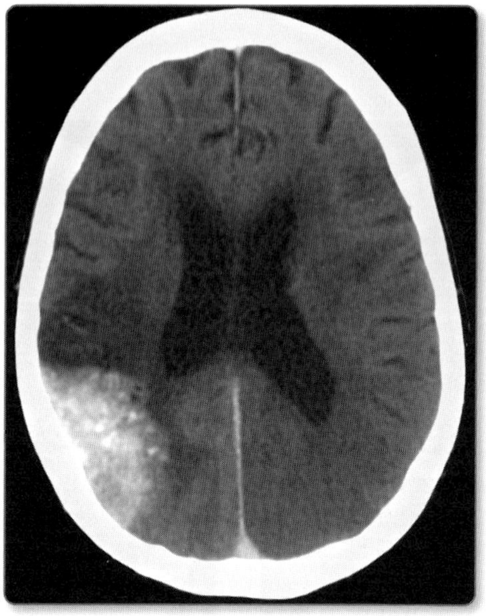

Suggested response

These are selected axial images from a CT brain scan, pre- and post-contrast. Firstly, there is a mass measuring several centimetres centred in the right parietal region. It appears to be extra-axial, with a broad base adjacent to the calvaria. It is heterogeneous but predominantly of high attenuation on pre-contrast imaging, and contains areas of calcification. There is patchy enhancement of the mass following contrast administration. In my usual practice, I would examine images on bony windows to assess for bony erosion or hyperostosis, but no gross bony destruction is evident on these images. There is surrounding low attenuation, which could represent vasogenic oedema. However, this is seen to extend to the cortex anterior to the mass and may conceivably represent an old infarct. There is no significant midline shift, although there appears to be mild effacement of the posterior horn of the right lateral ventricle.

There is also an abnormality in the left parieto-occipital region with homogeneous low density involving both grey and white matter and associated loss of sulcal definition. No mass is visible in that area. Appearances are consistent with a recent infarct. This finding is presumably related to the current clinical presentation and the indication for the CT scan. Further periventricular low attenuation is in keeping with small vessel disease.

To summarise, the most significant findings which I would convey to the referring clinicians are a recent left parieto-occipital infarct and a right-sided intracranial mass, appearances of which are most in keeping with a meningioma.

Diagnosis

Right-sided meningioma with recent left parieto-occipital infarct in a patient presenting with new right-sided weakness.

Tips: Acute imaging of stroke

Features of ischaemic stroke can be seen on unenhanced CT within 1–3 hours of arterial occlusion, but can be very subtle.

Key points

You may wish to mention the use of different window settings to assess for stroke or surface collection.

A number of potentially subtle findings that should be actively sought are:

- *Hyperdense artery sign:* This is usually seen in the middle cerebral artery (MCA) or its branches (look for the 'MCA dot sign' in the region of the Sylvian fissure). The hyperdense posterior cerebral artery and hyperdense basilar artery signs should also be looked for.
- *Basal ganglia obscuration:* The basal ganglia, in particular the lentiform nuclei, are liable to early damage due to supply by end vessels of the MCA, so look for subtle hypodensity.
- *Cortical ribbon sign (including insular ribbon sign):* Cytotoxic oedema causes loss of the normal grey–white matter differentiation, and may often be seen in the region of the insular ribbon.
- *Sulcal effacement:* Look for this and other manifestations of mass effect.

Remember to review the posterior fossa. Infarcts in the brainstem can be small and are often masked by artefact from the skull base, but look for asymmetry, particularly in an unconscious patient (MRI may be useful to further assess cases of suspected posterior fossa infarct). Each cerebellar hemisphere is supplied by three arteries, so there may be a wedge of affected cerebellum. The brainstem may be compressed by cytotoxic oedema from a cerebellar infarct, so it is important to check the cerebrospinal fluid spaces in the region of the foramen magnum.

If the abnormality does not correspond to a vascular territory, consider the possibility of a venous infarct (look at the dural venous sinuses). Multiple infarcts of varying ages suggest embolic phenomena (often in younger patients), e.g. of cardiac origin. Particularly in younger patients, consider also the possibility of arterial dissection.

Cerebral infarction

Stroke is one of the most frequently encountered pathologies by radiologists, so awareness of the common and subtle findings of cerebral infarction is important. Stroke is a huge topic and a detailed explanation is beyond the scope of this book, but it is vital to have a system for looking at CT scans of the brain in order to maximise your infarction detection rate. If there is no obvious abnormality, double check the review areas. Ensuring that there is no haemorrhage is crucial, particularly if faced with a patient being considered for thrombolysis. Make sure you are familiar with the current guidelines for thrombolysis and thrombectomy, which are likely to include CT angiography and may include perfusion CT depending on local arrangements.

Case 28

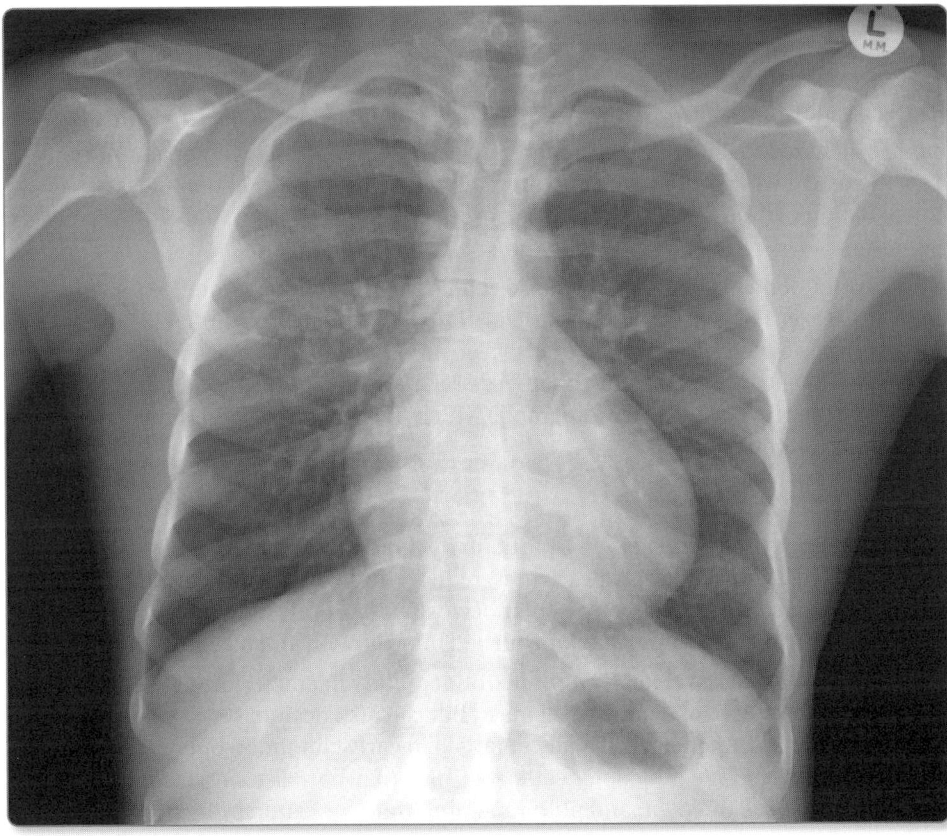

Suggested response

This is a frontal chest radiograph of a skeletally mature patient. The heart appears to be enlarged and there is some airspace opacification in the right mid-zone which may be infective, depending on symptoms. The lungs appear otherwise normal. However, I think that there are some subtle underlying skeletal abnormalities. A number of the anterior rib ends appear widened and the humeral heads may be slightly dense with some flattening of the contour of the left humerus. These findings are subtle and may be unrelated. Knowledge of the overall clinical picture would be relevant and it would be useful to review any available relevant previous imaging. However, in this case the combination of these skeletal abnormalities along with airspace opacification and cardiomegaly suggest an infective exacerbation of sickle cell disease.

Diagnosis

Sickle cell disease with an infective exacerbation. Avascular necrosis (AVN) in both shoulders (confirmed on MRI).

Tips: Sickle cell disease

It is debatable how realistic it is to make the underlying diagnosis from this radiograph, but it is included to illustrate the thought process of how to pull together and present a tricky case in which there is clearly more than just an acute infection. It is the constellation of findings that should suggest the diagnosis, rather than any one in isolation.

How frequently you encounter sickle cell disease (and other conditions such as Paget's disease, asbestos-related disease or HIV) will depend on your local population and the units in which you work. For a viva ensure that you become familiar with classic radiological cases that you do not see regularly in day-to-day practice. Ask senior colleagues to show you radiographs which they have collected from centres other than your own.

Key points

Look for a range of skeletal features, particularly those secondary to either marrow hyperplasia (e.g. widened marrow cavities, reduced bone density, expanded/thinned cortex, coarsened trabeculae) or vascular occlusion (e.g. bone infarcts, AVN, H-shaped vertebrae), but also any consequent disturbed bone growth and osteomyelitis.

Look also for extraskeletal features. Extramedullary haematopoiesis is an important differential for a paraspinal mass, but can also occur elsewhere (e.g. liver, spleen and skin). The spleen is usually enlarged in early childhood but becomes small and calcified in later life (autosplenectomy). There may be gallstones, evidence of a current crisis (e.g. infection and pulmonary infiltrate) or features due to vascular occlusion (e.g. cerebrovascular accident, renal infarct and pulmonary embolism).

Sickle cell disease

Sickle cell disease is an autosomal recessive haemoglobinopathy. Signs and symptoms develop as a consequence of abnormally shaped erythrocytes increasing the viscosity of blood and leading to the occlusion of small blood vessels (causing organ and skeletal damage). There is a significant risk of infection (which is the most common cause of death) as a consequence of loss of splenic function.

Case 29

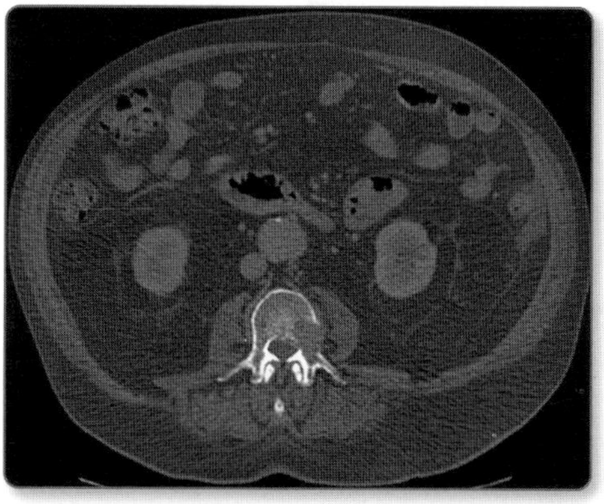

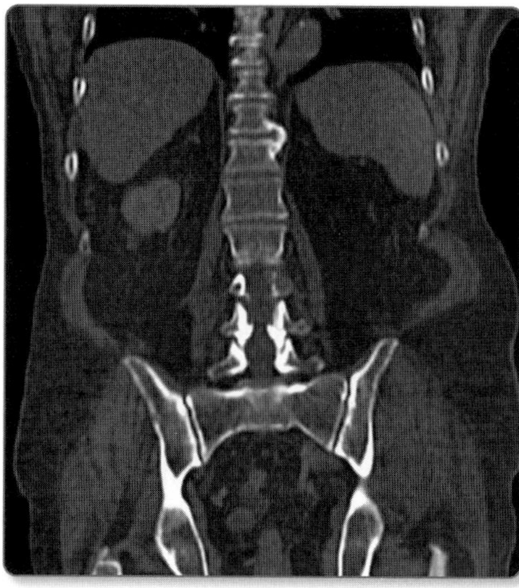

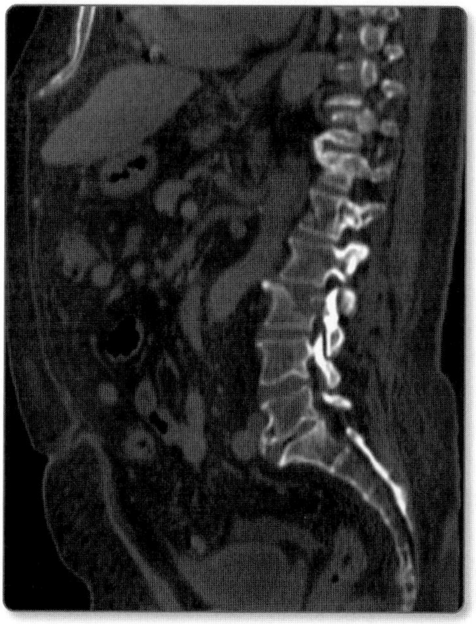

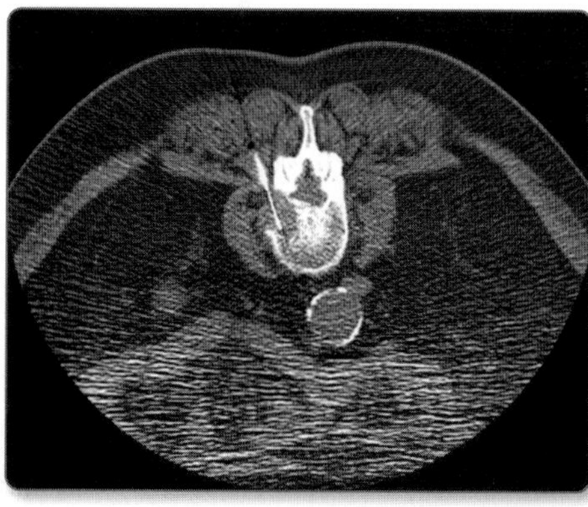

Suggested response

These are selected images from a CT scan. There is a well-defined lytic lesion in the left pedicle and left side of the vertebral body of L3. The cortical margins of the spinal canal appear to have been breached over a short segment on the axial images. I cannot see any other lesions on these images. In the final image, a CT-guided percutaneous intervention, possibly a biopsy, is being performed with the tip of a needle lying within the lesion.

The differential diagnosis depends on the age and past medical history of the patient, including whether there is a known history of a primary malignancy elsewhere. Given the degenerative disease elsewhere in the spine I assume that the patient is of middle age or older. If this is accurate then a metastasis, myeloma or lymphoma is even more likely than a primary bone lesion.

Diagnosis

Myeloma in L3 vertebra. The intervention is a diagnostic percutaneous biopsy.

Tips: A solitary spinal bone lesion

Although there are special considerations for lesions in the vertebral column, including encroachment into the spinal canal, use the same descriptive terms that you would use for any bone tumour (see Case 2).

Key points and differential diagnosis

Consider non-neoplastic causes such as haemangioma [a very common incidental finding; the internal matrix gives a characteristic 'pepper pot' (axial) or 'corduroy' (longitudinal) appearance], infection, Paget's disease and inflammatory causes including SAPHO (an acronym meaning synovitis, acne, pustulosis, hyperostosis and osteitis).

Consider the location of the lesion in the vertebra. Lesions found predominantly in the vertebral body include leukaemia, lymphoma, myeloma, metastasis and eosinophilic granuloma. Giant cell tumours mainly occur in the posterior elements. Aneurysmal bone cysts, haemangiomas and osteoid osteomas/osteoblastomas may be found in either the vertebral body or the posterior elements.

Age is a relevant factor. Primary vertebral tumours are rare in older patients. The most common primary vertebral tumours in children are osteoid osteoma/osteoblastoma, aneurysmal bone cyst and, rarely, Ewing's sarcoma. Lesions in younger patients (<21 years old) are almost always benign. Eosinophilic granuloma is the most common cause of vertebra plana in children, but the appearance of vertebra plana in adults should raise suspicions of a malignant process (e.g. myeloma or metastasis).

Myeloma

Solitary myeloma of bone (plasmacytoma) is a precursor to multiple myeloma, preceding the latter by up to two decades. It most commonly affects the spine (usually thoracolumbar), but is also seen in extravertebral locations including the ribs, pelvis and skull. Imaging appearances are variable and while it is often an expansile osteolytic lesion (mimicking renal cell carcinoma metastasis or a number of benign aetiologies), sclerotic forms of the disease may also occur.

Case 30

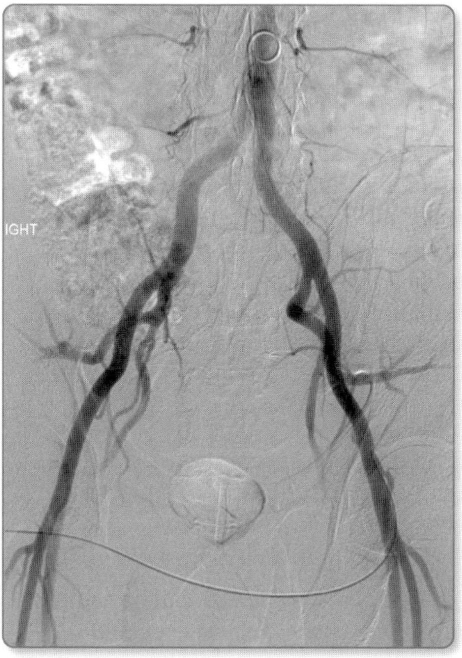

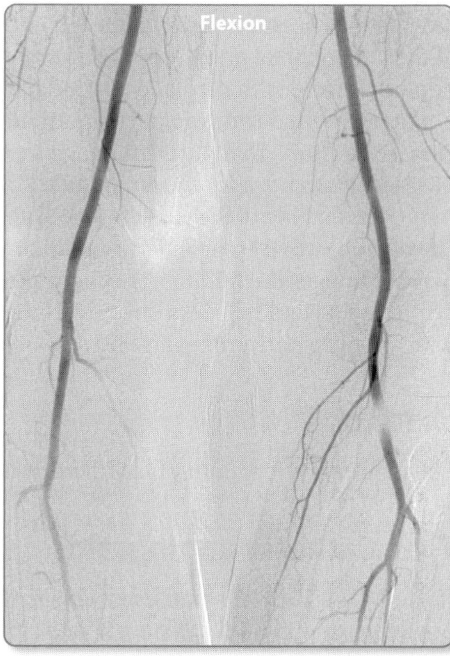

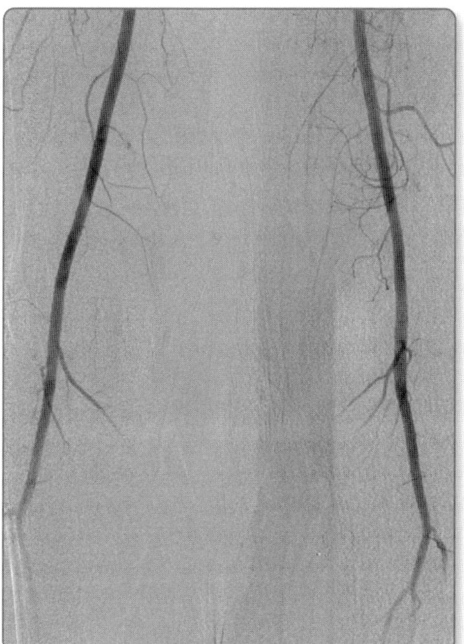

Suggested response

These are selected images from a catheter digital subtraction angiogram of the lower limbs showing the arterial system from the distal aorta to the upper calves. The catheter has been inserted via the left common femoral artery. There is an abnormality of the left popliteal artery. On the 'flexion' image, there is a filling defect in the mid-left popliteal artery with medial deviation of the vessel. On the subsequent view, the left popliteal artery is seen to opacify normally, and there is only minor deviation of the vessel. I presume that the third image was obtained with the leg held in the neutral position, to account for the apparent resolution of the filling defect. It would be useful to review imaging of the run-off vessels to assess for distal disease and, obviously, correlation with the clinical presentation would be desirable. However, on the basis of these images the findings are likely to represent left popliteal artery entrapment syndrome. I would discuss this case at the vascular multidisciplinary team meeting with a view to performing an MRI scan to assess for an underlying structural cause.

Diagnosis

Left popliteal artery entrapment syndrome in an adult male.

Tips: Catheter angiograms

If you do not know the name of a vessel, then the phrase 'a branch of' can be useful, but in an examination a certain level of anatomical knowledge will be expected.

Key points

Describe the study. Where is the access? Which vessels are being examined? Is there any annotation? Are images digitally subtracted or not?

Look for any catheters and balloons. Is there evidence of any previous interventions (e.g. stents, bypass graft, endarterectomy and embolisation coils)?

Look for abnormal vessels or abnormal filling of a normal vessel. If there is more than one image of the same area, then compare them carefully to assess the results of any intervention, including complications (e.g. rupture of a vessel, pseudoaneurysm, dissection, occlusion and embolus).

Differential diagnosis

Consider the types of pathologies that might arise in a viva: aortic pathologies (e.g. dissection and aortic stent-graft endoleak), haemorrhage (e.g. gastrointestinal, obstetric and post-traumatic), subclavian steal syndrome, popliteal artery entrapment syndrome, fibromuscular dysplasia (e.g. renal arteries), thromboembolic disease, hypervascular tumours (e.g. glomus, angiomyolipoma) and caroticocavernous fistula. If findings/history suggest thromboembolic disease (e.g. sudden onset of ischaemia), then echo/CT angiography of the heart and aorta may be needed to identify the source. This is not an exhaustive list.

Popliteal artery entrapment syndrome

Popliteal artery entrapment syndrome is uncommon but should be suspected in any younger patients, typically athletic men, who present with calf claudication. It arises when there is an abnormal relationship between the popliteal artery and muscle in the popliteal fossa. Normally, the popliteal vessels are surrounded by fat in the fossa (best depicted on axial T1-weighted MRI), but a slip of muscle or fibrous band may cause arterial compression. Angiographic findings are often nonspecific (e.g. popliteal artery occlusion), but medial arterial deviation or dynamic stenosis, manifested on forced plantar flexion or dorsiflexion in the presence of relevant symptoms, is strongly suggestive.

Case 31

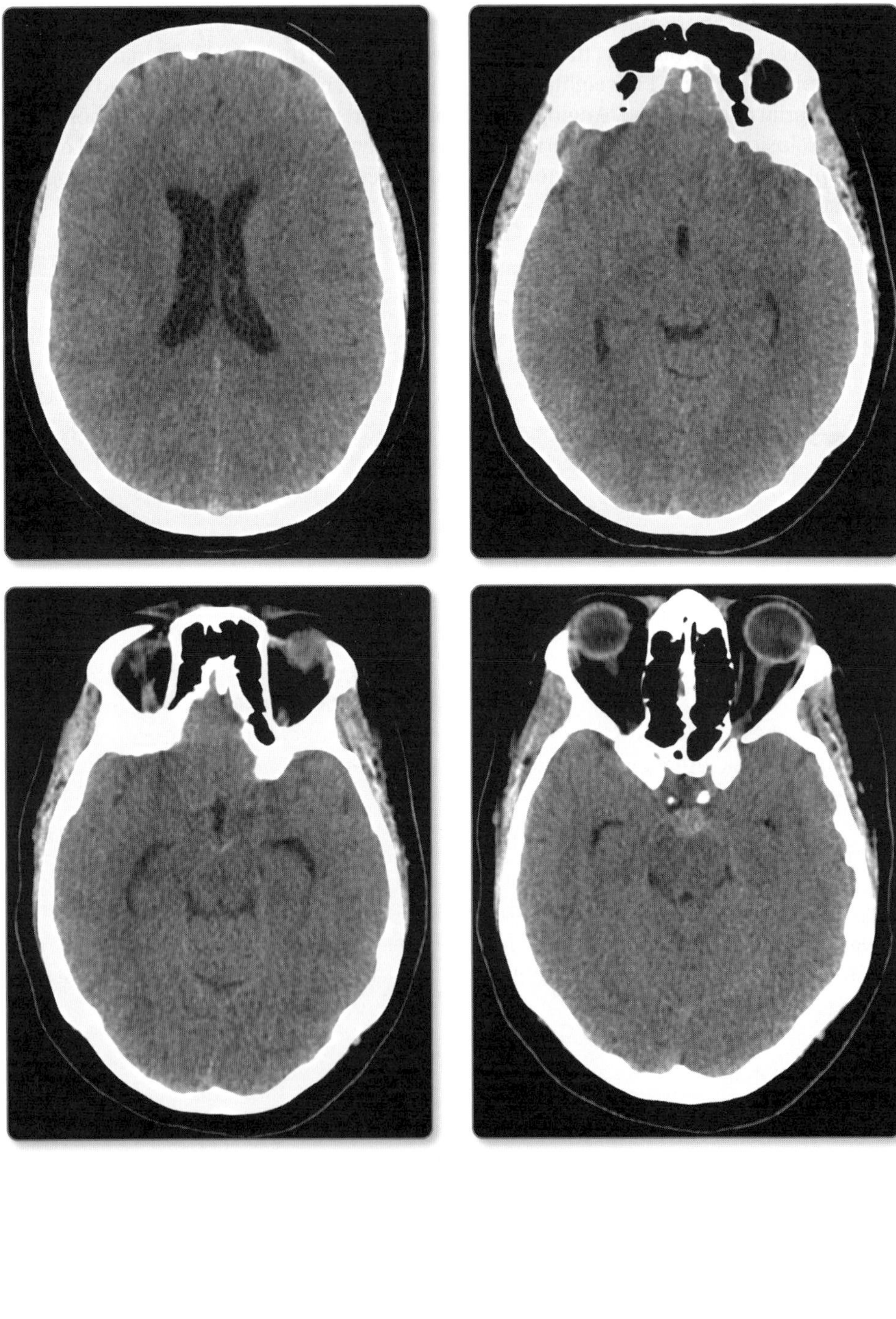

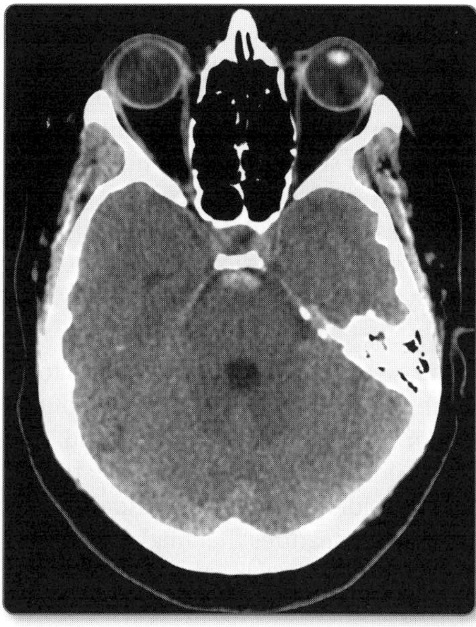

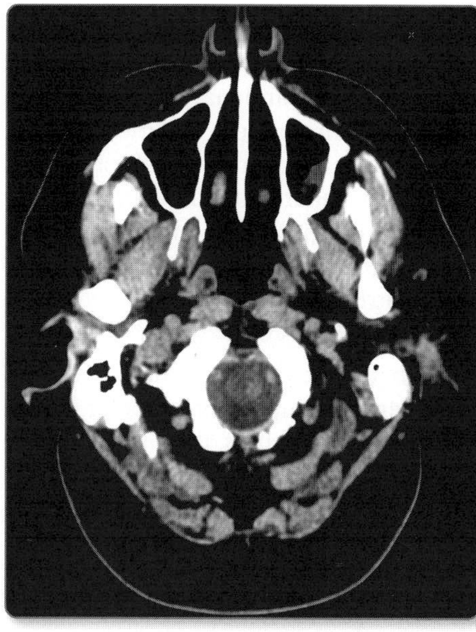

Suggested response

These are selected axial images from an unenhanced CT scan of the brain. Cerebral volume is preserved suggesting that this is a younger adult. High-attenuation material is evident in the prepontine cistern, extending anteriorly in the region of the cavernous sinuses. The lateral ventricles are more prominent than might be expected relative to the size of the sulci, suggesting the development of early hydrocephalus. The cerebrospinal fluid space at foramen magnum remains satisfactory. These appearances are likely to represent a recent subarachnoid haemorrhage; however, no obvious cause is identifiable in these images. In the first instance, I would want to scrutinise other images in the series on both brain and bone windows, looking for haemorrhage elsewhere and also for any evidence of trauma, such as calvarial fracture. In my ordinary clinical practice, if the patient is still on the CT table, immediate CT angiography might be considered to look for an intracranial aneurysm. In any event, I would discuss this case urgently with the referring clinical team and recommend getting a neurosurgical opinion.

Diagnosis

Subarachnoid haemorrhage in a young adult; no cause identified on CT angiography.

Tips: Intracranial haemorrhage

There may be several foci of haemorrhage, particularly in trauma, so beware of satisfaction of search!

Key points

First, try to identify where the blood is located. Extradural haematomas generally appear biconvex and may readily cross dural reflections such as the falx cerebri and tentorium cerebelli, but they do not cross undisrupted suture lines. Subdural haematomas are more typically crescentic and may cross suture lines, but not dural reflections. Subarachnoid haemorrhage may be focal, for instance at the site of trauma or a small bleed from an aneurysm, or more diffuse, as is seen with larger aneurysmal bleeds. Intracerebral haematomas may be secondary to hypertension or trauma. Intraventricular haemorrhage may occur secondary to haemorrhage elsewhere in the brain.

Subarachnoid haemorrhage can be very subtle, so paying particular attention to review areas is important. Look for hyperdensity in the basal cisterns, interhemispheric fissure, sylvian fissures, third ventricle, occipital horns of the lateral ventricles and foramen magnum. An increased blood load on one side is suggestive of an ipsilateral aneurysm (in the absence of trauma). Specifically consider if there is any evidence of trauma, looking for fractures and scalp swelling. Look for features that might suggest raised intracranial pressure, such as midline shift or herniation, crowding at the foramen magnum, or hydrocephalus.

If the history is that of a spontaneous bleed, then look for an underlying cause. The most common cause is ruptured aneurysm, so you may wish to consider suggesting performing CT angiography.

Subarachnoid haemorrhage

Remember that subarachnoid haemorrhage may be caused by trauma or may be secondary to an aneurysmal bleed (e.g. in a patient who collapses and hits his head). Detecting subarachnoid haemorrhage is a critically important role of the radiologist and the appearance of these bleeds can be extremely subtle. In a viva scenario, you are unlikely to face a CT of the brain showing only a miniscule amount of equivocal subarachnoid blood, but you should nonetheless ensure that you scrutinise the review areas highlighted above.

Trauma is a common cause of subarachnoid haemorrhage and in trauma cases there will often be extensive blood elsewhere. With spontaneous haemorrhage three-quarters of cases are due to an aneurysmal bleed (other causes include arteriovenous malformation and hypertension), so CT angiography should be performed. In the event that haemorrhage is secondary to an aneurysm, the aneurysm is typically found at bifurcations or branching points in the circle of Willis. There may be a role for MRI with gradient echo sequences in some cases if presentation has been delayed. However, this is controversial, so it is perhaps only worth mentioning if you are well versed in the topic.

Strong clinical suspicion of subarachnoid haemorrhage in the face of an apparently normal CT scan should result in a lumbar puncture being performed.

Case 32

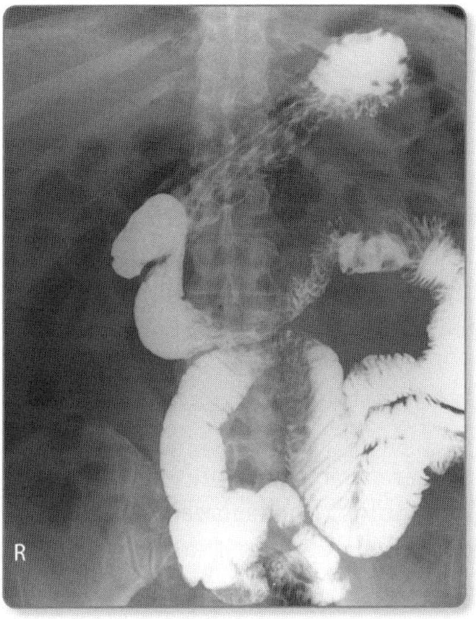

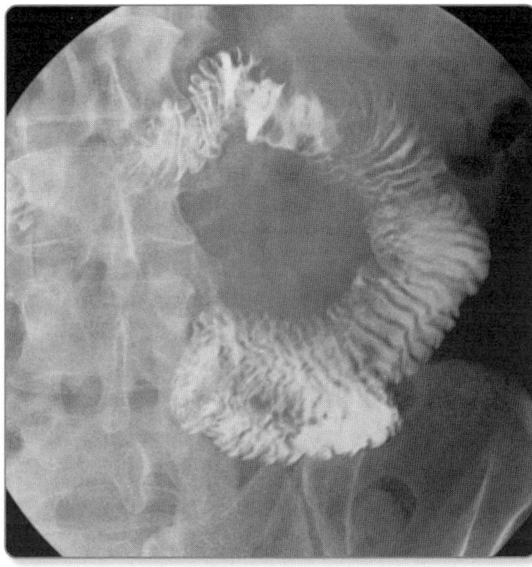

Suggested response

This is a pair of images from a barium follow-through examination. Both images demonstrate an apparently solitary focal abnormality at the duodenojejunal flexure. The mucosal fold pattern is obliterated over a short segment of 3 or 4 cm. It is replaced by a relatively featureless smooth pattern with a suggestion of nodularity inferiorly, although it is possible that this could be food debris. The calibre of the bowel lumen appears to be very slightly reduced but there is no tight stricture. There is no dilatation of the upstream segments of the duodenum to suggest obstruction.

Although the lesion is apparently solitary, I would examine the rest of the barium follow-through series carefully for the presence of synchronous lesions, and in particular I would carefully inspect the terminal ileum. Even if no other lesion is identified, if the patient is known to have a history of inflammatory bowel disease, then this lesion may represent a segment of Crohn's disease, although I do note the absence of stricturing or obvious ulceration. If the patient has a history of coeliac disease, and especially if diet control is poor, I would suggest lymphoma, which is a recognised complication. However, I note that mucosal fold pattern in the duodenum and jejunum appears to be normal. Otherwise, the differential diagnosis for an apparently solitary mucosal-based lesion in the small bowel is broad and includes malignant aetiologies such as adenocarcinoma or carcinoid tumour, benign aetiologies such as adenoma, haemangioma and lipoma, as well as inflammatory pathologies associated with connective tissue diseases and previous radiotherapy treatment. If this apparently mucosal-based lesion is indeed confirmed to be solitary, then definitive diagnosis could be sought by endoscopic inspection and biopsy, as the duodenojejunal flexure is usually accessible with conventional endoscopes. I would communicate these findings to the gastroenterology team.

Diagnosis

Non-Hodgkin's lymphoma at the duodenojejunal flexure.

Tips: Small bowel barium studies

You must be confident in your knowledge of the approach taken when performing a barium study of the small bowel, even if you have not performed many of these studies. You must also demonstrate that you are familiar with the common pathologies such as Crohn's disease, and that you are aware of the multitude of rarer pathologies which might be encountered.

Key points

It is important to consider the number of lesions that are visible. The presence of multiple lesions is more likely to indicate a benign pathology and is usually associated with Crohn's disease. Solitary lesions are more likely to be malignant (although small bowel malignancy is rare).

Determine whether the terminal ileum has been imaged. Crohn's disease is the most common cause of focal small bowel lesions and as the terminal ileum is affected in most patients with this disease, you should specifically state you would examine it. The terminal ileum is also relatively easy to access for endoscopic biopsy if histological diagnosis is required.

Next consider the space between bowel loops and look for any abnormal widening. Extrinsic pathologies may displace the loops; mesenteric fat hypertrophy is often seen in Crohn's disease.

If the case includes cross-sectional images, then look for enlarged lymph nodes and liver lesions, which suggest malignancy.

If you cannot decide the nature of a lesion, then use a template to structure your discussion. For instance, consider in turn extrinsic, submucosal, mucosal and intraluminal causes.

Small bowel barium studies

Crohn's disease is by far the most common cause of focal small bowel lesions. However, the prevalence of cases of the disease in examinations does not reflect real life, with more esoteric and unusual cases being far more common in the examination. During viva preparation, make a particular point of asking your seniors to show you small bowel studies. This is particularly important if you have not had much exposure to small bowel imaging during your training thus far. Ensure that you become familiar with the many and varied manifestations of Crohn's disease.

Case 33

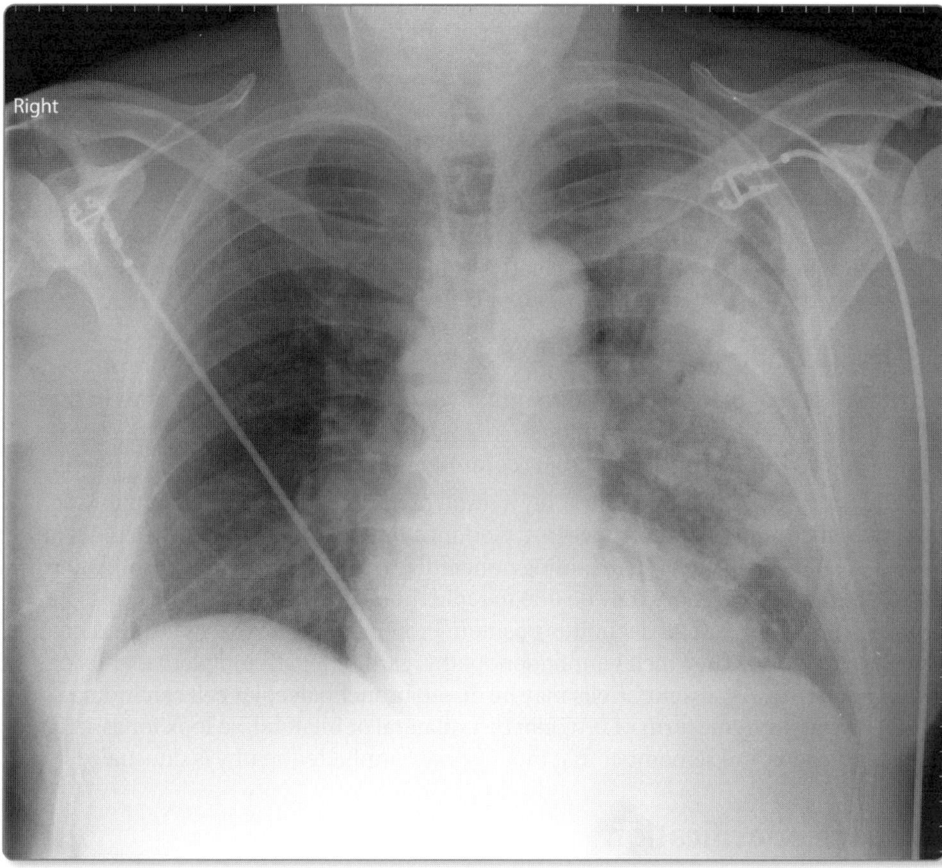

Suggested response

This is a frontal radiograph of an adult patient. Cardiac monitoring leads are noted.

There is a large area of airspace opacification in the left lung which contains air bronchograms. A small part of the left heart border is obscured, suggesting that some of this airspace disease is in the lingula, although I suspect that the majority is in the left lower lobe.

The left apex and right lung are clear, the mediastinal contour is otherwise normal and I do not see any abnormality of the thoracic wall.

There is a wide differential, but the most common cause of airspace disease is bronchial pneumonia. If this is in keeping with the clinical picture, I would report the radiograph and suggest repeating the radiograph in approximately 6 weeks to ensure radiological resolution as it is not currently possible to exclude an underlying tumour.

Diagnosis

Large area of airspace opacification in the left lung, mainly in the left lower lobe and lingula.

This was a case of pneumonia and the patient recovered with suitable antibiotic treatment. A repeat radiograph was normal.

Tips: Unilateral airspace opacification

Key points

The cardinal feature of airspace opacification is the presence of air bronchograms. Vessels and bronchial walls are not clearly visualised. The material within the air spaces may be pus, blood, fluid, protein or cells (see also *Case 10*).

Differential diagnosis

Acknowledge that there is a wide differential for this appearance. Seek clues in the clinical history and any other findings. Do not launch into an endless list of every cause you can think of and remember: common things are common!

The presence of blood is commonly a result of trauma, infarction or autoimmune diseases which cause haemorrhage (e.g. Goodpasture's syndrome). Fluid includes all causes of pulmonary oedema including noncardiac causes. Unilateral consolidation due to fluid in the airspaces may be due to rapid thoracocentesis, aspiration or prolonged lying in a lateral decubitus position. Protein in the air spaces is found in alveolar proteinosis (in which lymphadenopathy, cardiomegaly and pleural effusions are characteristically absent). Cells may be due to bronchoalveolar cell carcinoma (BAC). The pneumonic form of BAC can be unilateral or bilateral, so look for associated pleural effusions and remember that mediastinal lymphadenopathy is unusual.

Airspace opacification

Pneumonia is very common in clinical practice, as are many of the other causes of airspace opacification. It may be tempting to think that the examiner will not include simple cases of pneumonia so that you should instead be searching exclusively for esoteric causes. However, this is incorrect. The examiners are there to ensure that you are confident in dealing with a range of scenarios, both mundane and exotic. In cases such as this, the suggested management is just as important as the interpretation of the radiograph. In this case, failing to advise follow-up would run the risk of missing an underlying cancer.

Case 34

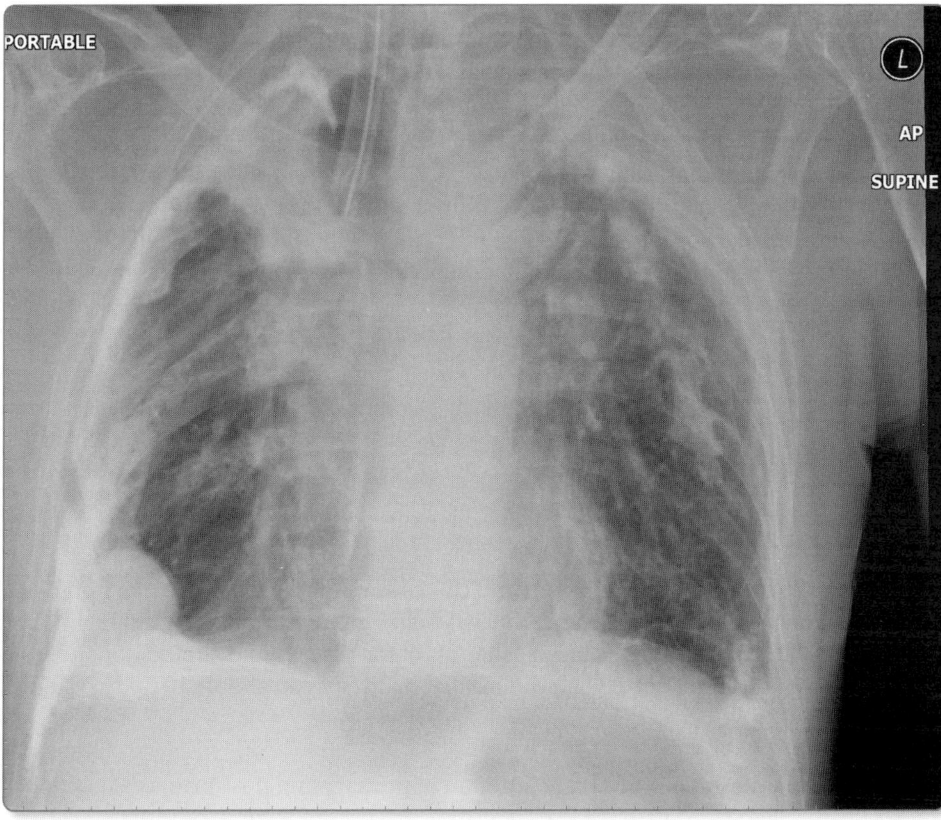

Suggested response

This is a rotated mobile supine radiograph of an adult patient.

The patient has been intubated and the tip of the endotracheal tube is projected over the distal trachea just above the carina. There is shift of the entire mediastinum, including the trachea, to the right due to volume loss in the right hemithorax. This is accompanied by extensive pleural calcification, which appears almost confluent laterally and inferiorly on the right. There is a rounded soft tissue density in the right costophrenic angle and further smaller areas of pleural calcification on the left.

The lung parenchyma is also abnormal with features of bronchiectasis in the lower zones, particularly on the right. Further opacification is visible in both apices, where volume loss is most marked, and there is an impression of a large apical cap on the right and patchy shadowing on the left with both airspace and interstitial characteristics.

In the left mid-zone, there is a thin, vertical opacity running parallel to the thoracic wall, raising the possibility of a pneumothorax. However, I cannot trace this further and think that there are lung markings peripheral to this, making a pneumothorax unlikely.

Distortion of the mediastinum and the supine projection limit interpretation of the mediastinal contour, but this limited assessment does not demonstrate any mediastinal masses. The bones appear normal.

At least some of these findings will be long-standing and are likely to reflect a distant history of tuberculosis. On this radiograph alone it is not possible to exclude even a large carcinoma in several places within the chest. Knowledge of the clinical presentation and a review of any available relevant previous imaging would be useful to determine if there is any new consolidation or if there has been progression of the fibrotic changes.

Diagnosis

Intubated patient who has old tuberculosis (TB) with loss of lung volume, particularly on the right. Stable over many years.

Tips: Tuberculosis

Tuberculosis can mimic many diseases and can cause such a wide range of pathologies that it can crop up in almost any case. The lists below are not exhaustive, but highlight various intra- and extra-thoracic manifestations of the disease and should hopefully act as a reminder to consider TB as a differential in diseases of almost all body systems.

Key points

The thoracic manifestations of TB are different in primary and post-primary infection.

In primary TB, the radiographic findings are often nonspecific with a normal chest radiograph in up to 15% of cases. When considering primary TB, specifically look for a possible (usually subpleural upper zone) Ghon focus.

Enlarged lymph nodes are common, particularly in children or those with HIV. Lymphadenopathy is most commonly unilateral and right-sided, and nodes often have a necrotic centre. Primary TB may cause atelectasis/consolidation, bronchiectasis and pleural effusions, particularly in adults. Miliary spread is more common in primary TB than in post-primary TB.

In post-primary TB, it is very unusual to have a normal chest radiograph. Other than in cases of immunosuppression such as HIV, there is usually cavitation with no nodal enlargement. Post-primary TB usually affects the upper lobes or apical segments of the lower lobes. If an effusion is present, then it is more likely to progress to an empyema than in primary TB.

The most common extrathoracic site for TB is in the genitourinary system, causing scarring, strictures or autonephrectomy when it affects the kidneys. Mural thickening and filling defects (due to granulomas) are seen when it affects the bladder and ureters, later progressing to strictures and scarring.

Other extrathoracic manifestations may be found almost anywhere, including in the musculoskeletal, neurological and gastrointestinal systems. When TB affects the musculoskeletal system, it may cause arthritis (especially in the hip), spondylitis/discitis, or osteomyelitis in any bone, particularly in the lower limb. Intracranial TB may cause meningitis or tuberculoma (which is associated with meningitis). In the gastrointestinal tract, it most commonly affects the ileocaecal region, may be ulcerative or hypertrophic and may mimic Crohn's disease.

Tuberculosis

Vivas commonly include chest radiographs showing chronic TB, but imaging showing acute infection is also often encountered. If you see a chest radiograph showing miliary disease, then you should indicate clearly that the possibility of miliary TB should be considered (the alternative is miliary metastases) and comment that this is an extremely contagious form of TB. You must state that the patient should be appropriately isolated from other patients, family and staff until that diagnosis is actively excluded.

Case 35

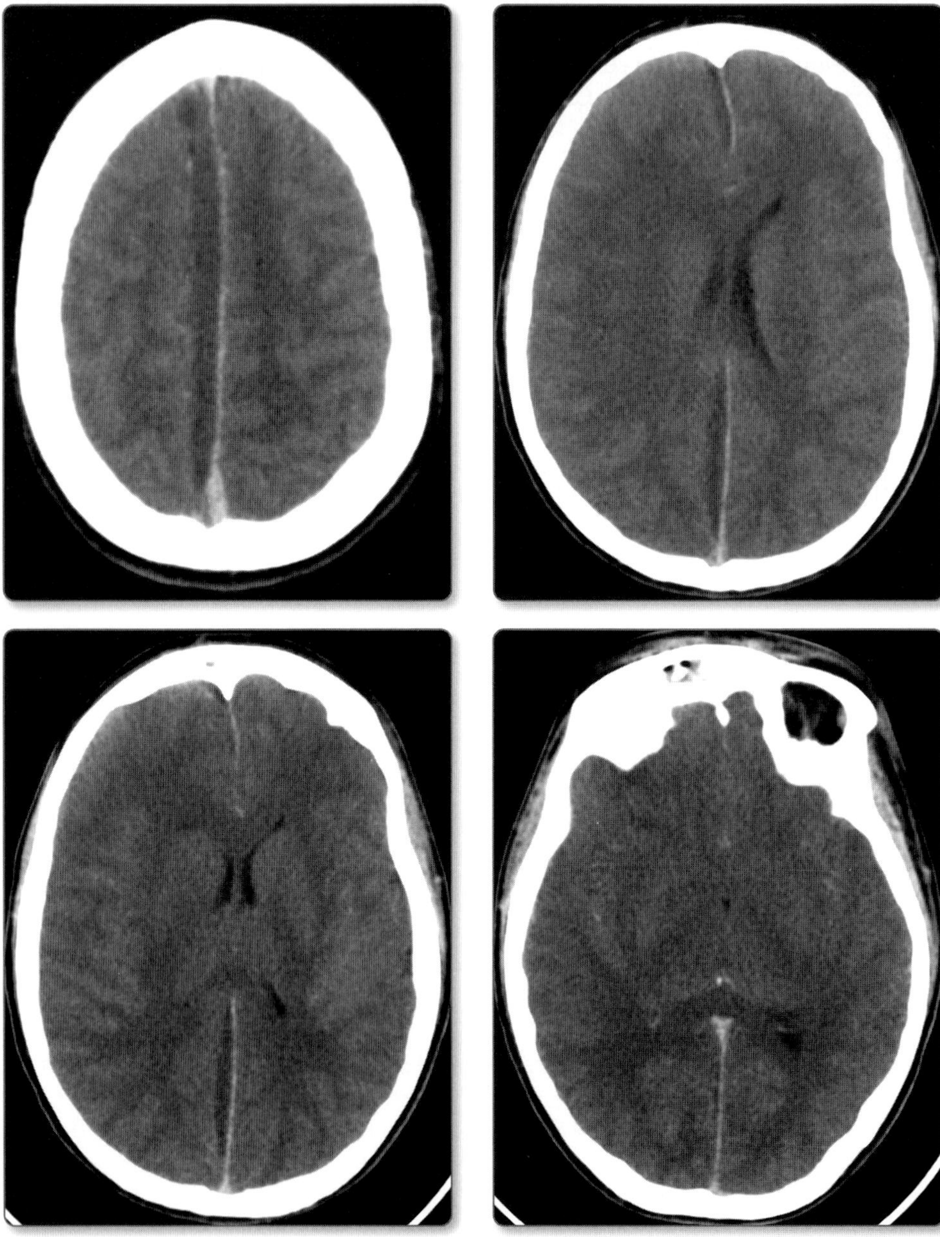

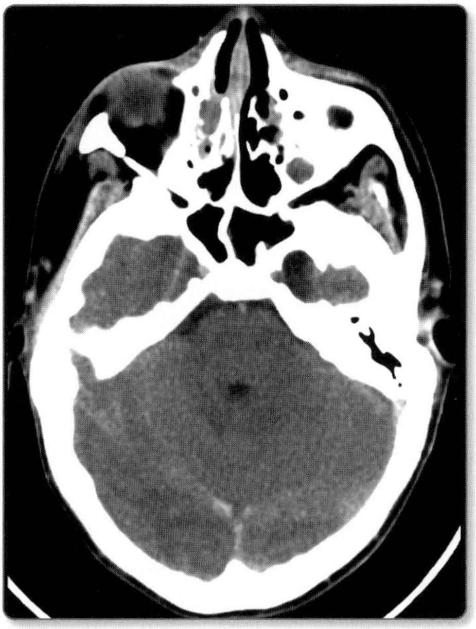

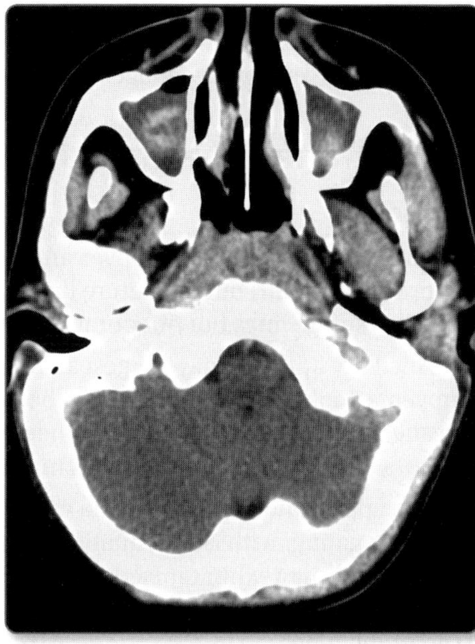

Suggested response

These are selected axial images from a post-contrast CT brain scan. A low attenuation collection, measuring approximately 1 cm in depth, extends along the right side of the falx cerebri and is most conspicuous near the vertex. There is an associated midline shift to the left. In my usual practice, I would measure both the depth of the collection and the extent of the midline shift. There appears to be minor enhancement along the right border of the collection. The visualised adjacent superior sagittal sinus appears to opacify normally. The small ventricles and lack of visualised sulci are more in keeping with a young brain than an excessively swollen brain, with grey–white matter differentiation being preserved.

Furthermore, there is evidence of extensive paranasal sinus disease, with high attenuation material evident in the visualised frontal, ethmoid and maxillary sinuses. In my usual practice I would evaluate the remaining images to assess for intracranial abscesses, evaluate the dural venous sinuses and ensure that the cerebrospinal fluid space at foramen magnum remains satisfactory, although no hydrocephalus is apparent in this case. I would also scrutinise imaging on bony windows to ensure that there are no fractures.

The most likely explanation for these findings is subdural empyema secondary to extensive paranasal sinus disease, particularly if the patient is unwell with features of sepsis (e.g. pyrexia and leucocytosis). A less likely explanation, relevant if this is an afebrile patient with a history of previous trauma, would be chronic subdural haematoma. Subdural empyema has a high mortality rate and I would discuss this case with the neurosurgical team as a matter of urgency.

Diagnosis

Subdural empyema in a teenager with sinusitis.

Tips: Intracranial extra-axial collection

Key points

Extradural collections are biconvex and cross dural reflections (e.g. falx cerebri, tentorium cerebelli) but not suture lines, whereas subdural collections are crescentic and cross suture lines but not dural reflections.

Ancillary findings may suggest an underlying diagnosis. If there is subdural empyema, look for dural sinus thrombosis or paranasal sinus disease, but do not be caught out by a high-attenuation haemorrhage in the sinuses following trauma. Subdural haematomas or hygromas may be associated with calvarial fractures.

The appearance of haematoma varies with age from hyperattenuating to hypoattenuating, with isoattenuation occurring at about 1 week. Acute-on-chronic haematomas may exhibit mixed attenuation. Subdural hygroma exhibits the same attenuation as cerebrospinal fluid and subdural empyema may be isoattenuating or hypoattenuating.

Subdural empyema

Subdural empyema can be very subtle, particularly if isoattenuating, and may only be evident on manipulation of the CT window settings (the authors suggest using window width 150, level 75, rather than conventional brain window settings, to more satisfactorily evaluate the subdural spaces). Intravenous contrast renders subdural empyema more conspicuous as it causes a thin rim of enhancement between the collection and the brain parenchyma. There may be infarction, cerebritis or abscess formation in adjacent brain tissue. The most common cause of subdural empyema in young children is meningitis. In these patients, hypoattenuating subdural collections could be reactive effusions rather than empyema. Subdural empyema usually occurs in older children and adults as a consequence of infection in the middle ear, paranasal sinuses or mastoid air cells.

Case 36

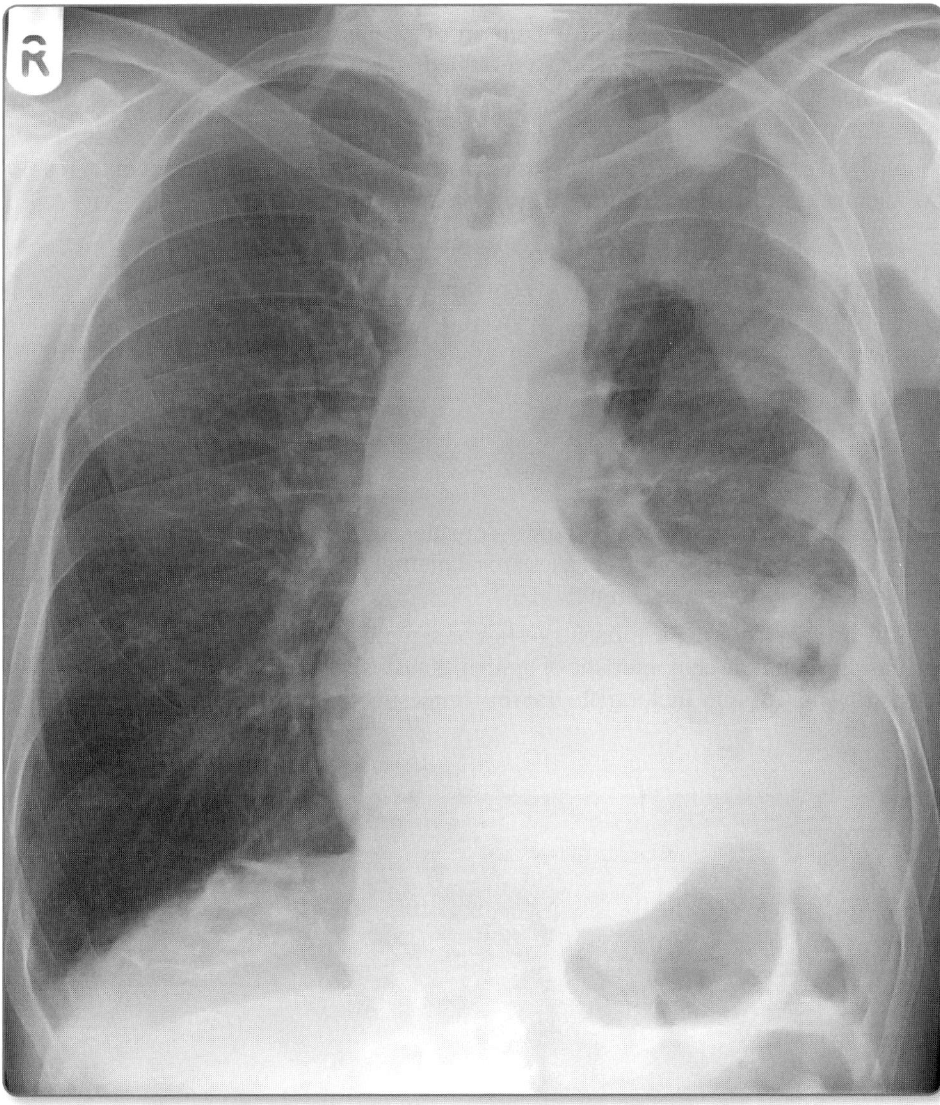

Suggested response

This is a frontal chest radiograph of a skeletally mature patient. The most striking abnormalities are evident in the left hemithorax where there is loss of volume compared with the right side. There is left-sided multifocal lobulated opacification which is predominantly peripheral in distribution, with aeration of the most central parahilar lung. The left base is not clearly visualised. The right lung is hyperinflated with an irregular area of calcification projected over the right hemidiaphragm, likely to represent a pleural plaque. There is no convincing bony destruction. The opacification in the left hemithorax is likely to be pleural in origin, the most likely differential diagnoses being malignant mesothelioma (particularly in light of the calcified pleural plaques) or pleural metastases. Loss of clarity of the left base may also be due to pleural disease, but could represent superadded infection or pleural effusion.

Review of any available relevant previous imaging would be useful to assess for change, but if this is a first presentation, an urgent respiratory referral and CT scan should be performed, with a view to discussion at the relevant multidisciplinary team (MDT) meeting and consideration of biopsy to obtain a tissue diagnosis.

Diagnosis

Left-sided malignant mesothelioma in an adult patient (see **Figure 1** from the same patient).

Tips: Pleural thickening

Key points

Post-traumatic fibrothorax may occur, so consider a history of trauma (including surgery). Tuberculosis typically causes apical pleural thickening, whereas chronic empyema causes basal thickening.

The presence of calcification suggests a benign diagnosis. Bilateral involvement, including plaques, is characteristic of benign asbestos-related disease. Features suggesting malignancy include pleural rind (encasing the lung), nodular pleural

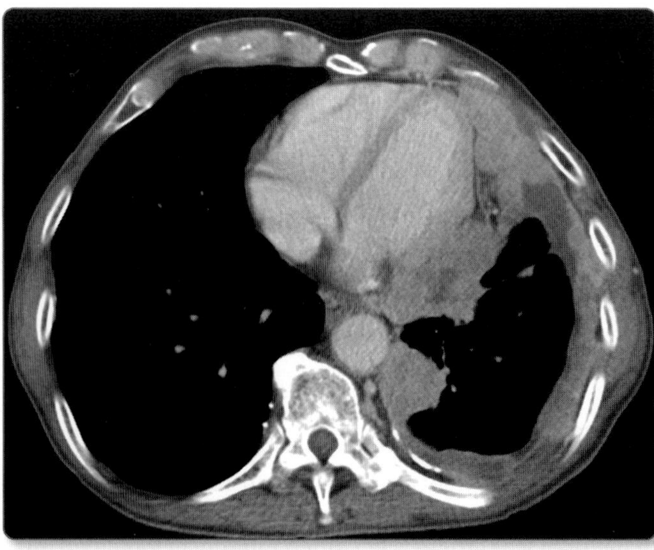

Figure 1 Axial CT from the same patient, confirming diffuse pleural thickening.

thickening, parietal pleural thickening of >1 cm and mediastinal pleural involvement.

Pleural metastases are far more common than mesothelioma, but they may be impossible to differentiate from one another if there is diffuse pleural thickening (unless an underlying primary adenocarcinoma is apparent, e.g. lung or breast). Metastases are typically nodular but this feature may be obscured by malignant pleural effusion.

Malignant mesothelioma

Malignant mesothelioma and benign mesothelioma are two distinct entities, the latter having no association with asbestos exposure. Malignant mesothelioma has a latent period of around 20–40 years following asbestos exposure. There is usually extensive pleural thickening **(Figure 1)** with associated pleural plaque disease manifesting in half of patients and often with an exudative pleural effusion. Isolated pleural thickening or effusion is also well documented. A pleural rind can form around the affected lung causing a 'frozen lung'. Circumferential encasement, with spread along the fissures and involving pericardium and mediastinum, occurs at a late stage. Bear in mind that malignant mesothelioma can also involve the peritoneum and include this in your differential diagnoses when faced with peritoneal-based pathologies in a viva. Remember that lung cancer is still far more common than malignant mesothelioma in patients with a history of asbestos exposure, especially if they are smokers.

Case 37

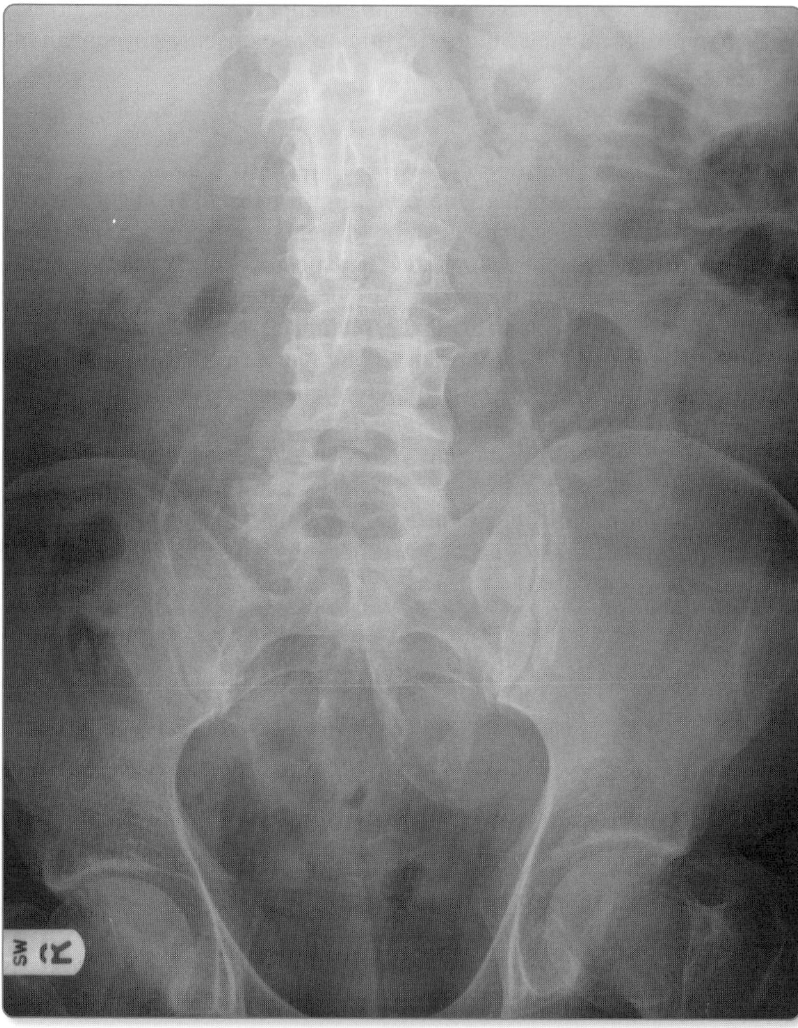

Suggested response

This is an abdominal radiograph of an adult patient. There is curvilinear calcification projected over the lateral margin of the psoas shadows and sacroiliac joints bilaterally.

There is also a background of some degenerative changes in the spine and both hips. The bowel gas pattern is nonspecific.

The findings are highly suggestive of a very large aortic aneurysm. This diagnosis may already be known, but in any event, if the patient is presenting with abdominal pain, I would urgently discuss the case with the referring clinician with a view to arranging further appropriate imaging. An ultrasound could confirm that there is a large aneurysm, but assuming that an intervention is being considered, then a CT scan is likely to be required to assess the suitability of the aneurysm for open or endovascular repair.

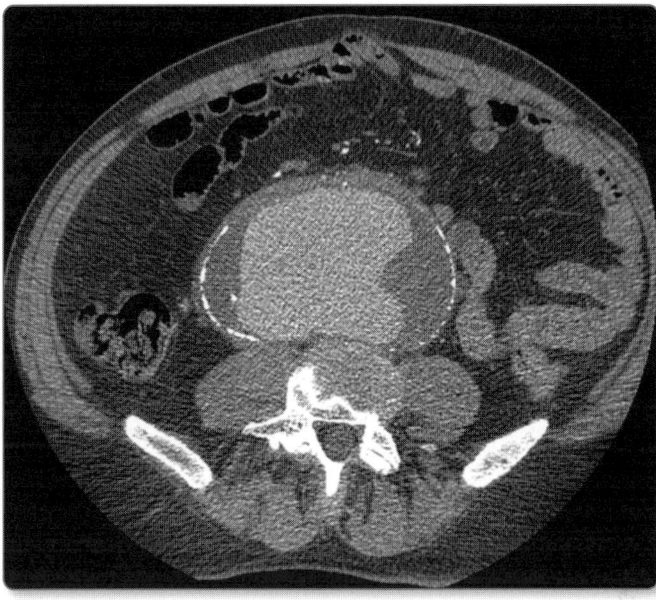

Suggested response

This is an image from a CT scan of the abdomen which confirms the presence of a very large aortic aneurysm. I would routinely review the whole study, but there are no convincing signs of rupture or impending rupture on this image. I would again discuss the patient with the referring clinician to formulate a management plan.

Diagnosis

Very large unruptured abdominal aortic aneurysm (AAA).

Tips: Calcifications in the abdomen or pelvis

Key points

Descriptive terms for calcifications include curvilinear, punctuate, solid, popcorn and rounded. They may comprise recognisable structures (teeth and bones). If calcification is widespread, consider an underlying metabolic disorder such as renal failure, hyperparathyroidism or diabetes.

Differential diagnosis

Common vascular calcifications include AAA and splenic artery aneurysm. Renal, adrenal and vesical calcifications include calculi, old infection, infarction or aneurysms. Hepatobiliary calcifications include gallbladder wall disease, gallstones and pancreatic calcification. Uterine calcifications are usually fibroids, but a fetal skeleton may be seen. Adnexal calcifications are usually related to dermoid tumours: the presence of teeth is rare but a radiological classic and, therefore, a common viva radiograph. A wide variety of soft tissue calcifications may be identified; phleboliths and calcified lymph nodes are common.

Abdominal aortic aneurysm

On every abdominal radiograph, you should look for calcification in the wall of an abdominal aortic aneurysm. Scrutinise the psoas major outlines. These outlines are normally evident on a radiograph as lines of fatty density which demarcate the lateral aspects of the muscles. However, in retroperitoneal pathologies (e.g. secondary to haemorrhage from aortic aneurysm rupture), one or both outlines may be obscured.

Case 38

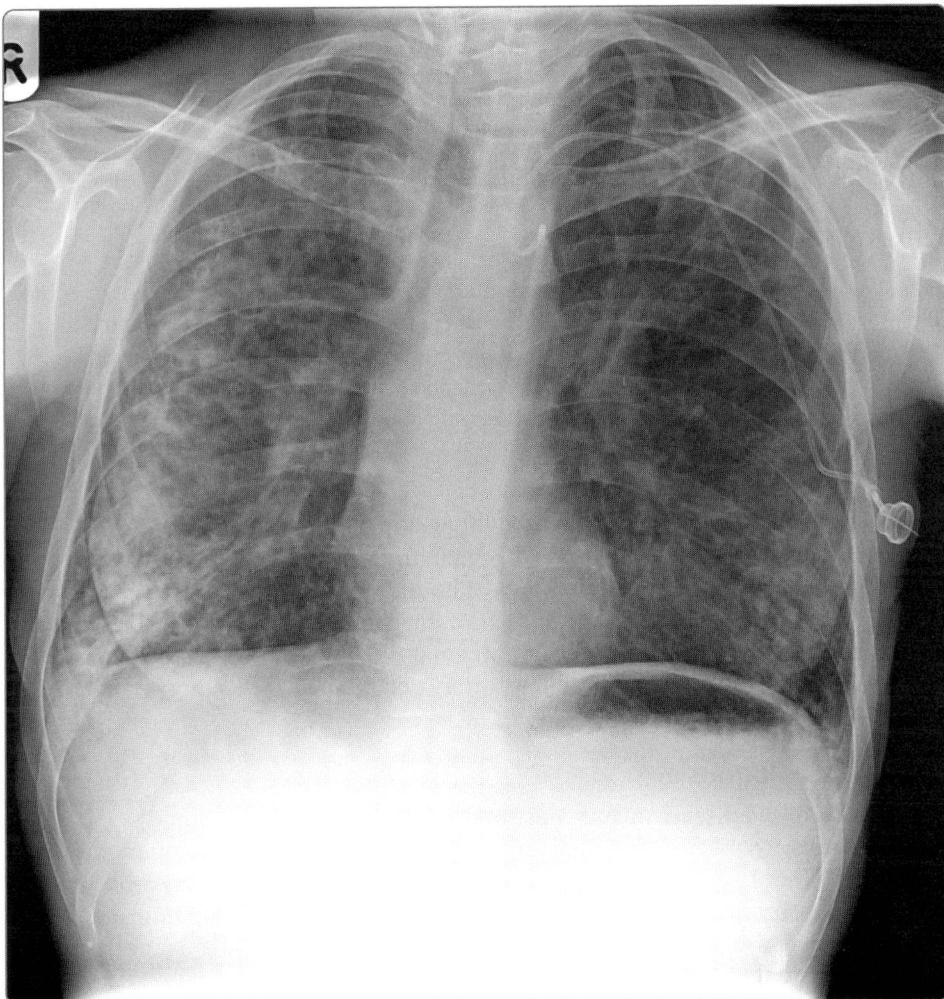

Suggested response

This is a frontal chest radiograph of a skeletally mature female. A left-sided vascular access port device is present. The line follows an unusual track as it passes inferior to the medial end of the clavicle and the tip of the line is not projected in a typical location. Despite the degree of radiograph rotation, the tip of the line is projected just to the left of the vertebral column over the lower descending aorta; an aortic placement cannot be excluded on the basis of the current radiograph alone. This is unlikely, but if there is any uncertainty then I would advise the clinicians to check a blood gas measurement via the port to confirm venous blood. It is more likely to lie in a left-sided superior vena cava or mediastinal collateral vessel. Review of previous imaging and reports should clarify this. The lungs are grossly abnormal. There is bronchial wall thickening and a widespread pulmonary infiltrate, most marked on the right side and predominantly peripheral in distribution, albeit with relative sparing of the extreme periphery/subpleural lung. The heart is not enlarged but the central pulmonary vasculature is prominent and consistent with chronic lung changes. These findings are most likely to represent cystic fibrosis. It would be useful to review previous imaging to assess for change, particularly if there has been a clinical deterioration. I cannot see a pneumothorax.

Diagnosis

Teenager with cystic fibrosis (CF) and vascular access port placement in a hypertrophied left internal thoracic vein (unusual venous access location necessitated by extensive central venous occlusion caused by previous venous access devices).

Tips: Bronchiectasis

Key points

Hyperinflation is the earliest change in CF, but volume loss is the characteristic appearance in later stages. Thick-walled, nontapering bronchi produce 'tram line' shadows. Mucous-filled bronchi may appear nodular (if seen 'end on') or tubular (if seen in long axis). Cystic bronchiectasis is associated with the classical 'bunch of grapes' appearance. The hila may be prominent due to lymphadenopathy associated with chronic infection and/or pulmonary artery enlargement, reflecting pulmonary hypertension in late-stage disease.

Differential diagnosis

Causes of localised disease include post-obstructive and post-pneumonic bronchiectasis. Characteristic patterns may be seen in allergic bronchopulmonary aspergillosis (perihilar/upper lobe) or bronchiectasis associated with mycobacterial infection. 'Dry bronchiectasis' is upper lobe bronchiectasis without sputum production and is caused by TB. 'Lady Windermere syndrome' is lingular or right middle lobe bronchiectasis caused by *Mycobacterium avium* complex.

Causes of diffuse disease include CF, Kartagener's syndrome (immotile cilia syndrome), immunodeficiencies and post-pneumonic bronchiectasis (following childhood infections).

Other features to look for in diffuse disease include situs inversus, indicating Kartagener's syndrome. Pneumothorax precipitated by airway obstruction is common in CF because of the associated viscous secretions. Long-term vascular access devices may be present (e.g. vascular access port) and there may be an enteral feeding tube (e.g. gastrostomy). The thoracic spine may reveal features of osteoporosis (kyphosis/vertebral fractures), a condition commonly seen in CF due to poor nutrition and steroid use.

Cystic fibrosis

Cystic fibrosis is a common autosomal recessive disease with reduced life expectancy, predominantly as a consequence of pulmonary complications. Thoracic manifestations should be well known to viva candidates, but bear in mind that it is a multisystem disease characterised by exocrine gland dysfunction. Gastrointestinal findings include meconium ileus (or meconium ileus equivalent syndrome in older patients), jejunisation of the colon, distal intestinal obstruction syndrome (DIOS) and pneumatosis intestinalis. Pancreatic insufficiency is seen in the majority of cases and results in malabsorption, although endocrine function is preserved until a late stage. Pancreatic fibrosis leads to diabetes mellitus and cholestasis predisposes to gallstone formation. Hepatic steatosis and fibrosis are common; the latter may lead to portal hypertension.

Case 39

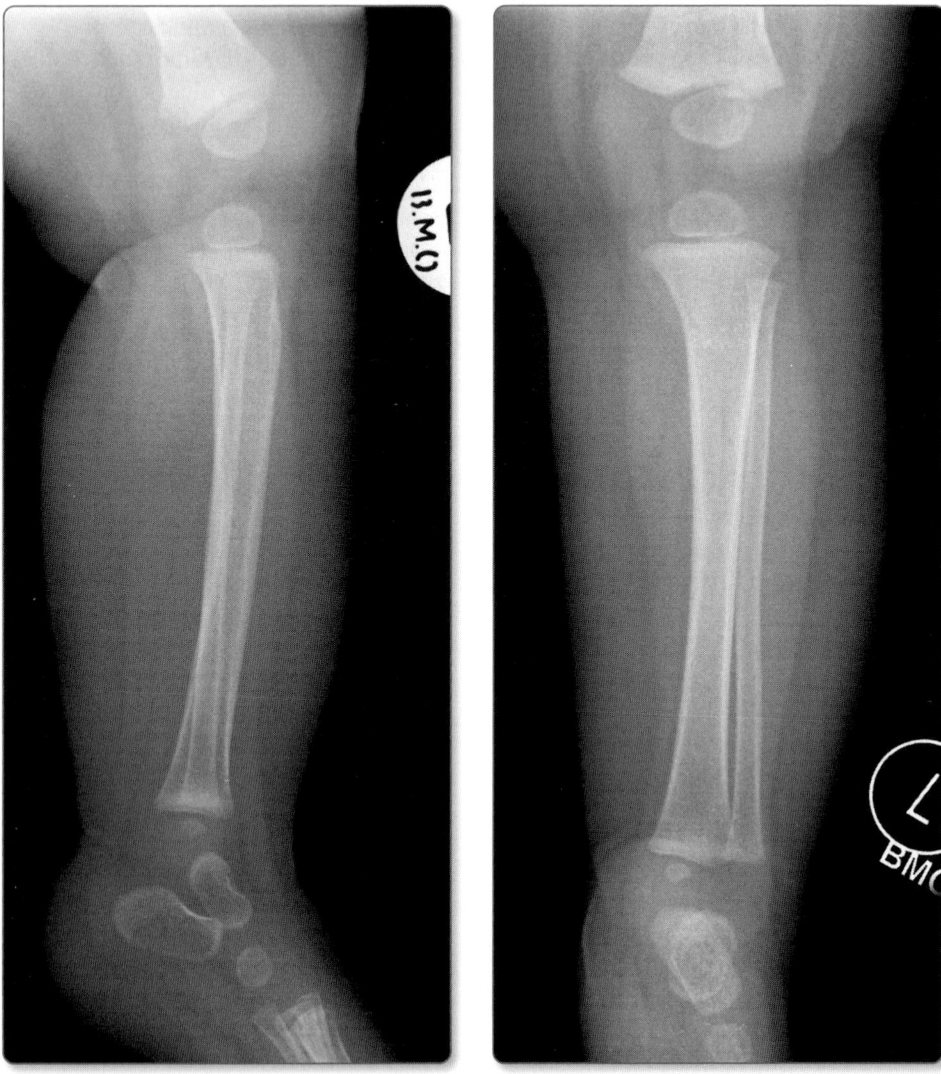

Suggested response

These are anteroposterior and lateral views of the left lower leg in a young child. The age would clearly be relevant here but the stage of osseous development in these radiographs suggests a child of no more than a few months of age. I do not see an abnormality of the tibia or fibula, but there is an unusual appearance of the distal femur which is suspicious for a fracture.

This would be an unusual injury to occur accidentally at this age as the child is unlikely to be walking yet. This injury raises the possibility of inflicted injury [nonaccidental injury, (NAI)]. In the first instance, I would recommend immediately continuing the examination to obtain anteroposterior and lateral views of the femur and would recommend keeping the child under observation in the department until the subsequent radiographs can also be reviewed to confirm these findings.

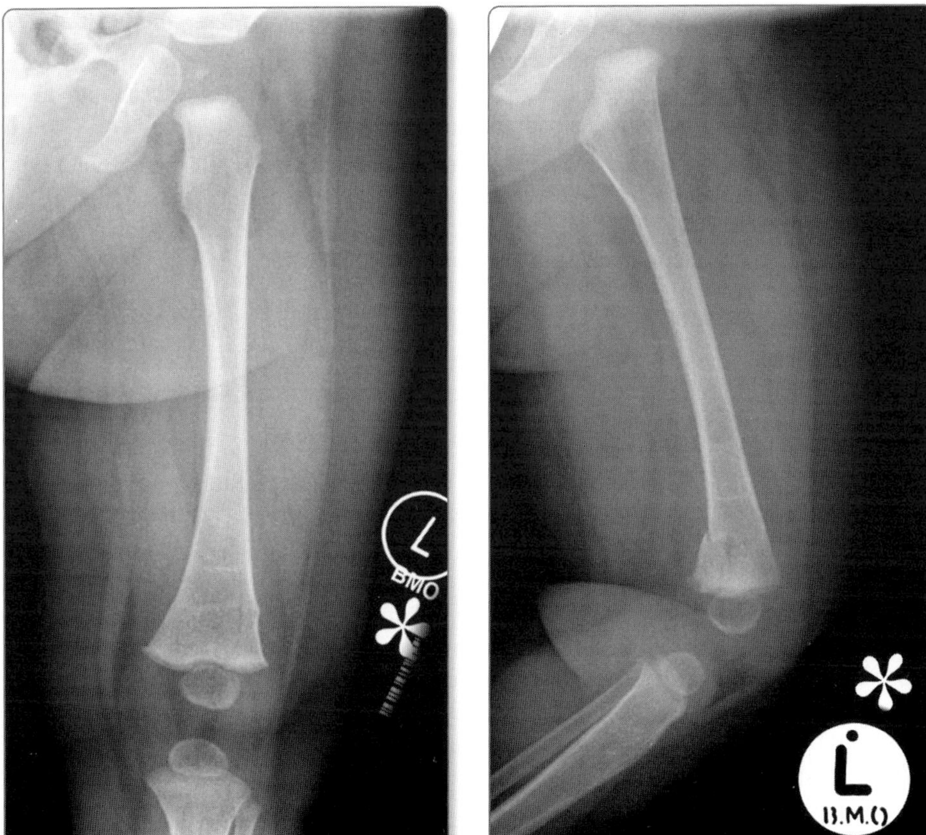

Suggested response

These are anteroposterior and lateral views of the left femur which confirm the impression of a fracture of the distal femur. The fracture extends from the posterior lateral margin of the distal femur into the physis.

I would follow the local policy for protecting children when they are recognised as being at risk through possible inflicted injury. In my institution, this would involve telephoning the designated senior emergency department staff or paediatrician on-call to discuss the findings, while ensuring that the child remained under observation in hospital.

Diagnosis

Distal femoral fracture in an 8-month-old child. No history of injury was available.

Tips: Possible inflicted injury

Key points

Consider the possibility of inflicted injury when presented with any paediatric radiograph. 'Normal' fractures and other conditions may be due to inflicted injury, which is increasingly superseding the term nonaccidental injury. Skeletal surveys are performed to protocol, but only form one part of the assessment. They should be reported by experts and are typically double reported.

Look out for multiple or asymmetrical fractures of varying ages, metaphyseal corner fractures, isolated spiral fractures of the femoral or humeral diaphysis, extensive periosteal reaction or callus formation, cortical hyperostosis extending to the physis, separation of the distal epiphysis, and evidence of head trauma.

Differential diagnosis

Osteogenesis imperfecta is associated with multiple fractures and exuberant callus. More unusual differentials include infantile cortical hyperostosis, scurvy, congenital syphilis and copper deficiency.

Inflicted injury

It can be difficult to know when to mention inflicted injury, both in a report and in a viva scenario, but failing to raise the possibility when faced with suspicious patterns of trauma (particularly in very young children who are not yet walking) has far-reaching implications. This would make an interesting discussion topic in an examination. Protocols for this scenario differ from department to department, so ensure that you know your local policy (there will be one – ask your senior colleagues) and be prepared to explain how you would act in a particular situation.

Case 40

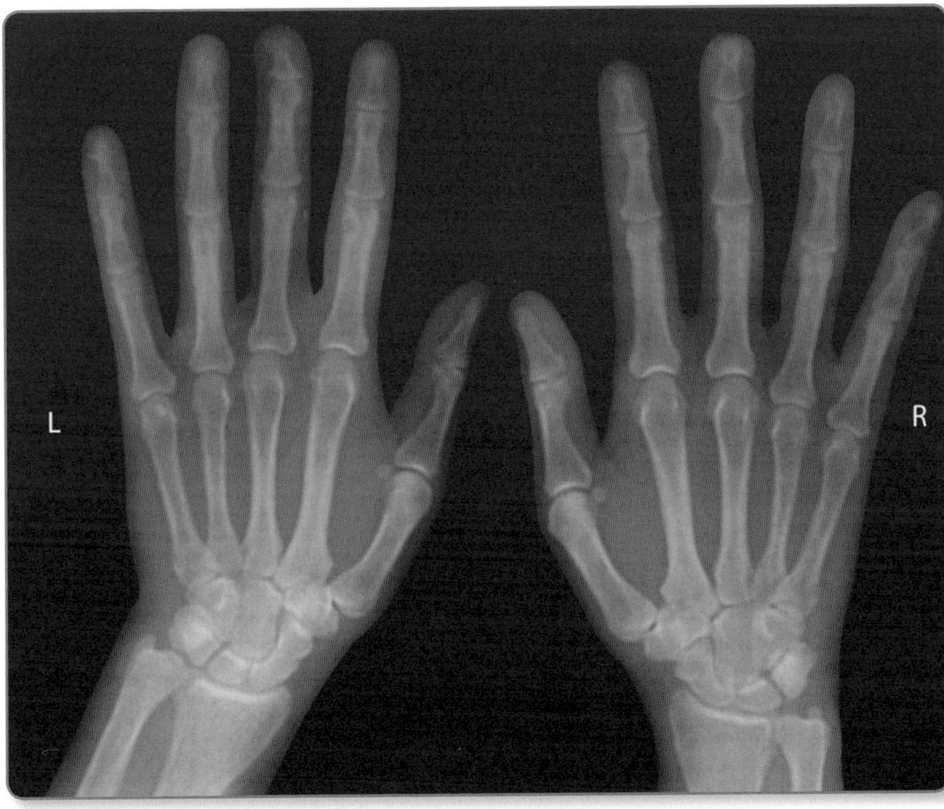

Suggested response

This is a dorsipalmar view of both hands.

There is subperiosteal bone resorption which is most marked in the right hand on the radial border of the middle phalanx of the middle finger. It is also present elsewhere, for instance on the ulnar border of the middle phalanx of the left middle finger.

In addition, there is a small well-defined lucent lesion in the proximal phalanx of the left index finger at the ulnar border of the distal diaphysis.

The bone density is normal and I cannot identify any fracture.

Appearances are those of hyperparathyroidism with a brown tumour.

Diagnosis

Hyperparathyroidism with brown tumour in proximal phalanx of left index finger.

Tips: Hyperparathyroidism

Hyperparathyroidism has multisystem manifestations: the so-called 'bones, stones and abdominal groans'.

Key points

Skeletal manifestations are characterised by osteopaenia and subperiosteal bone resorption, classically on the radial sides of phalanges and maximal in the middle finger middle phalanx, but also occurring around the sacroiliac joints, lateral clavicles and elsewhere. Primary hyperparathyroidism is associated with brown tumours (look for a pathological fracture) and chondrocalcinosis. Secondary hyperparathyroidism is associated with soft tissue calcifications and osteosclerosis including 'rugger jersey' spine.

Extraskeletal manifestations are common in the abdomen. There may be generalised vascular calcification. The genitourinary system may be affected by renal calculus formation and nephrocalcinosis. The gastrointestinal tract may be affected by peptic ulceration, calcific pancreatitis and constipation.

Hyperparathyroidism

Hyperparathyroidism may be primary [usually due to a parathyroid adenoma secreting parathyroid hormone (PTH) inappropriately], secondary ('appropriate' PTH production in the context of chronic renal failure) or tertiary (autonomous, inappropriate production of PTH complicating secondary hyperparathyroidism). If suspecting hyperparathyroidism on imaging grounds, you should recommend measuring serum calcium, phosphate, alkaline phosphatase and PTH. Phosphate levels will be elevated in secondary and tertiary forms due to renal failure.

Case 41

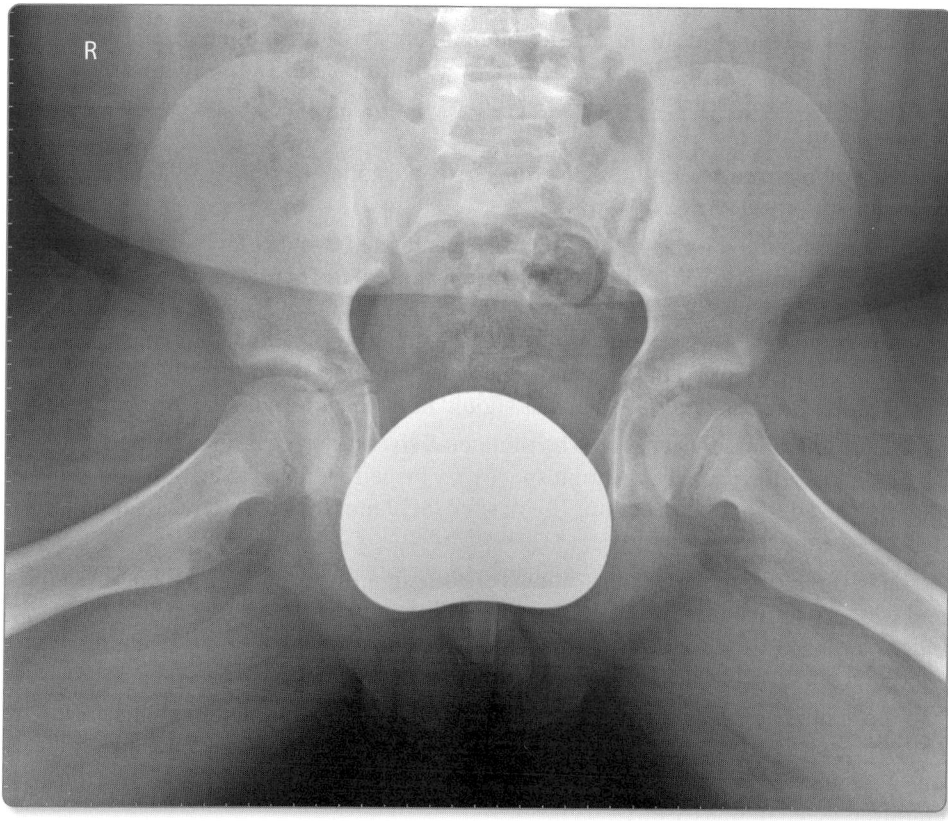

Suggested response

This is a 'frog's leg' lateral view of the pelvis of a skeletally immature male patient. The stage of osseous development is most in keeping with a young adolescent patient, although I would routinely correlate the appearance with the patient's age. The left upper femoral epiphysis is seen to have slipped medially. The epiphysis itself is of smooth contour with no features to suggest avascular necrosis. The right hip appears normal.

The rest of the visible skeleton is unremarkable. The appearance is of a left-slipped upper femoral epiphysis. I would discuss this case with the orthopaedic surgical team as a matter of urgency.

Diagnosis

Left slipped upper femoral epiphysis (SUFE) in a teenage male.

Tips: Paediatric hip radiographs

Key points

The single most important thing in the history is the patient's age. Developmental dysplasia of the hip tends to present in infancy, septic arthritis under 3 years of age (though it can present at any age), Perthes' disease from 2 to 12 years (with a mean of 7 years) and SUFE from 8 to 17 years (with a mean of 11 years for girls and 13 years for boys).

It is not uncommon for these disorders (except septic arthritis) to be bilateral, so do not be falsely reassured by symmetry!

Developmental dysplasia of the hip is characterised by a shallow acetabulum, disruption of Shenton's line and delayed ossification of the femoral epiphysis (normally evident by the 8th month postpartum). In your mind, divide each hip into four quadrants by drawing an imaginary vertical line through the lateral margin of the acetabulum and a horizontal line through the superolateral margin of the triradiate cartilage. The normal femoral epiphysis should lie in the inferomedial quadrant.

Septic arthritis is most likely to be unilateral, so comparing both sides is particularly useful. Initially, the joint space may be widened due to an effusion but later narrowed due to destruction. The normal fat planes may be displaced and there may be periarticular osteopaenia.

In Perthes' disease, the early findings are of a small sclerotic femoral epiphysis and widened joint space (this usually remains widened with no articular destruction, differentiating it from septic arthritis). Later in the disease, subchondral fracture (with a radiolucent crescent) and femoral head fragmentation may develop.

The features of SUFE are physeal widening, an apparently smaller epiphysis (a consequence of dorsal tilt) and increased metaphyseal density (early healing). The line of Klein, which follows the upper femoral neck contour, does not intersect the epiphysis (seen in this case).

Slipped upper femoral epiphysis

Slipped upper femoral epiphysis is an orthopaedic emergency with possible complications including avascular necrosis, chondrolysis and leg length discrepancy if not detected and treated in a timely manner. The typical patient is an overweight prepubertal teenage boy. It is easily missed, in part due to its often misleading clinical presentation (e.g. knee pain) and potentially subtle findings on radiographs. Sometimes minor physeal widening is the only appreciable sign. It is commonly bilateral, although slips are not necessarily synchronous. Radiographic abnormalities are usually most conspicuous on 'frog's leg' lateral views, although the positioning required to obtain this view can itself cause further slippage.

Case 42

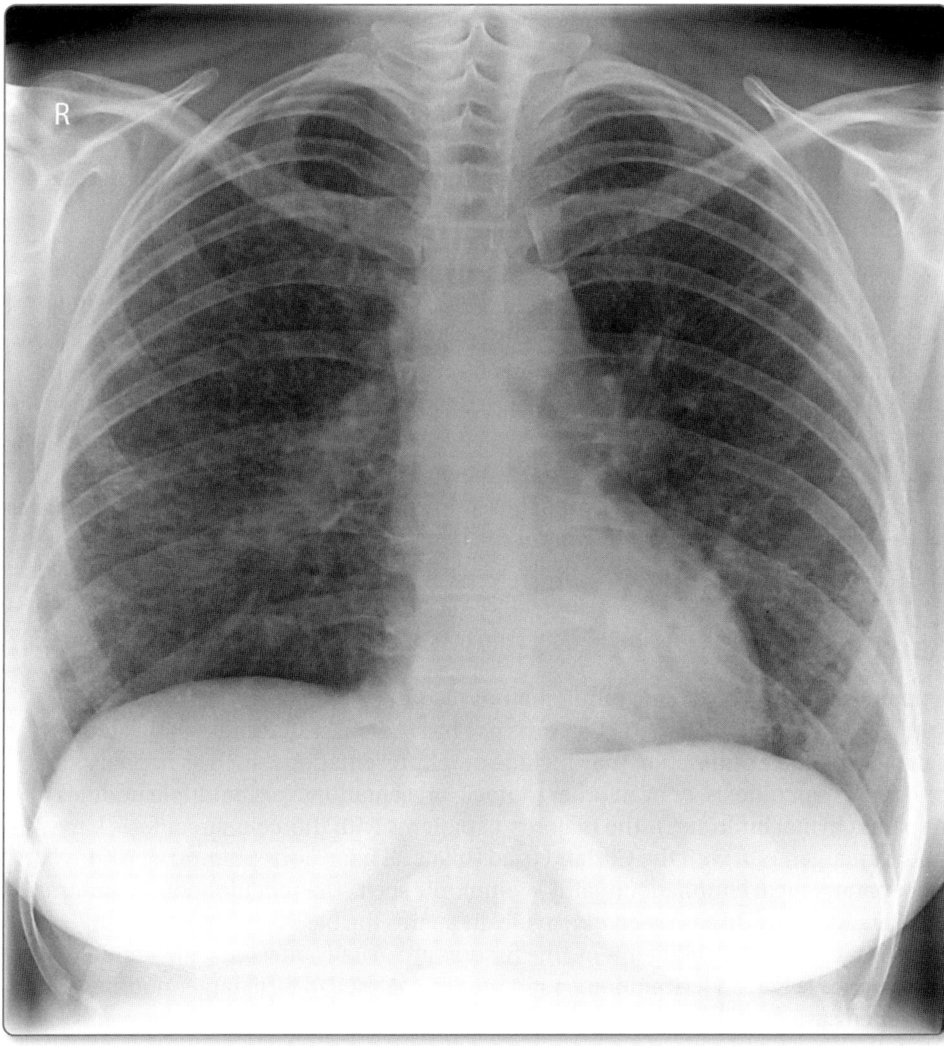

Suggested response

This is a frontal chest radiograph of a skeletally mature female patient. There is diffuse bilateral lung disease with extensive interstitial shadowing which involves all zones but with relative sparing of the costophrenic angles. Lung volumes are preserved and there is no pneumothorax. Both hila are bulky and irregular without visible calcification. There is no convincing widening of the right paratracheal stripe. The heart size is normal.

Features are strongly suggestive of sarcoidosis. If this is the initial presentation, then respiratory referral is advised with a view to high-resolution CT scanning of the chest for further assessment.

Diagnosis

A 33-year-old female with sarcoidosis.

Tips: Bilateral hilar enlargement

Key points

It can be difficult to distinguish pulmonary arteries from lymphadenopathy. Nodes typically have more irregular, 'bumpy' outlines, whereas arteries have smooth outlines and can be traced away from the hilar point.

Infections (including TB and viral infections) are far more likely to give unilateral hilar enlargement. Lymphoma or metastases can cause either unilateral or bilateral hilar enlargement.

Hilar calcification can help to narrow the differential diagnosis, but a lack of nodal calcification does not exclude any diagnosis. The presence of nodal calcification makes silicosis, sarcoidosis and treated lymphoma (typically asymmetrical lymphadenopathy with 'eggshell' calcification) more likely.

Sarcoidosis

Sarcoidosis is a multisystem granulomatous disorder which is most common in young women. The image shown in this case has the classic findings of pulmonary sarcoidosis. The examination may include other presentations, such as hepatosplenic or osseous sarcoidosis, or even other thoracic presentations (e.g. multiple nodules or parenchymal infiltrates). The majority of patients with thoracic sarcoidosis have nodal enlargement, with the Garland triad (bilateral hilar, aortopulmonary and right paratracheal lymphadenopathy) commonly seen. The reticulonodular pattern of interstitial lung disease seen here typically spares the bases and can occur in the absence of nodal enlargement. The fissures are usually affected with a nodular appearance **(Figure 1)**. Granulomas sometimes coalesce to form larger nodules which may then cavitate. Fibrosis represents the end-stage of the process.

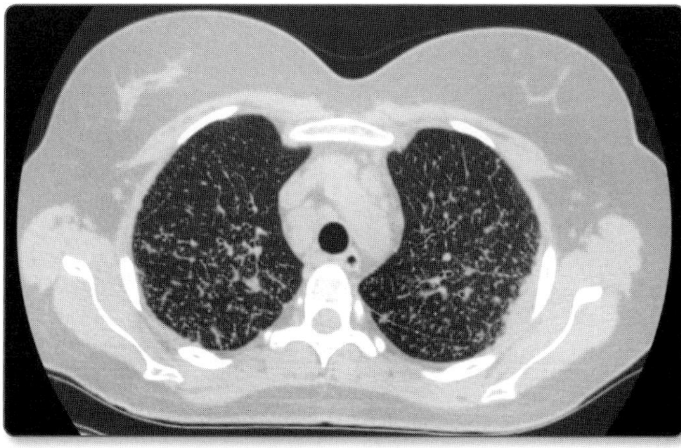

Figure 1 Axial CT in this patient demonstrating multiple tiny nodules and nodularity of the fissure on lung windows. Mediastinal lymphadenopathy is also visible.

Case 43

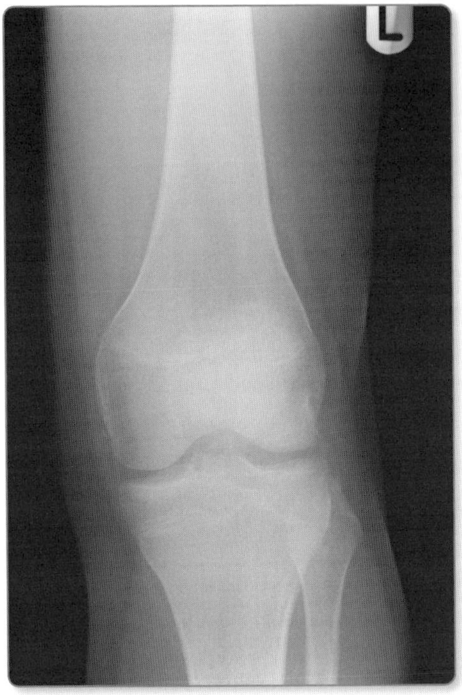

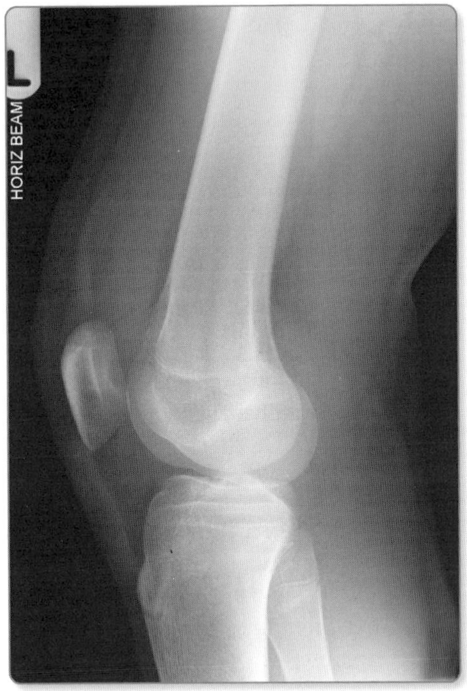

Suggested response

These are frontal and lateral radiographs of the left knee of a skeletally immature patient. There is a lipohaemarthrosis, indicating an intra-articular fracture. Several bony abnormalities are evident. Firstly, a small fragment is projected adjacent to the medial femoral condyle. Another fracture fragment is projected over the fibular head, adjacent to the lateral tibial plateau. A further fracture is evident through the medial tibial spine, the full extent of which is not clearly visualised, with a possible intra-articular osseous loose body projected superolateral to this. No convincing tibial plateau flattening is identified. This is a highly significant cluster of findings with the main injury being consistent with a Segond fracture, making injuries such as ligamentous and meniscal disruption highly likely. I would discuss this case with the orthopaedic surgical team with a view to an urgent MRI scan for further evaluation of the soft tissue injuries.

Diagnosis

Segond fracture in a 16-year-old patient.

Tips: Knee trauma

Key points

Look at the soft tissues. Is there a lipohaemarthrosis (intra-articular fracture) or haemarthrosis/effusion (many causes)? What about the supra- and infrapatellar contours (quadriceps/patellar tendon rupture – position of the patella is also indicative)?

Look at all bony contours. Osteochondral fractures of the femoral condyles can be easily missed! Beware of bony fragments projected over the fibular head, as in this case. The LATeral tibial plateau should be fLAT and the medial concave. If both are concave, suspect a lateral tibial plateau fracture (more common than medial).

If there is a proximal fibular fracture, there is the possibility of a Maisonneuve fracture, hence clinical examination and possibly imaging of the ankle joint is necessary.

Segond fracture

The Segond fracture is a significant injury caused by abnormal internal rotation and varus stresses on the knee. It can be radiographically subtle and refers to a vertical avulsion fracture from the lateral tibia, just inferior to the plateau. Associated tears in the anterior cruciate ligament, menisci (particularly medial) and the lateral capsular ligament are very common. CT may help to define the extent of any fracture and any co-existing fractures, whereas MRI is more useful in assessing ligamentous and meniscal injury as well as bone oedema.

Case 44

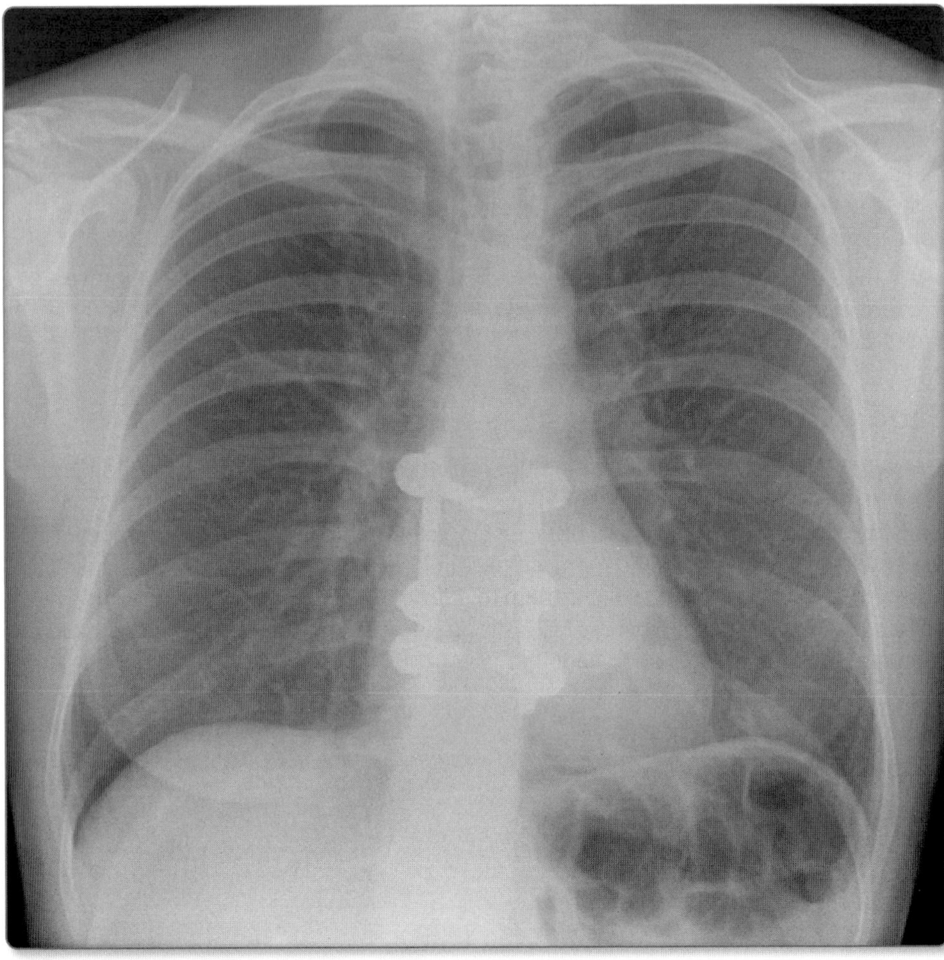

Suggested response

This is a posteroanterior chest radiograph of an adult female patient.

There has been previous spinal surgery with fusion of three lower thoracic vertebrae. At this level there is a rounded mass projected behind the heart. It is not possible to distinguish the medial border of this mass from the vertebral column.

The lungs appear otherwise clear and the mediastinal contour is otherwise normal. The remaining bones of the thoracic wall are also normal.

The differential for the mass projected behind the heart is wide as it could be in lung or arising from the anterior or middle mediastinum, but the previous spinal surgery and the appearance of the medial border of the mass are most suggestive of a paravertebral location.

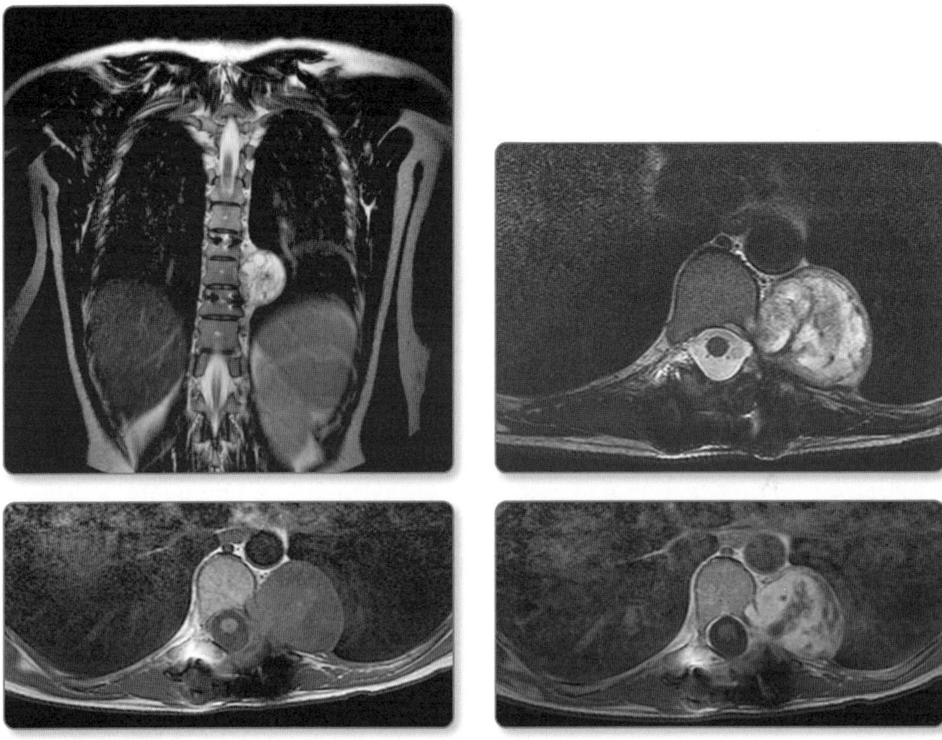

Suggested response

These are selected images from an MRI study. This shows that the mass appears to arise from the lateral margin of the spinal column and involves the neural exit foramen, at which point its margins are poorly defined. By contrast, the remaining margins are rounded and well-defined. The mass is heterogeneous but predominantly T2 hyperintense and T1 isointense relative to muscle. It largely enhances with a small crescentic cystic area laterally and some nonenhancing, presumably necrotic, foci centrally. The position makes a neural or epineural tumour the most likely explanation.

Diagnosis

Recurrent nerve sheath tumour following previous resection and spinal stabilisation.

Tips: A paraspinal mass

Key points

Ensure that you scrutinise the paraspinal lines on every chest radiograph. Suspect a paraspinal mass when the thickness of the left paraspinal soft tissues exceeds the width of the adjacent pedicle (often much less prominent than in the case above) or if there is any right paraspinal soft tissue.

Look for features suggesting a neural tumour, e.g. widening of the neural exit foramen, posterior vertebral scalloping and other features to suggest neurofibromatosis. Around one-third of paediatric mediastinal masses are located in the posterior mediastinum and 95% of these are neurogenic.

See Case 1 for more tips for mediastinal masses.

Differential diagnoses

True spinal/paraspinal masses include bony pathologies, neural tumours, abscesses and extramedullary haematopoiesis. However also consider the other anatomical structures which lie in the posterior mediastinum [e.g. blood vessels (aorta and azygos vein), oesophagus and thoracic duct] and also diaphragmatic herniae (e.g. Bochdalek and hiatus hernia) which may mimic paraspinal masses.

Nerve sheath tumours

Peripheral nerve sheath tumours can be either benign (neurinoma, schwannoma and neurofibroma) or malignant (malignant schwannoma). Spinal neurofibromas are usually seen in patients who have neurofibromatosis type 1 so scrutinise imaging for other manifestations of this disease (skin nodules can be subtle and can even mimic pulmonary nodules).

Case 45

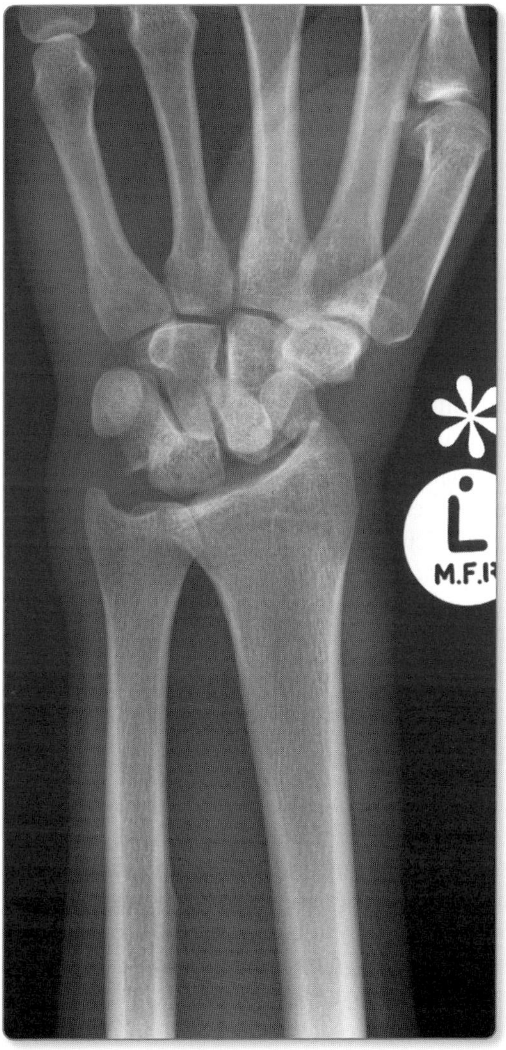

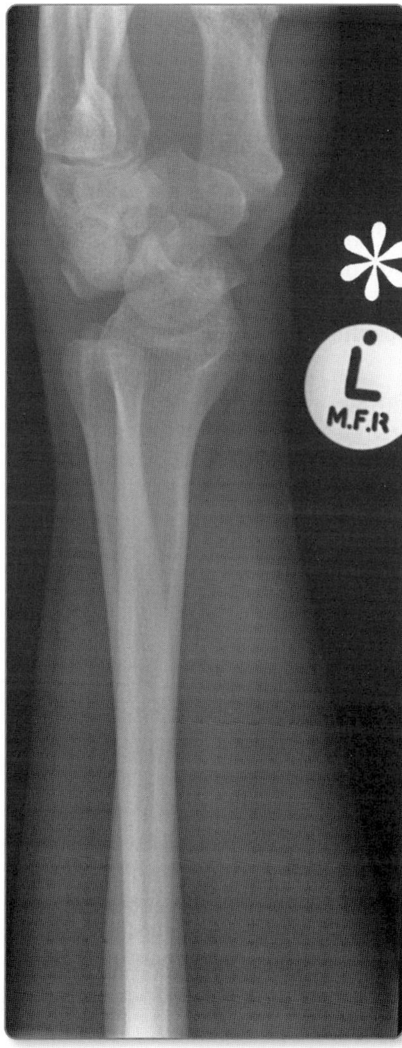

Suggested response

These are dorsipalmar and lateral radiographs of the left wrist of a skeletally mature patient. The alignment of the lunate is normal relative to the radius, but there is dorsal dislocation of the capitate. There is an associated fracture through the waist of the scaphoid. Findings are consistent with a trans-scaphoid perilunate fracture/dislocation. I would confirm that this injury had been recognised and promptly reduced and would urgently contact the referring clinician if this was not the case.

Diagnosis

Trans-scaphoid perilunate fracture/dislocation of the wrist.

Tips: Hand/wrist trauma

Key points

Look round the cortical margins of each and every bone. Buckle fractures, in particular, can be very subtle. If there is a radial or ulnar injury, think about the joint above/below (Monteggia/Galeazzi fracture/dislocations).

Think about the carpus in terms of proximal and distal rows. Look at three smooth arcs outlining the proximal and distal margins of the proximal row and the proximal margin of the distal row. Most (>90%) of carpal fractures involve the triquetrum or scaphoid.

On lateral views, look at/for the alignment (capitate on lunate on radius should form a straight line), triquetral fracture and infilling of the normal concavity of the soft tissues of the dorsum of the wrist (this raises suspicion for a subtle fracture).

On dorsi-palmar views, look for scapholunate separation ('Terry Thomas'/ 'Madonna' signs) – normal distance < 2 mm in skeletally mature patients – or overlap, which may suggest dislocation (often less conspicuous on lateral views), classically at metacarpophalangeal joints or within the carpus.

Be suspicious in a viva if the views are more limited than you would expect in normal practice; this is often a clue that there is a subtle finding that will be better seen on the remainder of the series that has not (yet) been shown.

Lunate and perilunate dislocations

These are generally easily detected (particularly on the lateral view), assuming the viewer has a sound knowledge of the wrist joint anatomy. There should be no excuses for struggling with this type of case if encountered in a viva or in everyday practice. In lunate dislocation, the radius and capitate remain aligned while the lunate is dislocated anteriorly. Perilunate dislocations commonly occur in combination with a scaphoid fracture: as seen in this case, the radius and lunate remain normally aligned while the capitate and remainder of the carpus is dislocated posteriorly.

Case 46

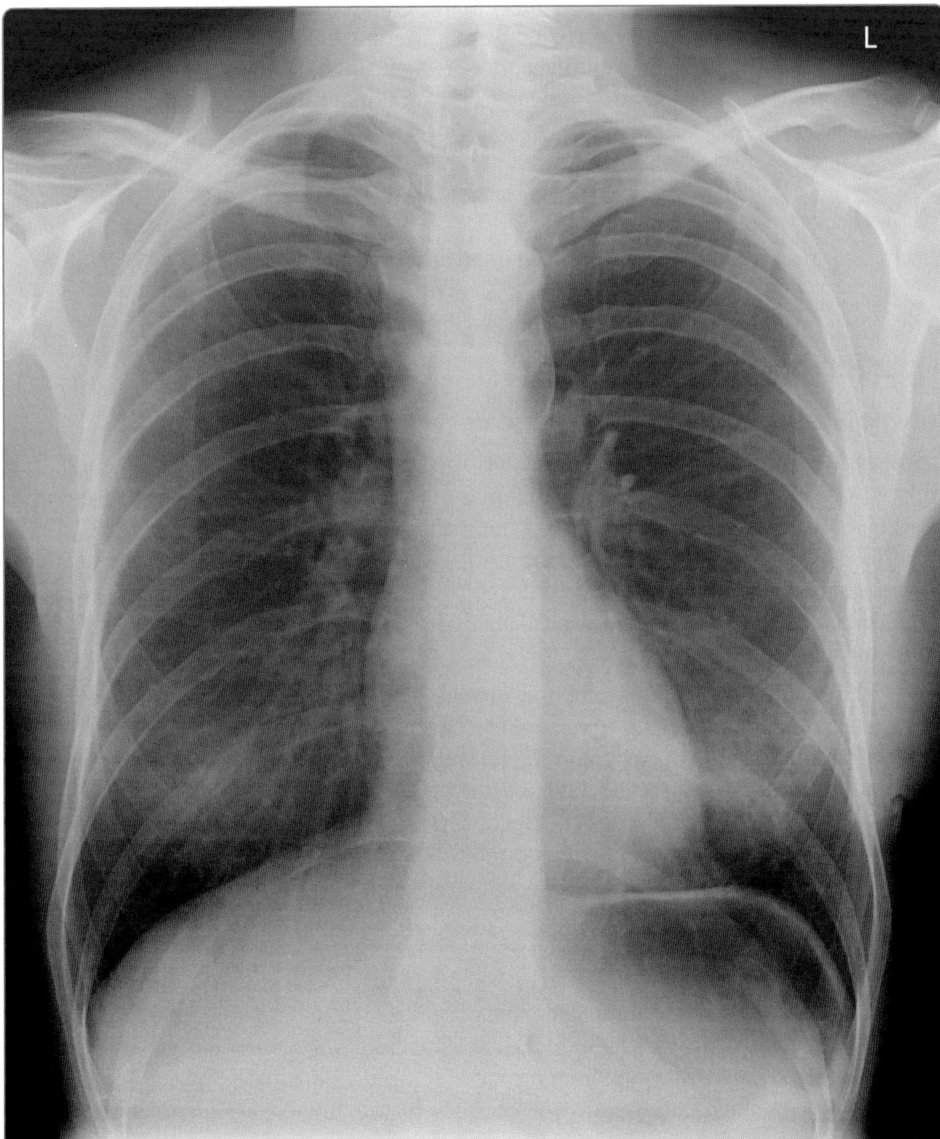

Suggested response

This is a frontal chest radiograph of a skeletally mature patient. The first abnormality I have identified is an abnormal contour of the left-sided aortic knuckle with a 'figure 3' configuration. The mediastinum is otherwise within normal limits, in particular the heart is not enlarged and the cardiac apex is left-sided. Notching of the inferior aspects of the posterior ribs in the mid-thorax is evident and is most conspicuous in the fifth to seventh ribs bilaterally. Symmetrical bilateral increased density in the lower zones is likely to reflect overlying breast tissue and there is no lung abnormality. The combination of abnormal aortic contour and inferior rib notching bilaterally is likely to represent aortic coarctation. If there is no known diagnosis of coarctation, then referral to cardiology with a view to cross-sectional imaging to delineate the anatomy is advised.

Diagnosis

Residual or recurrent aortic coarctation in an adult female with previous coarctation repair.

Tips: Rib notching

Key points and differential diagnosis

Consider whether it is the superior or inferior surfaces of the ribs that are notched. If inferior, consider the structures passing under the ribs, i.e. within the neurovascular bundle. Causes may be neurogenic (e.g. neurofibromatosis; this may involve superior and inferior surfaces, i.e. 'ribbon ribs'), arterial (e.g. coarctation and aortic thrombosis; usually bilateral) or venous (e.g. obstruction of the superior vena cava). If superior, it is unrelated to anatomical structures (e.g. metabolic disorders and connective tissue diseases).

Unilateral inferior rib notching may also be seen, with varying distributions. In some circumstances, this can be caused by coarctation (if right-sided notching, by coarctation proximal to the origin of the left subclavian artery or if there is a right aortic arch with an anomalous left subclavian artery; if left-sided notching, when there is an anomalous right subclavian artery). Subclavian artery obstruction can cause ipsilateral upper rib notching (this is usually postoperative, e.g. Blalock–Taussig shunt).

Aortic coarctation

Infantile aortic coarctation involves a long segment of the aorta and is commonly associated with cardiac anomalies. A more typical viva case is an adult with coarctation. This involves a more focal segment of the aorta, usually without cardiac anomalies, and may be detected incidentally on imaging since symptoms are often absent. The classical 'figure 3' sign on chest radiography (or, conversely, the 'reverse 3' sign on contrast swallow) corresponds to the segmental narrowing separating the superiorly placed aortic arch or enlarged left subclavian artery from the inferiorly placed poststenotic aortic dilatation. Inferior rib notching is seen posteriorly, involving the third to ninth ribs bilaterally (with certain caveats highlighted above), as a result of hypertrophy of the posterior intercostal arteries. The upper two ribs are spared because the intercostal arteries arise from the subclavian arteries. Cardiac enlargement may be seen in affected children but does not usually occur in adults.

Case 47

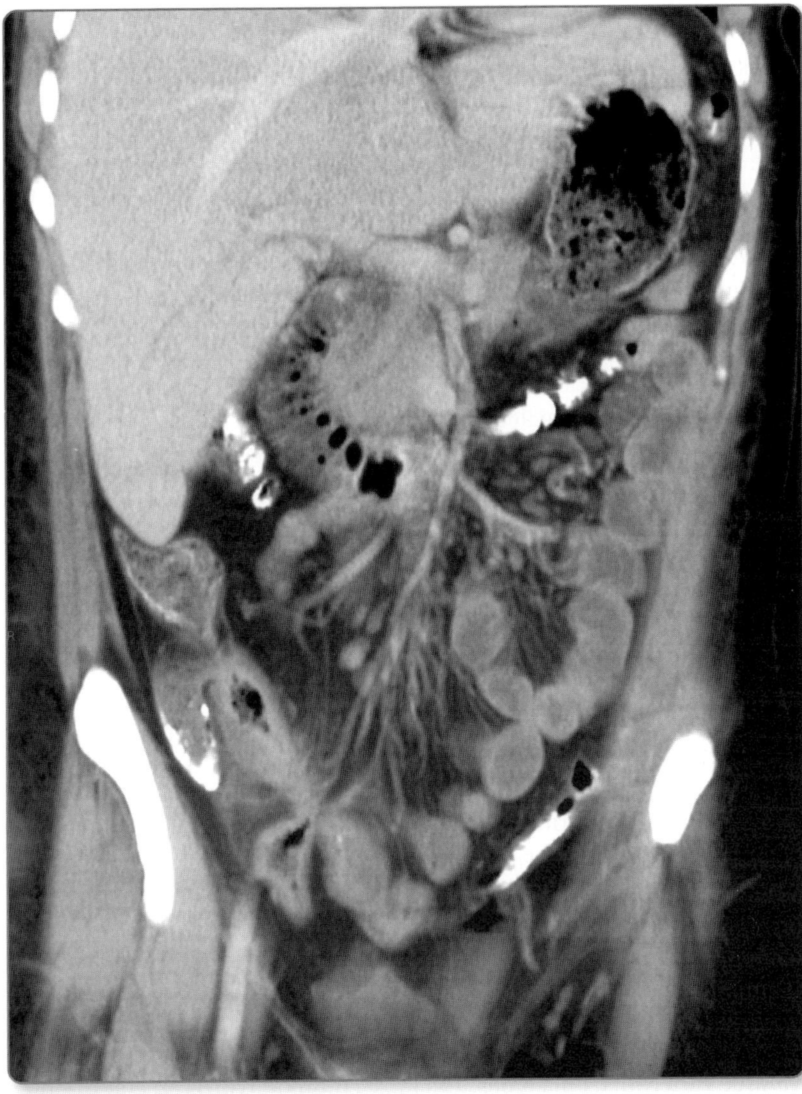

Suggested response

This is a coronally reformatted CT image of the abdomen which demonstrates an abnormal appearance in the right lower quadrant. There is high-attenuation material in the caecum, transverse and descending colon, presumably positive contrast, perhaps from a prior gastrointestinal contrast study. The wall of the terminal ileum is thickened and the surrounding mesenteric fat is streaky, suggesting inflammation.

An acute angle at the inferior aspect of this abnormal fat, inferior to the caecal pole, suggests the presence of some free fluid. These inflammatory changes are accompanied by enlarged lymph nodes lying along the line of the ileocolic vessels in the mesentery. There is an abnormal convergence of the distal ileal loops forming a clover-leaf appearance in the right pelvis. This appearance suggests a cicatrising process causing adherence of adjacent bowel loops. Clearly I would normally review the rest of the scan. However, taken together with the changes in the terminal ileum, the appearances on this single image most strongly suggest a diagnosis of Crohn's disease with involvement of the terminal ileum and an entero-enteric fistula between distal small bowel loops. If the patient is known to have inflammatory bowel disease, then this diagnosis can be made with confidence. If there is no prior history, then I would communicate these findings to the gastroenterology team who may wish to perform endoscopic inspection and biopsy of the terminal ileum.

Diagnosis

Crohn's disease of the terminal ileum with entero-enteric fistula.

Tips: A gastrointestinal fistula

Key points

The actual fistula track itself may not be demonstrated but the presence of a fistula may be inferred by other features. For instance, ingested contrast may demonstrate opacification of the sigmoid colon before contrast has traversed the rest of the large bowel, indicating the presence of an enterocolic fistula. Gas bubbles in the bladder on a CT scan which also demonstrates abnormal sigmoid colon adjacent to the bladder wall suggests the presence of a colovesical fistula.

Precise delineation of fistula tracts and also determination of the underlying cause of a fistula (in particular discriminating between benign and malignant aetiologies) using diagnostic imaging may be challenging and it may be relevant to convey these facts to the examiner.

Cross-sectional imaging, barium studies and endoscopic examinations may be useful to clarify findings. Endoscopic or percutaneous biopsy may be considered.

Gastrointestinal tract fistulation

There is a wide variety of fistula types. The most common type is an entero-enteric fistula caused by Crohn's disease, but almost any combination of adjacent luminal structures may be connected by a fistula. If the underlying diagnosis is not Crohn's disease, then malignancy or non-Crohn's chronic inflammatory disease may be the cause.

Case 48

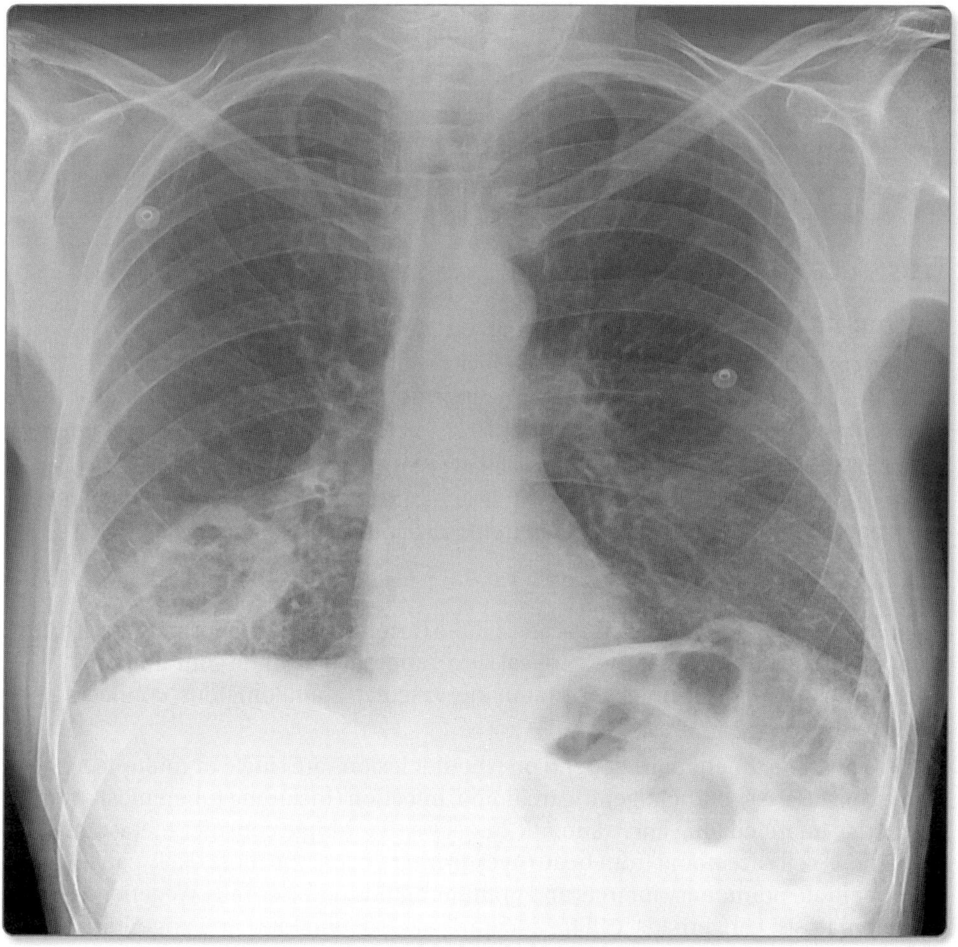

Suggested response

This is a frontal chest radiograph of a skeletally mature patient. Projected in the right lower zone is a large, well-defined, rounded opacity, with its medial aspect projected over the inferior right hilum. The opacity has a thick wall with central cavitation. The internal cavity margins are irregular and there is an impression of an air-fluid level within the cavity. There is no appreciable bony destruction in relation to the lesion or elsewhere on the radiograph. There is some airspace opacification medial to the lesion, but no further focal lung lesions are identified. The hila are not enlarged.

In the first instance, I would want to review any available relevant previous imaging. The range of differential diagnoses for this appearance is very wide and is critically dependent on the overall clinical picture, but assuming that this is not a stable finding, the most important differential diagnosis is a cavitating lung neoplasm, most likely squamous cell carcinoma. This merits an urgent respiratory referral with a view to bronchoscopic evaluation, a staging CT scan and if the presumptive diagnosis remains lung cancer, then discussion in the lung cancer multidisciplinary team meeting.

Diagnosis

Cavitating bronchogenic carcinoma in a male smoker.

Tips: A cavitating lung lesion

Key points

The 'air-crescent' sign (air separating the cavity wall from an inner mass) implies infection, but is occasionally seen in bronchogenic carcinoma. Remember that mycetoma can form in a cavitating tumour.

Look at the wall of the lesion. Thin-walled (<4 mm) lesions are benign in the vast majority of cases. Thick-walled (>16 mm) lesions are strongly suggestive of malignancy. Spiculated/irregular inner and outer margins also indicate malignancy.

Differential diagnosis

Pulmonary nodules of most causes can cavitate (arteriovenous malformations are the main exception). Remember the 'surgical sieve' approach to guide your thinking, i.e. causes can be neoplastic, infective, traumatic, vascular, granulomatous, connective tissue disease, etc.

The possible differentials depend on whether lesions are single or multiple. If single consider, e.g. bronchogenic carcinoma, infection (including tuberculosis and *S. aureus*), infarcted lung and traumatic lung cyst. If multiple consider metastases (squamous cell carcinoma from head/neck primary being the most likely cause), septic emboli, pulmonary infarcts and granulomatous diseases (e.g. Wegener's granulomatosis, Langerhans' cell histiocytosis and rheumatoid). In Langerhans' cell histiocytosis there are multiple lesions and the natural history of a single lesion is progression from a solid nodule to a cavitating nodule to a thick-walled cyst to a thin-walled cyst (a combination of findings may be seen at any one time).

Cavitating tumours

There is a vast differential diagnosis for a cavitating pulmonary mass, but morphology of the cavity wall is a useful means of assessing the likelihood of the mass being malignant. Cavitation in primary bronchogenic carcinoma is most commonly seen in squamous cell carcinoma **(Figure 1)** and confers a worse prognosis. The presence of cavitation effectively excludes a diagnosis of small cell carcinoma. Other primary lung tumours can cavitate, including lymphoma and Kaposi's sarcoma.

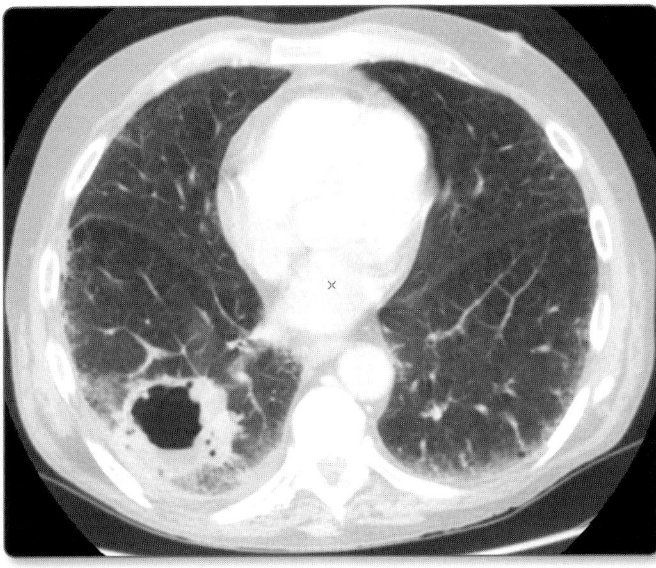

Figure 1 Axial CT on lung windows from this case demonstrating a cavitating right lower lobe bronchogenic carcinoma.

Case 49

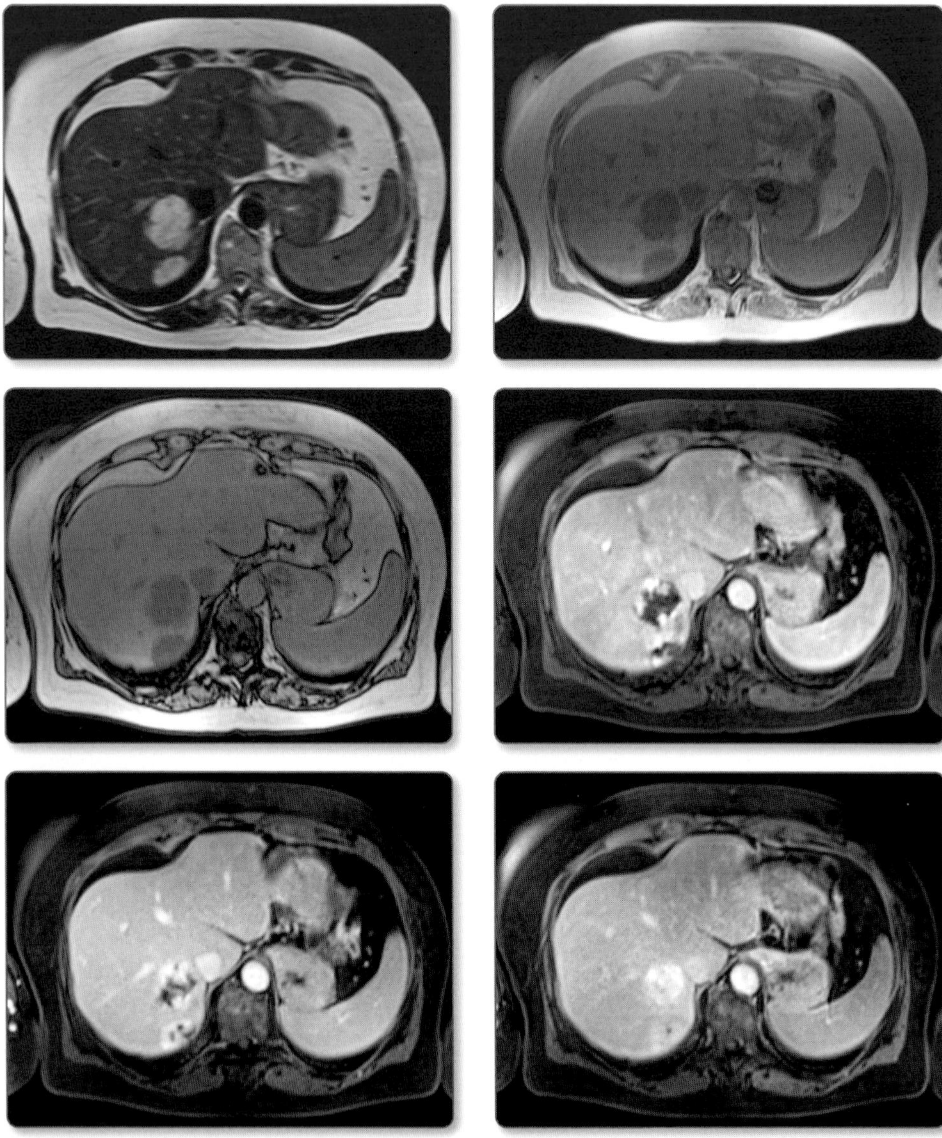

Suggested response

This is a series of axial MRI images of the liver, all taken at the same level. There are two discrete focal liver lesions, each measuring 3–4 cm across. On the T2-weighted image, both the lesions exhibit relatively uniform high-signal intensity. There are two noncontrast T1-weighted images, one of which exhibits the Indian ink artefact characteristic of out-of-phase images. On both of these noncontrast T1-weighted images, the lesions exhibit low-signal intensity. There is no conspicuous loss of signal intensity on the out-of-phase image. The three post-gadolinium images appear to be acquired during arterial, portal venous and delayed phases. In these sequences, the lesions exhibit progressive centripetal enhancement which is initially marginal and irregular, but which becomes more homogeneous and uniform over time. There is no evidence of a central scar on either the T2-weighted image or the post-contrast images. The lesions are rounded and well-defined with clear margins and no changes apparent in the surrounding liver parenchyma. The background liver appears homogeneous with no evidence of macronodular cirrhosis. I also note that the spleen is not enlarged on this image.

In summary, there are two focal lesions in an otherwise apparently normal liver with no evidence of cirrhosis. The native tissue signal and post-contrast characteristics exhibited by the lesions are characteristic for benign cavernous haemangiomas.

Diagnosis

Multiple benign cavernous haemangiomas in the liver.

Tips: Lesions in the liver

Because of the substantial overlap between the MRI characteristics of many different types of focal liver lesion it is likely that you will be presented with classical characteristic appearances rather than an equivocal mixture of radiological and clinical features. although it is possible atypical findings will become a topic for questions from the examiner.

If you are not convinced that the lesions exhibit classical diagnostic appearances, then it is important that you indicate that the confidence of diagnosis is very much dependent on the full clinical picture of the patient, as well as the imaging findings. For instance, a new solitary 3 cm slightly arterialised lesion in a 19-year-old female patient on the oral contraceptive pill is likely to be an adenoma, whereas a radiologically identical lesion in an older, alcoholic patient with chronic hepatitis B status is most likely to be an hepatocellular carcinoma (HCC). Lesions that are not absolutely classical should be considered for biopsy or follow-up imaging, depending on the overall clinical picture.

Key points

When describing liver lesions, consider whether they are solitary or multiple, their site, their approximate size, whether they have a central scar and what their enhancement characteristics are. The background state of the liver is important because the presence or absence of cirrhosis has substantial influence on the likely nature of any focal liver lesions. Extrahepatic findings may point to a particular diagnosis: splenomegaly, ascites and varices suggest portal hypertension and lymphadenopathy suggests malignancy.

If a central scar is present, then describe it, but do not let this feature guide your diagnosis too much. HCC, for instance, may have a distinct central scar, while a focal nodular hyperplasia lesion may have no scar.

If you are asked to interpret imaging performed using specialist hepatic contrast agents, then 'hepatocyte-specific' agents are used to identify bile leaks and to improve the specificity of focal liver lesion characteristics. Iron oxide agents are used to identify small liver metastases and to aid discrimination between hepatoid liver lesions that contain Kupffer cells (focal nodular hyperplasia) and those that do not (HCC and adenoma).

Differential diagnoses

Pure cysts and benign cavernous haemangiomas may exhibit cast-iron diagnostic characteristics on noninvasive imaging. All other types of focal liver lesions may exhibit a range of appearances with particular overlap between hepatocyte-derived (hepatoid) lesions (focal nodular hyperplasia, regenerating nodule, adenoma and HCC).

Arterialised contrast enhancement may help to distinguish hepatoid lesions and metastases from neuroendocrine-derived tumours of the bowel and pancreas, such as carcinoid tumours.

If HCC is suspected, then indicate your awareness that serum alpha-fetoprotein is usually elevated in this condition, but that a low level does not exclude the diagnosis. It is widely believed that biopsy of a lesion that may be a treatable HCC is contraindicated because of fears about 'seeding' of the tumour. Therefore, many clinicians will proceed directly to surgical resection.

Liver haemangiomas

Cavernous haemangiomas in the liver are extremely common and are often incidental findings. They are often well visualised at ultrasound and are typically well-defined high-reflectivity lesions in the periphery of the liver (although they may be isoreflective or of low reflectivity compared to fatty liver). The majority show some posterior acoustic enhancement. They may have atypical features which make their appearance on ultrasound nonspecific. The typical features on CT and MRI, with filling in of the lesion from the periphery, are as described above. They usually have a very low rate of complications and intervention is rarely required.

Case 50

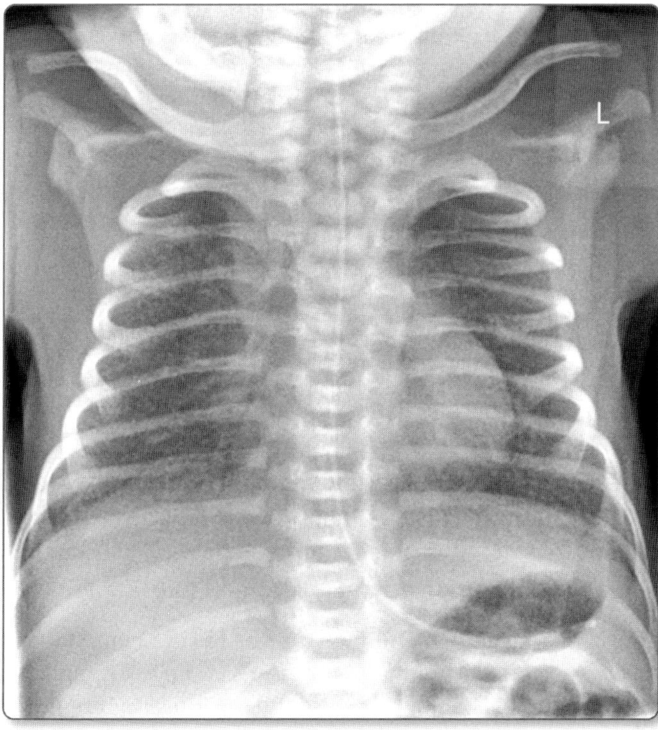

Suggested response

This is a chest radiograph of an infant. Given the nonvisualisation of the proximal humeral epiphyses, this is likely to be a neonate, possibly premature.

A nasogastric tube appears to be in an appropriate position. Lung volumes appear reduced bilaterally and there is diffuse granularity with multiple air bronchograms. There is no convincing pneumothorax or pleural effusion. The cardiothymic contour is within normal limits.

If this is a premature neonate, then the most likely diagnosis is respiratory distress syndrome. Appearances could also represent transient tachypnoea of the newborn, particularly in a term baby. Diffuse pneumonia is also a possibility, particularly if the baby presents with a clinical picture of sepsis.

Diagnosis

Respiratory distress syndrome (RDS) in a premature neonate in the first day of life.

Tips: Neonatal chest radiographs

Key points

The gestational age is key in formulating a differential diagnosis. RDS is most commonly seen in premature neonates and neonatal pneumonia is most commonly seen in premature/term neonates. Transient tachypnoea of the newborn (TTN) is most commonly seen in term neonates and meconium aspiration is most commonly seen in term/post-term neonates.

Look at the lung volumes and decide if they are increased, normal or decreased. If they are increased then this would suggest meconium aspiration, giving increased volume due to air trapping. If normal, then TTN or neonatal pneumonia is most likely. If decreased, then RDS is more likely.

Air bronchograms are not a feature in meconium aspiration since there is airways obstruction, but are prominent in RDS which gives airways distension.

Pneumothoraces may be secondary to meconium aspiration or complications of intubation. Pleural effusions are more commonly associated with meconium aspiration and transient tachypnoea of the newborn than the other conditions above.

Do not forget to assess the cardiothymic silhouette and examine the heart and pulmonary vasculature for evidence of congenital heart disease.

Respiratory distress syndrome

Sometimes referred to as hyaline membrane disease or surfactant deficiency syndrome, RDS typically affects premature neonates in the few hours after birth and results from an inability to sufficiently expand the lungs. Symptoms peak after 1–2 days before gradually improving. The features in this case are typical, with low volume lungs (unless intubated) and diffuse granular or reticulogranular shadowing which may become confluent. Air bronchograms are prominent. RDS often resolves spontaneously within 7–10 days. In an intubated baby, carefully evaluate for signs of complications of ventilation (including pneumothorax and pulmonary interstitial emphysema).

Case 51

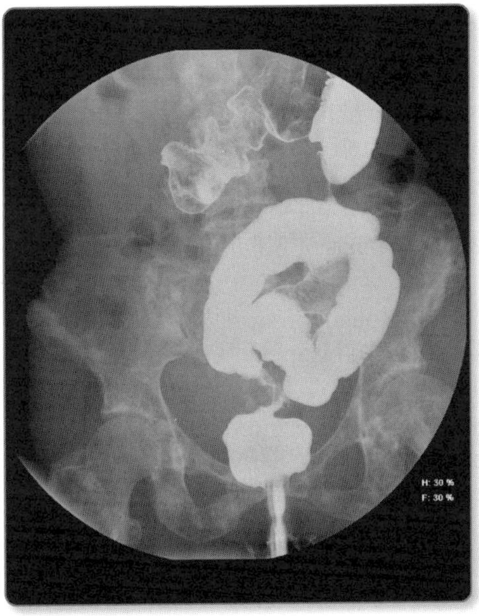

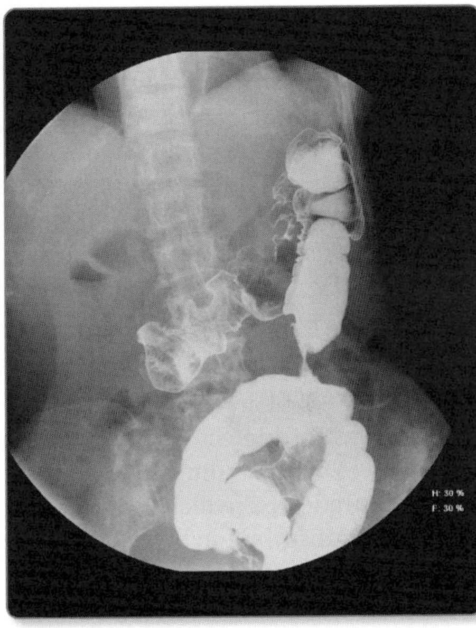

Suggested response

These are two spot images from a contrast enema examination, with the rectum and visualised colon predominantly seen in single contrast only. The first thing to note is that on these images contrast is not seen to pass beyond the mid-transverse colon. If this was the proximal limit of passage of contrast, it may reflect complete obstruction. There are at least two further strictures in the visualised bowel and a large irregular filling defect in the distal transverse colon.

There are also widespread sclerotic bony lesions throughout the pelvis, most in keeping with metastases.

Although synchronous colorectal malignancies may manifest in this way, or the colonic and bony lesions may be unrelated, I suspect that the appearance is more likely to be due to colonic and sclerotic bony metastases from one of a number of potential primary lesions, including colorectal, breast and prostate carcinoma. Review of any available relevant previous imaging would be useful to help to clarify this, but if this is the initial presentation then the case should be discussed with the referring clinicians with a view to further investigation. CT scanning is a possibility in the first instance, ideally after the patient passes the majority of the very dense contrast which has just been inserted for this study, or more urgently but with the potential for more artefact if they are very unwell.

Diagnosis

Adult female with breast cancer and colorectal and sclerotic bone metastases.

Tips: Strictures on a contrast enema

Key points

When considering strictures, think in terms of broad groups of differentials, i.e. neoplastic processes, inflammatory or infective processes, extrinsic processes.

Neoplastic processes may be primary, such as the classical 'apple core' lesion caused by an annular carcinoma, and there may be synchronous or secondary lesions elsewhere. Secondary neoplastic processes often have an intra-abdominal source, but may be due to haematogenous spread (for instance in breast cancer, as in this case) or lymphatic spread. Synchronous primary lesions are more common if there is a predisposing factor such as familial polyposis or inflammatory bowel disease (IBD).

Colonic lymphoma is less common than lymphoma of the stomach or small bowel and usually involves the caecum. It has a variety of imaging appearances including circumferential thickening.

Inflammatory/infective processes usually have smoother, more tapered appearances than tumours. IBD should be considered, particularly if long segments of colon are affected (which is not usually the case in malignancy). Remember the difference in distribution between ulcerative colitis and Crohn's disease. Multifocal strictures with normal intervening bowel will not be ulcerative colitis, which is continuous from the rectum proximally. Radiotherapy strictures tend to occur years after treatment so do not be put off by a distant history.

Extrinsic processes include other intra-abdominal inflammatory processes, such as pancreatitis and endometriosis.

Ancillary findings may suggest a particular diagnosis. Bone metastases or radiotherapy changes (well-defined edges to bony changes or bone tumours in previously irradiated bone) may point to radiotherapy as a cause. Sacroiliitis may be associated with IBD.

Iatrogenic findings such as a stoma (which could reflect previous bowel resection), nephrectomy (suggesting renal cell carcinoma), brachytherapy pellets in the pelvis (indicating prostate carcinoma) and pancreatic calcification (which points to chronic pancreatitis) may all be useful in narrowing the differential.

Colonic metastases

Metastases can reach the colon in a number of ways. Spread from other abdominopelvic malignancies is not uncommon, be it via intraperitoneal seeding, direct invasion from an adjacent tumour or along reflections of mesentery. Haematogenous spread can also occur, with breast carcinoma representing the most common primary tumour. Symptoms arising as a result of colonic metastases may be the initial presentation of breast cancer although, conversely, they may be a late finding occurring years after initial presentation and treatment. They usually cause thickening of a long segment of colon. Haematogenous spread may also give rise to submucosal metastases which manifest as 'target lesions' (also seen in the stomach).

Case 52

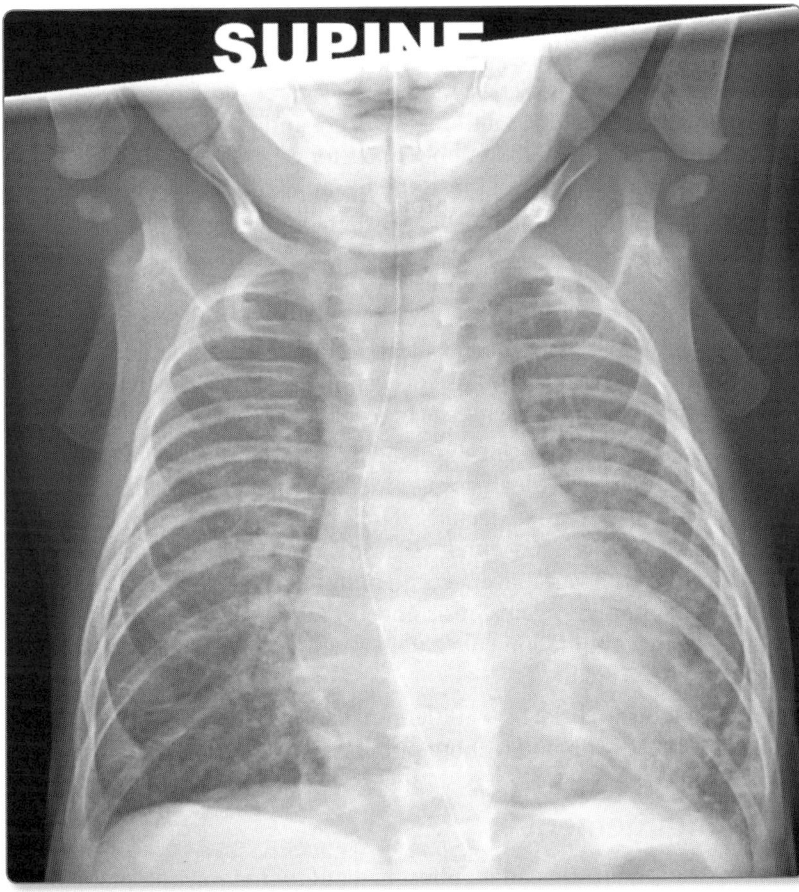

Suggested response

This is a supine chest radiograph of an infant. There is a nasogastric tube, the tip of which is projected in the distal oesophagus; this should be advanced into the stomach. I also note that the middle part of this tube is deviated to the right as it passes behind the heart. In addition, there is splaying of the carina. This combination of findings is consistent with left atrial enlargement and, allowing for the projection and age of the patient, there is also probably generalised cardiomegaly in addition to the left atrial enlargement. There is perihilar haziness bilaterally and increased interstitial markings which are most conspicuous in the right lower zone. While the lung findings could be infective changes, in the context of all the other findings they most likely represent interstitial pulmonary oedema. I would discuss this with the referring clinicians, but further assessment with echocardiography would be useful in the first instance because the cluster of findings suggest congenital mitral valve disease.

Diagnosis

Two-month-old girl with mitral regurgitation and pulmonary hypertension.

Tips: Congenital heart disease

Making a specific diagnosis on a chest radiograph is rarely possible. However, several congenital heart diseases (such as tetralogy of Fallot and transposition of the great vessels) have classic findings and therefore make for very testable subjects in the viva setting. You should be aware of these and be familiar with the corrective surgical procedures which may be identifiable on a chest radiograph (e.g. Blalock–Taussig shunt).

Key points

Clinical features are essential for diagnosis. Important features include cyanosis, heart failure and age. The most common cause of cyanotic heart disease in the neonate is transposition of the great vessels, whereas in older children it is tetralogy of Fallot.

Findings suggesting a significant shunt include cardiomegaly and altered pulmonary vascular markings (decreased or increased). Right-to-left shunts (which are suggested by cyanosis) lead to decreased pulmonary vascular markings, whereas left-to-right shunts are associated with increased pulmonary vascular markings. Shunts may be mixed with variable effects on pulmonary vascularity. Cardiomegaly is a consequence of pumping against resistance. For example, it will develop in cases of tricuspid atresia in combination with a tight atrial septal defect, but not if the defect is large.

Ensure that you have a brief list of differential possibilities for cyanotic and acyanotic heart disease, with and without pulmonary plethora.

Left atrial enlargement

Enlargement of the left atrium can manifest in a number of ways on plain film. Splaying of the carina is classical. The oesophagus is displaced posteriorly and to the right, seen here because of the nasogastric tube (this was historically evaluated with contrast swallow examinations). A 'double density' sign may be evident through the right upper heart border caused by the right side of the enlarged left atrium becoming visible. Both chronic mitral regurgitation and mitral stenosis can give an enlarged left atrium with wall calcification so look at the left ventricle. Regurgitation leads to left ventricular enlargement as a consequence of increased diastolic volume. In mitral stenosis, the left ventricle is not enlarged and the aorta is small.

Case 53

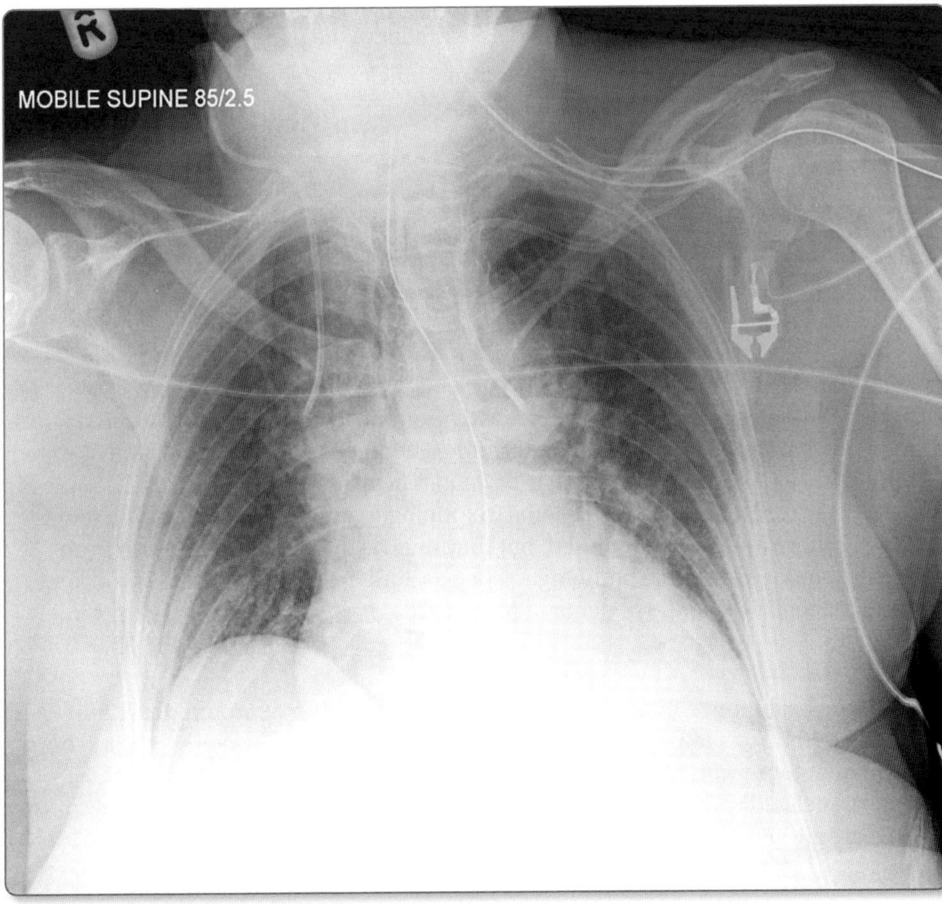

Suggested response

This is a mobile supine chest radiograph of a skeletally mature patient. There are features to suggest that this patient is unwell: vascular lines, cardiac monitoring leads, oxygen tubing and an enteric feeding tube are visible. A right internal jugular venous catheter is evident, the tip of which is projected in a satisfactory position in the region of the brachiocephalic venous confluence. A vascular line is also present on the left. Although the superior aspect of the line is projected in the region of the subclavian vein, it takes an unusual course inferiorly with the tip being projected over the aortic arch. While tip position in a vein is not excluded, for example if the tip is in a small vein or if there is aberrant venous anatomy, appearances should be considered suspicious for inadvertent arterial cannulation.

An enteric tube is also noted, I suspect it passes below the diaphragm given appearances in the left upper quadrant of the abdomen but I would routinely manipulate the image to better assess the tube. No pneumothorax is identified. The lungs appear clear, although patient rotation and limited inspiration in combination with the supine projection limit detailed assessment of the parenchyma.

I would discuss this case with the referring clinicians urgently, highlighting the potential arterial location of the left-sided vascular line. They may wish to confirm the line tip placement using blood gas analysis in the first instance.

Diagnosis

Incorrectly sited left subclavian venous catheter (inadvertent subclavian artery cannulation) in a post-laparotomy patient.

Tips: Chest radiographs in the ITU

ITU chest radiographs can be confusing, with multiple lines and tubes. Your first effort must be to identify each device and determine whether or not each is correctly located. The prevalence of line misplacement is far higher in vivas than it is in real life. Supine films may be hard to interpret. Pulmonary pathologies in intensive care unit patients are often diffuse and easily identified, but they may be difficult to distinguish from each other. Indeed, multiple pathologies such as adult respiratory distress syndrome, pneumonia and pulmonary oedema may co-exist.

Key points

An endotracheal tube (ETT) tip should lie in the mid-trachea at around the T2–T4 level. The finding of a low-lying ETT tip (at the carina or in the bronchus) should be immediately communicated to the clinician who is caring for the patient. High ETT tips are associated with an increased risk of aspiration pneumonia or laryngeal spasm (vocal cords lie at C5/C6 level).

Central venous catheters may have been inserted in the jugular, subclavian, femoral or peripheral veins. Determine whether or not the catheter follows its expected course and whether the tip is projected over a vein.

Enteral tubes include gastrostomy feeding tubes, nasogastric and nasojejunal tubes and Sengstaken–Blakemore tubes. Inadvertent bronchial placement of a nasogastric tube is common but potentially fatal. This finding should be immediately communicated to the clinician who is caring for the patient. Many departments have a way of checking tube position when the radiograph is acquired and you should be familiar with what happens in your institution.

The tip of an intercostal chest drain may be projected too medially with the heart and mediastinal structures at risk of injury. If the tip is too peripheral, the side holes – which should lie in the pleural cavity – may instead lie outside, in the chest wall. Kinking of the drain may preclude adequate function.

A range of monitoring devices may be observed including oesophageal Doppler probes for cardiac output monitoring (the tip should lie in the mid-oesophagus), temperature probes and ECG leads. Cardiac pacing leads may be in place for monitoring and rhythm stabilisation.

The principal complications of chest lines and tubes are pneumothorax, pneumomediastinum, pneumoperitoneum and pneumonia/lobar collapse.

Inadvertent subclavian artery cannulation

The subclavian vein is frequently used for venous catheter insertion, primarily due to its lower infection rate compared with the jugular vein approach. An uncommon but important complication is inadvertent subclavian artery cannulation. This is often recognised immediately, but the radiologist has an important role in identifying those cases which have gone undetected and interventional radiology input may be necessary when removing the line due to a high risk of haemorrhage at this non-compressible site. You may not always be correct in suspecting arterial placement of a central venous catheter (e.g. when the line tip lies in a left-sided superior vena cava (SVC) or in a collateral vessel, as in Case 38), but raising the possibility with clinicians (advising blood gas analysis to help determine whether the line is intra-arterial or intravenous, if needed) would be considered safe practice.

Case 54

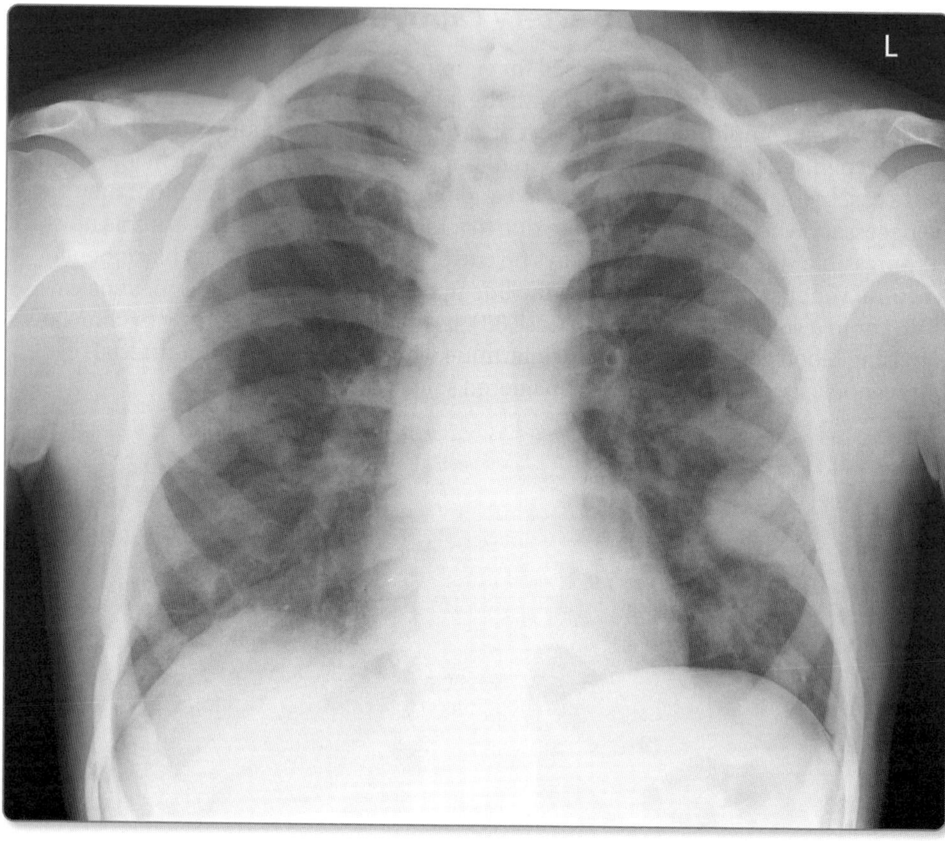

Suggested response

This is a frontal chest radiograph of a skeletally mature patient. There are two striking features on this film. The first is the presence of multiple rounded opacities of varying sizes projected in both lungs, in keeping with large pulmonary nodules. The second is the impression of widespread bony sclerosis. The visualised lungs in the mid zones both appear to be of normal density, hence this appearance is not likely to be due to an underpenetrated radiograph and is likely to reflect true bony sclerosis.

Although the combination of pulmonary nodules and bony sclerosis may be unrelated, unifying diagnoses such as metastatic malignancy should be considered. If this is a male patient, metastatic prostate cancer should be considered, although pulmonary metastases are uncommon in this condition. No breast shadows are evident. However, the film could represent a female patient who has undergone a bilateral mastectomy and has metastatic breast cancer. Haematological malignancies should also be considered. Review of any available relevant previous imaging and the patient's medical history would help to determine the diagnosis. If this is an initial presentation, then the range of possibilities should be discussed with the referring clinician with a view to establishing a diagnosis and undertaking staging of any malignancy.

Diagnosis

Metastatic prostate cancer with skeletal and pulmonary metastases.

Tips: Diffuse bony sclerosis

Consider the possibility that technical factors such as an underpenetrated chest radiograph may explain the appearance. If the lungs are of normal density then underpenetration is unlikely.

Differential diagnosis

Metabolic causes include renal osteodystrophy associated with secondary hyperparathyroidism. This tends to affect the axial skeleton and may be accompanied by other indicators of renal failure such as a haemodialysis line or a peritoneal dialysis catheter. Look for other features of hyperparathyroidism such as brown tumours, subperiosteal resorption and soft tissue calcification.

Neoplastic causes include sclerotic bony metastases which, when advanced, can be so diffuse that they might be mistaken for generalised sclerosis. There may be evidence of bone destruction which would support this diagnosis (scapular metastases may be very subtle) or there may be extraskeletal manifestations of malignancy such as focal pulmonary lesions or widening of the paratracheal stripe. The breast shadows and axillae may provide clues that indicate previous breast surgery.

Esoteric causes (including osteopetrosis, mastocytosis and diffuse Paget's disease) are not uncommon in viva-type teaching collections.

Metastatic prostate cancer

Pulmonary metastases are considerably less common than skeletal metastases in prostate cancer although they may coexist, as in this case. Bone scintigraphy is indicated in cases of prostate cancer in which there is a high Gleason score or elevated prostate-specific antigen level, or if the patient has symptoms suggestive of the presence of skeletal metastases. This may result in a 'superscan' appearance (as seen for this case in **Figure 1**), which is a nonspecific finding in which there is diffusely increased skeletal radionuclide uptake but reduced renal and soft tissue uptake.

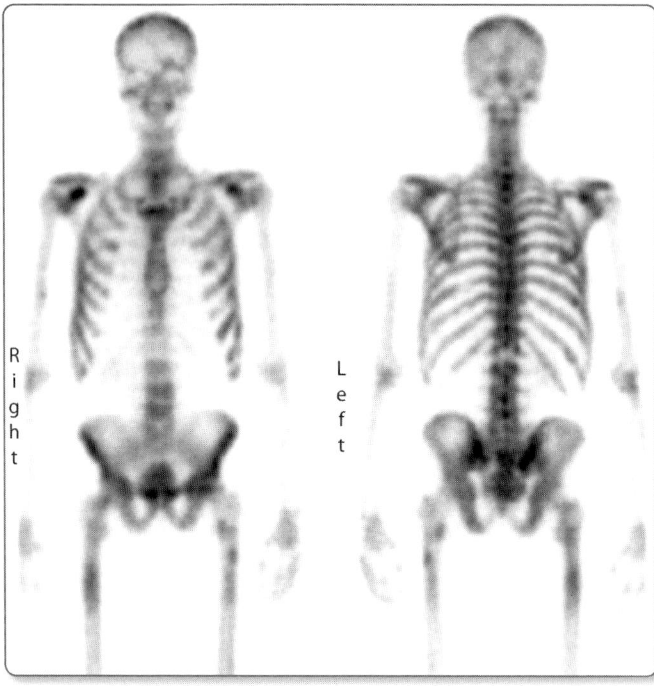

Figure 1 Bone scintigraphy for this case, showing a 'superscan' as a result of diffuse osteoblastic metastases.

Case 55

Perfusion

(K Counts)	Posterior Left	Right
	002K	034K
Total	002K	034K
(% Ratios)	Left	Right
	4.50	95.50
Total	4.50	95.50

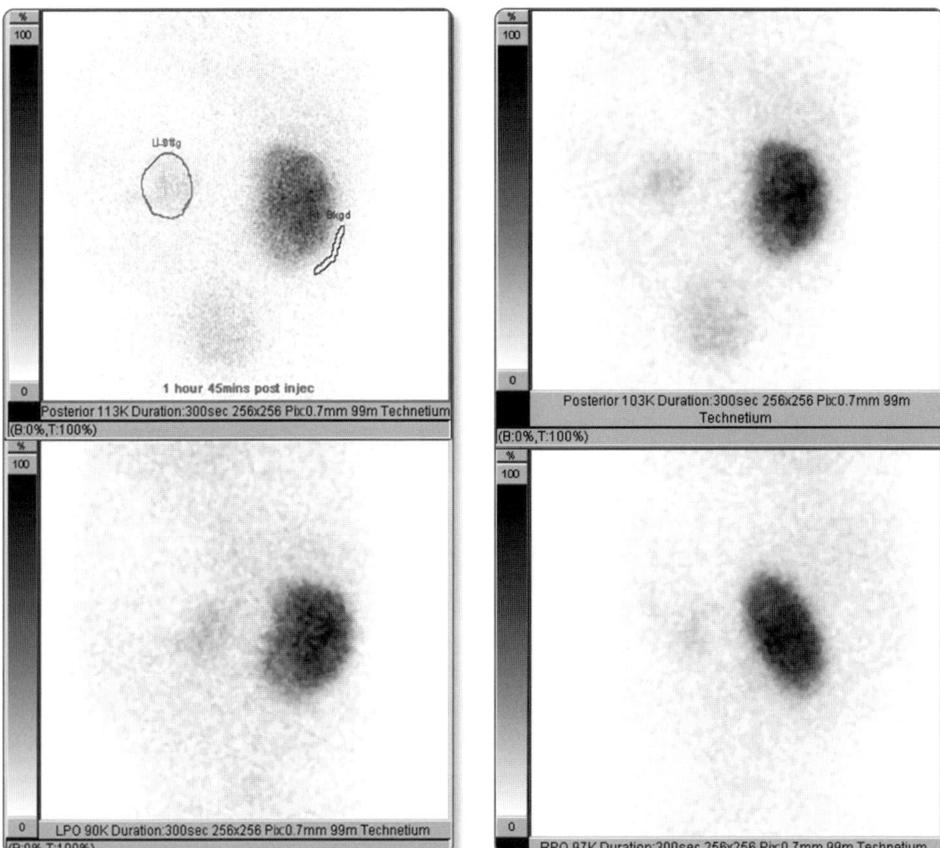

Suggested response

These are selected images from a renal dimercaptosuccinic acid (DMSA) scan. There is a marked discrepancy in tracer uptake between the two kidneys, with increased tracer uptake on the right side compared with the left. The differential renal function is 95.5% (right) and 4.5% (left) at 1 hour 45 minutes following injection. It is difficult to estimate the size of the left kidney given the global reduction in tracer uptake. Tracer uptake is fairly uniform in the right kidney. Differential diagnosis possibilities include obstruction, multicystic dysplastic kidney (particularly if a young patient) and renal artery stenosis (particularly if an adult patient). Renal ultrasound is likely to be an appropriate next investigation depending on these and other clinical factors.

Suggested response

These are selected renal ultrasound images. Appearances on the right suggest a normal kidney in a very young child, measuring 5 cm in length. As suggested on renal scintigraphy, the left kidney is grossly abnormal. It measures 6 cm in length and contains multiple large cysts, predominantly cortically based with minimal normal renal cortex. The appearances are most in keeping with a left-sided multicystic dysplastic kidney.

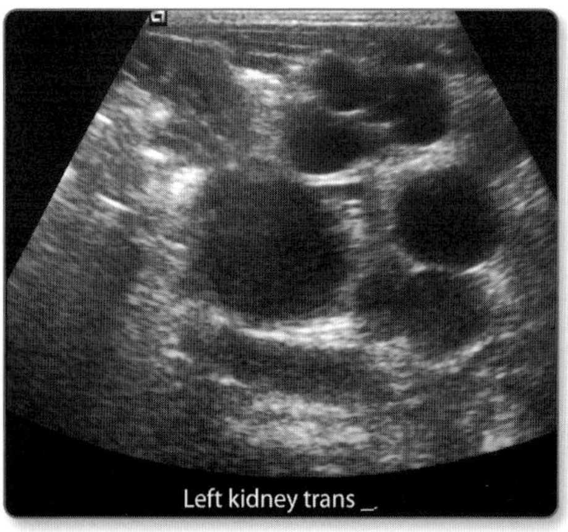

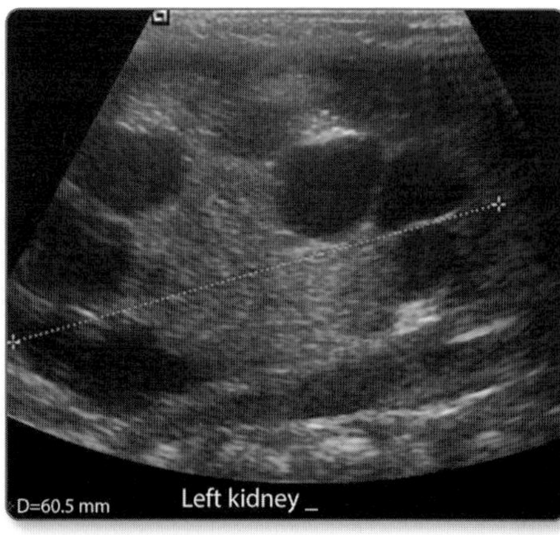

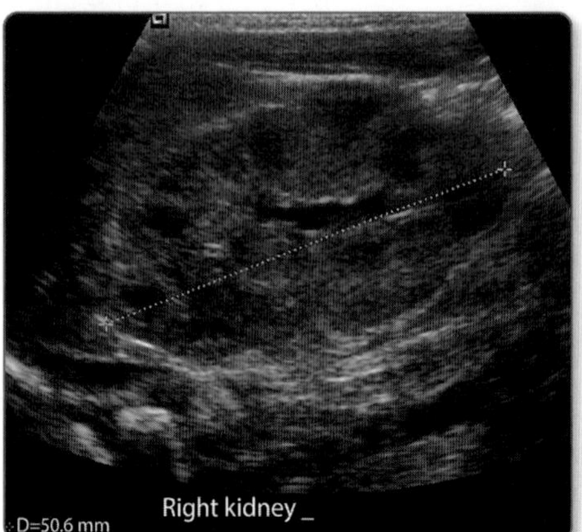

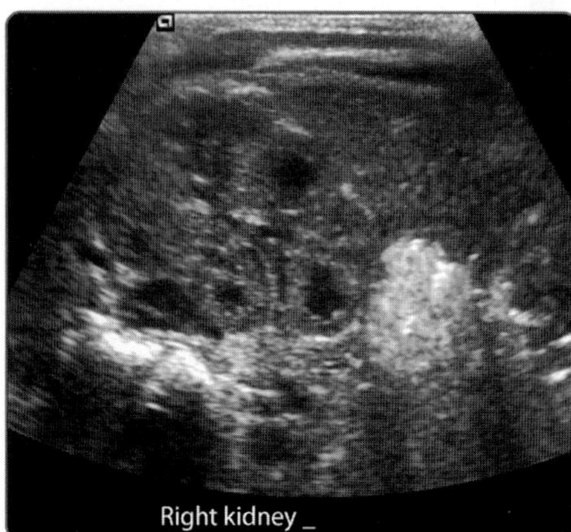

Diagnosis

Multicystic dysplastic kidney (MCDK) in a 14-day-old infant.

Tips: Congenital renal disorders

There is a wide range of congenital renal structural disorders. Some are discussed in other sections of this book.

Differential diagnosis

Apparent nonvisualisation of one kidney may be caused by unilateral renal agenesis, in which case the single kidney is usually large. This disorder is often associated with extrarenal (cardiac and gastrointestinal) anomalies. Alternatively, a kidney may lie in an ectopic location in the pelvis (or even the chest). In crossed-fused renal ectopia, both kidneys lie fused together on one side (usually the left) each with one ureter entering the bladder in the normal locations on each side. Supernumerary kidneys are usually seen on the left (i.e. two left and one right kidney).

Unusual renal contours include the wide midline location of renal fusion disorders such as horseshoe kidney and pancake kidney. Enlarged renal outlines are observed with crossed-fused renal ectopia, duplex kidney (which may be exacerbated by hydronephrosis) and MCDK, or may be a consequence of compensatory hypertrophy related to contralateral renal disease.

The cysts of MCDK are large and visible on ultrasound. Bilateral MCDK is incompatible with life due to associated pulmonary hypoplasia. Unilateral MCDK is commonly associated with contralateral urinary tract abnormalities such as vesicoureteric reflux and pelviureteric junction obstruction, but not with extrarenal abnormalities. The cysts of autosomal recessive (infantile) polycystic kidney disease (ARPCKD) are too small to visualise on ultrasound (1–2 mm). In this condition, both kidneys are enlarged and extrarenal manifestations are common, including hepatic and pancreatic fibrosis.

Multicystic dysplastic kidney

Multicystic dysplastic kidney is a congenital disorder that should be very familiar to aspiring radiologists, being the second most common cause of neonatal abdominal masses. It may be diagnosed on antenatal imaging. Various types have been described including a classic type (various sizes of noncommunicating cysts, randomly distributed, with no renal function) and a hydronephrotic type (dilated renal pelvis surrounded by cysts, possibly with some renal function). The latter can mimic pelviureteric junction obstruction and may need renal scintigraphy to help clarify. Affected kidneys are large in infancy but regress with age; small kidneys may be detected incidentally in adulthood.

Case 56

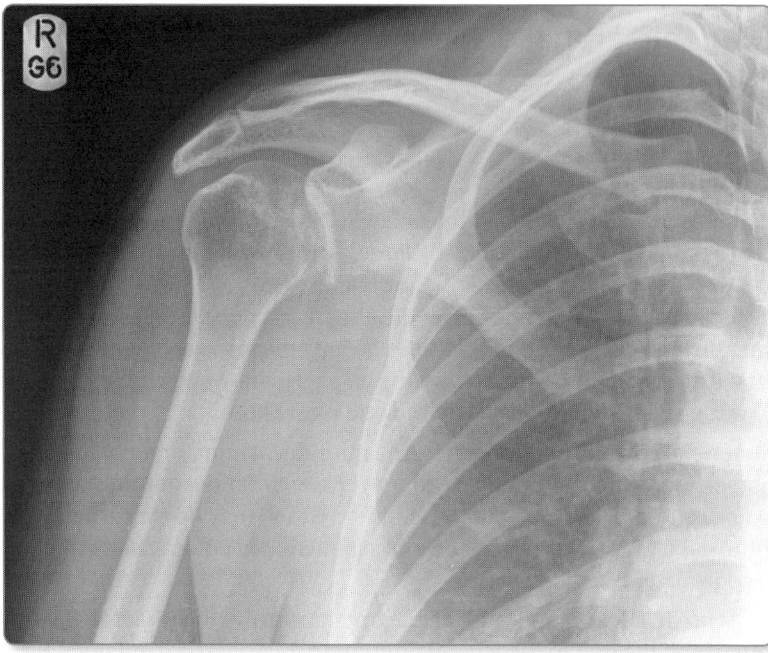

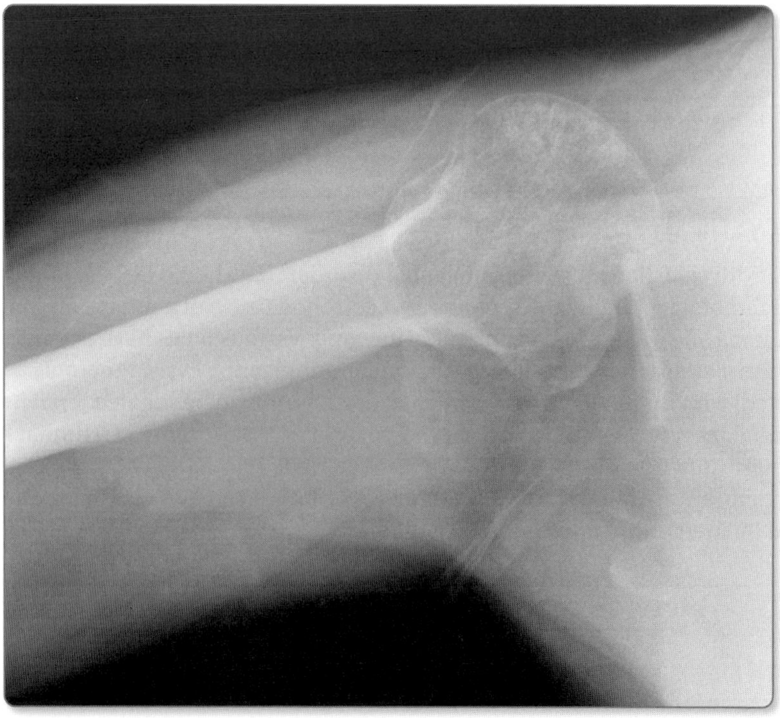

Suggested response

These are anteroposterior and axial views of the right shoulder of a skeletally mature patient.

The humeral head does not articulate normally with the glenoid but is displaced posteriorly and impacted on the posterior margin of the glenoid with a large reverse Hill–Sachs defect in the humerus. There is sclerosis around the margins of the defect suggesting that it is long-standing.

The acromioclavicular joint is normal, the visible lung is clear and there are no fractures elsewhere.

In conclusion, there is an impacted posterior dislocation of the humerus which appears to be long-standing. I would correlate the findings with the clinical history and contact the referring clinician as surgical reduction is likely to be required.

Diagnosis

Delayed (3 months) presentation of impacted posterior dislocation with very large reverse Hill–Sachs defect.

Tips: Shoulder trauma

Key points

The type of radiographic view is important. Dislocations may be hard to appreciate on an anteroposterior view alone. Remember that the curved articular surfaces of the glenoid fossa and the humeral head should be congruent. The apparent size of the humeral head should 'fit' in the glenoid fossa. If dislocated, it may appear magnified or minified relative to the glenoid fossa depending on the direction of the dislocation and of the X-ray beam. In general, it is wise to avoid commenting too much on joint alignment on a single view. It may be prudent to say 'Although the glenohumeral joint appears congruent on this anteroposterior view, it would be my usual practice to review this film in conjunction with a second view'.

There are many alternative views including the Y view, axial view, and the Garth (axial oblique) view. If possible, try to become familiar with the interpretation of different views. At the very least become comfortable identifying anterior and posterior orientations.

A checklist for shoulder radiographs might include consideration of dislocation (including the acromioclavicular joint), fracture (including Hill–Sachs, reverse Hill–Sachs and bony Bankart defects and pathological fractures), the subacromial space (normal >6 mm), rotator cuff calcification, erosive lesions (particularly at the ends of clavicles), the glenohumeral joint space, soft tissue abnormalities and lung findings including mass, pneumothorax or the sequelae of trauma.

Shoulder dislocation

The glenohumeral joint is the most commonly dislocated joint in the body and you should be well versed in the features of each direction of dislocation. Anterior dislocation occurs by far the most often. Although less common in real life, posterior dislocation is disproportionately more likely to appear in a viva. In everyday practice, it is frequently missed on initial imaging (look for the 'rim sign', in which the distance between the humeral head and anterior glenoid rim increases to >6 mm, and reverse Hill–Sachs defects). Bear in mind that the shoulder can also dislocate inferiorly or superiorly.

Case 57

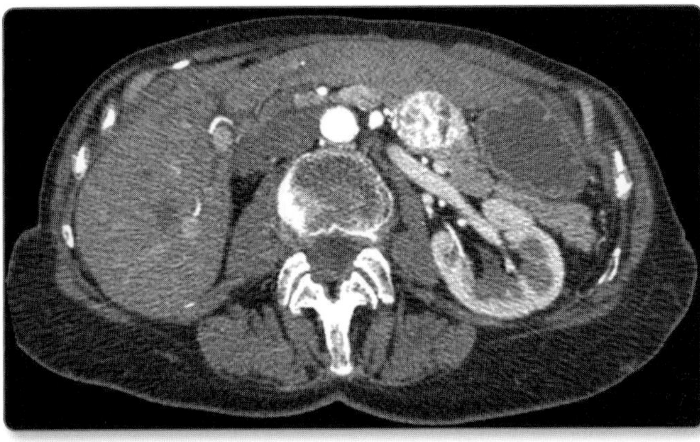

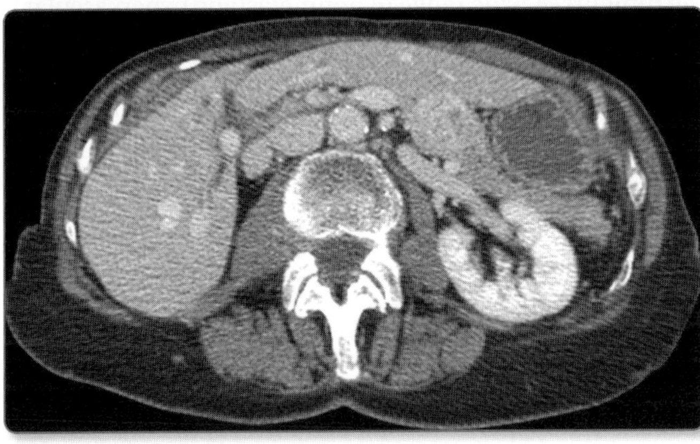

Suggested response

These are selected images from an abdominal CT scan, with one image in the arterial phase and another in the nephrographic or perhaps portal venous phase.

There is a mass in the body of the pancreas which enhances avidly on the arterial phase image and appears more vascular than the adjacent pancreatic tissue. The lesion remains hyperenhanced on the later image but the contrast is less pronounced.

These images are through the mid-pole of the left kidney and I note that the right kidney is not visible. It could be present lower in the abdomen and I would routinely review the entire study to look for it. However, I suspect that there has been a previous nephrectomy and I would correlate this with any available clinical history. If previous nephrectomy is confirmed, then the findings are most in keeping with a hypervascular metastasis to the pancreas from a renal cell carcinoma (RCC). Other causes of hypervascular metastases include thyroid carcinoma and melanoma. Another possibility is a primary islet cell tumour.

Diagnosis

Renal cell carcinoma metastasis to the pancreas. Previous right nephrectomy.

Tips: Metastatic renal cell carcinoma

Key points

Renal cell carcinoma metastases to bone may be aggressive and rapidly progressive. They are most commonly seen in vertebrae, ribs, pelvis and the proximal long bones. They are often solitary and characteristically exhibit a bubbly/expansile appearance. A surrounding soft tissue mass is common. The principal differential for this appearance at multiple sites is metastatic thyroid carcinoma.

Differential diagnosis

Renal cell carcinoma metastases are typically hypervascular. Other hypervascular metastases include thyroid carcinoma, melanoma, choriocarcinoma and neuroendocrine tumours. A wide range of nonmetastatic hypervascular lesions may be encountered in different organs. In the liver, benign hypervascular lesions include haemangiomas and hepatoid neoplasms (focal nodular hyperplasia, adenoma and hepatocellular carcinoma). In the pancreas, islet cell tumours and microcystic adenomas may be hypervascular. Renal oncocytomas and angiomyolipomas are typically hypervascular, as are adrenal phaeochromocytomas and neuroblastomas. Hypervascular arteriovenous malformations and paragangliomas may be encountered in almost any location.

Metastatic renal cell carcinoma

Metastases are frequently seen at the initial presentation of RCC, most commonly in the lungs and bones. In later stages of disease, it metastasises to lymph nodes and the liver. RCC metastases should feature prominently in differential diagnosis lists when certain features are present, i.e. characteristically hypervascular masses and expansile/bubbly bony lesions that present many years after treatment of the primary lesion.

Case 58

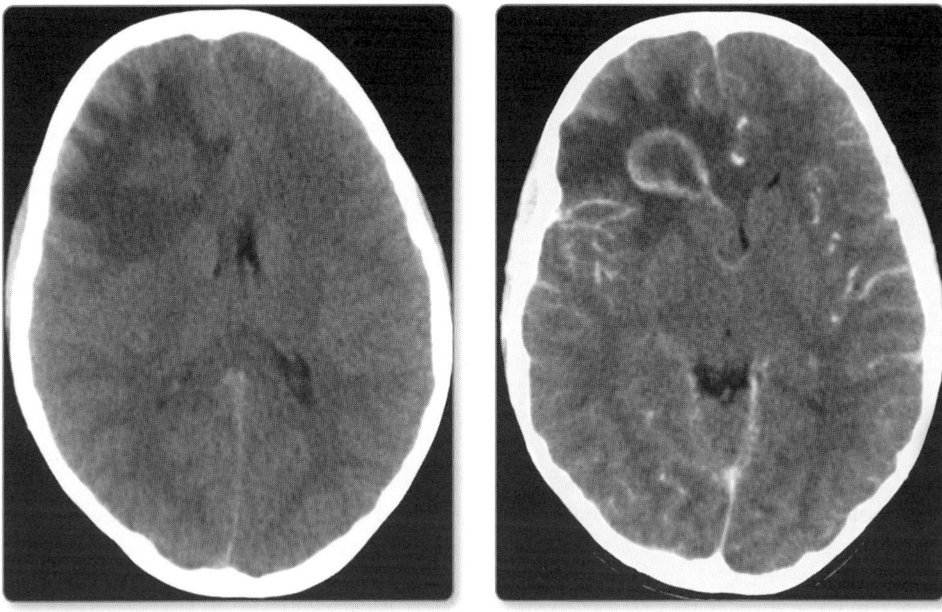

Suggested response

These are selected axial views from a CT scan of the brain performed pre- and post-contrast. There is extensive low attenuation within the white matter of the right frontal lobe, with an ovoid area internally which has the same attenuation as grey matter and measures several centimetres in diameter. This exhibits peripheral enhancement following contrast administration. There is mass effect, with effacement of the frontal horn of the right lateral ventricle and midline shift to the left of approximately 1cm. I would routinely review the remainder of the study, in particular to assess the cerebrospinal fluid spaces and paranasal sinuses and to look for further lesions. The preservation of cerebral parenchymal volume suggests that this is a younger patient.

In summary, there is an apparently solitary lesion in the right frontal lobe with surrounding hypoattenuation, consistent with vasogenic oedema, and mass effect. The differential diagnosis is contingent on the clinical presentation. If the patient is relatively young, pyrexial or has sinusitis, then I would favour a diagnosis of cerebral abscess. If the patient is otherwise well, then a primary brain tumour could also have this appearance. If the patient is known to have a primary malignancy elsewhere, then this would increase suspicions for a metastatic deposit.

The wall appears generally thin and the lesion 'points' towards the ventricular system, so on the basis of the imaging alone I would favour the diagnosis of a cerebral abscess.

Regardless of the diagnosis, I would discuss this case with the neurosurgical team urgently. If diagnostic doubt persists, then MRI with diffusion-weighted imaging may help to narrow the differential diagnosis.

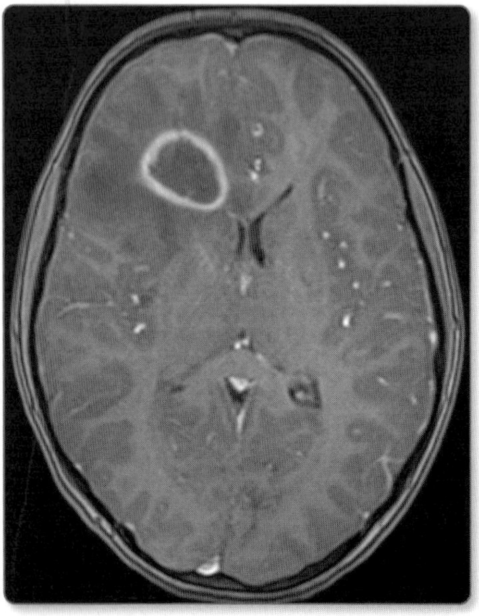

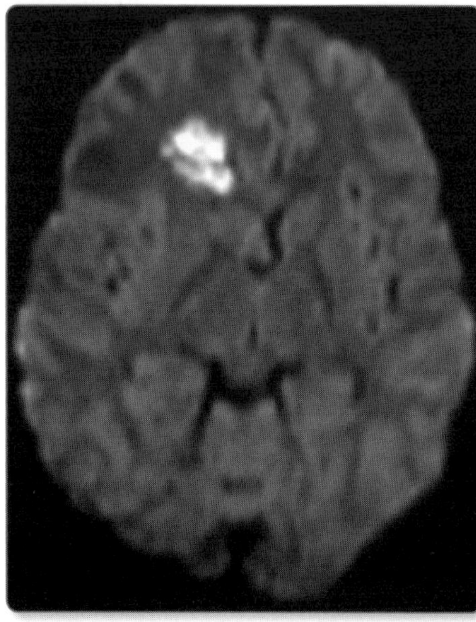

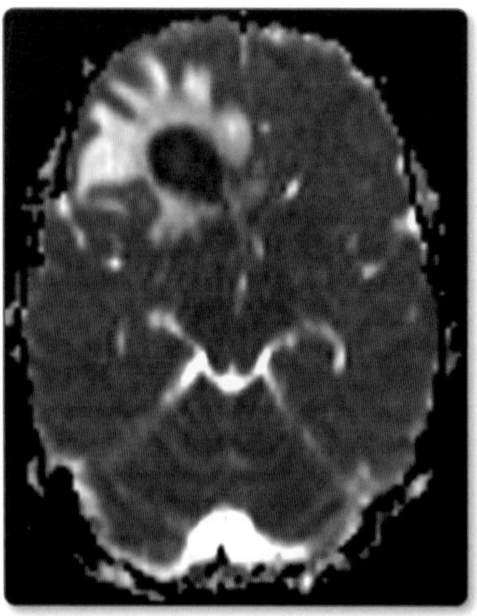

Suggested response

These are selected MRI images with axial T1 post-contrast and diffusion-weighted imaging (DWI) with corresponding apparent diffusion coefficient (ADC) map. This confirms the right frontal lobe lesion, with low signal on T1 both internally and surrounding the lesion, again consistent with vasogenic oedema. The wall is of increased signal on the post-gadolinium images and if this was not present on the pre-contrast images, it must represent enhancement.

The frontal horn of the right lateral ventricle is again shown to be effaced. DWI and ADC show the lesion to exhibit restricted diffusion. This is more in keeping with an abscess than a tumour, although occasionally a tumour may have this appearance. I would again discuss this with the neurosurgical team to further guide management.

Diagnosis

Cerebral abscess in an 11-year-old child.

Tips: An intracranial ring-enhancing lesion

Key points

A range of different pathologies including abscesses, primary or secondary tumours, demyelination, infarcts and haematoma (with peripheral enhancement when the blood–brain barrier breaks down) can cause solitary or multiple ring-enhancing cerebral lesions. The clinical presentation is key to diagnosis. Therefore, use conditional differential diagnoses in a viva such as: 'If the patient is pyrexial/has sinusitis....' (abscess), 'If there is a known primary malignancy...' (metastasis) or 'If there was a history of trauma...' (haematoma).

Ninety percent of solitary intracranial masses in patients with a known primary malignancy turn out to be cerebral metastases.

Differential diagnosis

Metastases and abscesses are both usually found at the corticomedullary junctions. Although metastases typically have thicker walls than abscesses, distinguishing tumour from abscess is a common problem in both daily clinical practice and examinations.

Untreated lymphoma and low-grade glioma (WHO Grade 1) are typically solid and do not usually exhibit ring enhancement. Cystic or necrotic tumours and abscesses may appear identical on conventional imaging, with ring enhancement around a low-density centre and with surrounding vasogenic oedema. Diffusion-weighted MRI may help to clarify the nature of a lesion. An abscess typically shows restricted diffusion centrally (high DWI signal and low ADC signal) whereas a necrotic tumour more usually shows facilitated diffusion centrally (low DWI signal and high ADC signal). Haemorrhage into a cystic tumour can give a confusing appearance. In the event of uncertainty, tumours are more likely to mimic abscesses (i.e. have restricted diffusion) than abscesses are to be mistaken for tumours.

Cerebral abscess

Infection can spread to the central nervous system locally (e.g. by direct spread or venous reflux), so ensure that you scrutinise the paranasal sinuses (see also Case 35), mastoid air cells and orbits if faced with cerebral lesions. Haematogenous spread from elsewhere (e.g. lungs or heart) may also be causative, so a review of available chest imaging may be helpful if an underlying cause is not apparent on imaging of the brain. As seen in this case, abscesses give characteristic DWI findings, although spectroscopy could also be employed to clarify the diagnosis.

Case 59

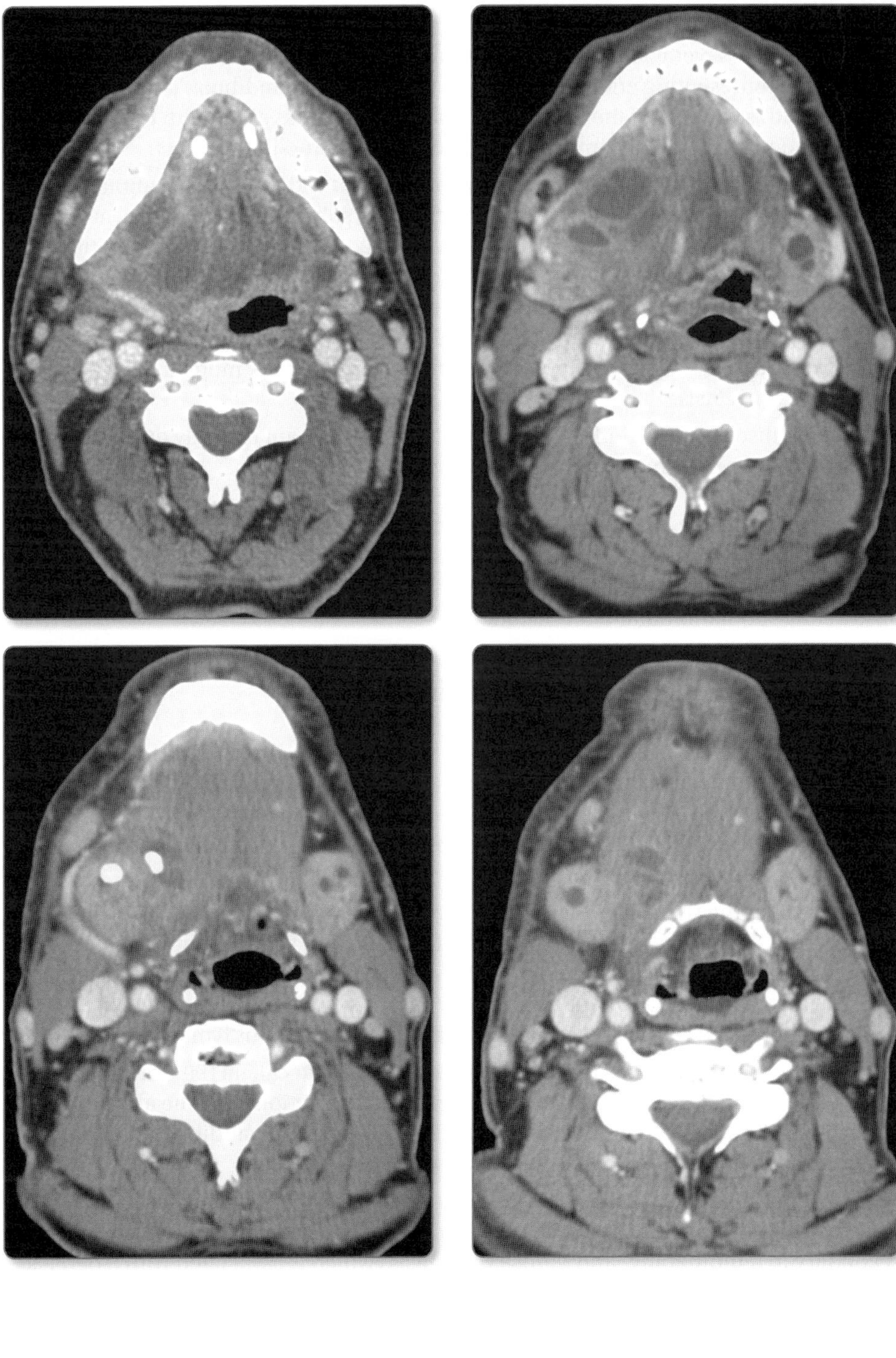

Suggested response

These are selected images from a post-contrast axial CT scan of the neck. Several abnormalities are present. In the submental region, a well-defined ovoid subcentimetre calcific lesion is evident on either side of the midline. In the right submandibular region, there are several low-attenuation areas with peripheral high attenuation, presumably representing enhancement, and the right submandibular gland itself is enlarged with stranding of the surrounding fat. There is mass effect with deviation to the left, and possibly slight compression, of the upper aerodigestive tract.

At least one rounded low-attenuation area is present within the right submandibular gland itself, with two ovoid calcific lesions in the right submandibular region, at least one of which is in the gland. Several small low-attenuation areas are evident in the left submandibular gland, although there is no significant fat stranding. Findings are most in keeping with obstructing calculi in the distal submandibular ducts bilaterally, with further right submandibular gland calculi, abscess formation and probable co-existing obstructive sialectasis. Appearances in the left gland are more in keeping with obstructive sialectasis.

I would discuss these findings with the ENT surgical team urgently due to the risk of mortality from a submandibular space abscess.

Diagnosis

Adult male patient with right submandibular space abscess formation and bilateral obstructing submandibular duct calculi.

Tips: Salivary gland abnormalities

Key points

Tumours are more common in the parotid gland than the submandibular gland. In adults, the larger the salivary gland, the greater the chance that a mass within it will be benign. In children, the larger the salivary gland, the greater the chance that a mass within it will be malignant.

Remember the rule of 80s for parotid gland masses: 80% are benign, 80% are pleomorphic adenomas (there is a potential for malignant transformation but 80% of these remain benign if untreated) and 80% are found in the (larger) superficial lobe. Primary lymphoma can manifest in the parotids but is almost never seen in the submandibular and sublingual glands (only the parotid contains lymphoid tissue).

The submandibular gland/duct is more predisposed to calculi (90% of which are radio-opaque) than the parotids due to more viscous secretions and the angulation of the duct. The submandibular gland and duct are in the submandibular space – an important conduit for spread of infection and other diseases.

If faced with a sialogram in an examination, then look for filling defects (representing air bubbles or calculi), strictures (which may be postinflammatory or secondary to radiotherapy) and diffuse sialectasis (which is associated with Sjögren's syndrome). While MR is now used routinely, conventional sialography may include control and postsialagogue (to stimulate saliva production) images as well as those with contrast within the ducts.

Submandibular abscess

Abscess formation can occur in the submandibular gland itself (e.g. in severe infective sialadenitis) but often occurs in the submandibular space secondary to spread from elsewhere in the head and neck (commonly from dental infections). Ludwig's angina is a potentially fatal type of severe cellulitis that typically occurs a few days after mandibular dental extraction. It manifests as swelling in the submandibular and sublingual regions that can spread to other neck spaces and cause compromise of the airways. Accordingly, imaging for suspected submandibular space abscess formation should be performed urgently (contrast-enhanced CT being the examination of choice, as in this case).

Case 60

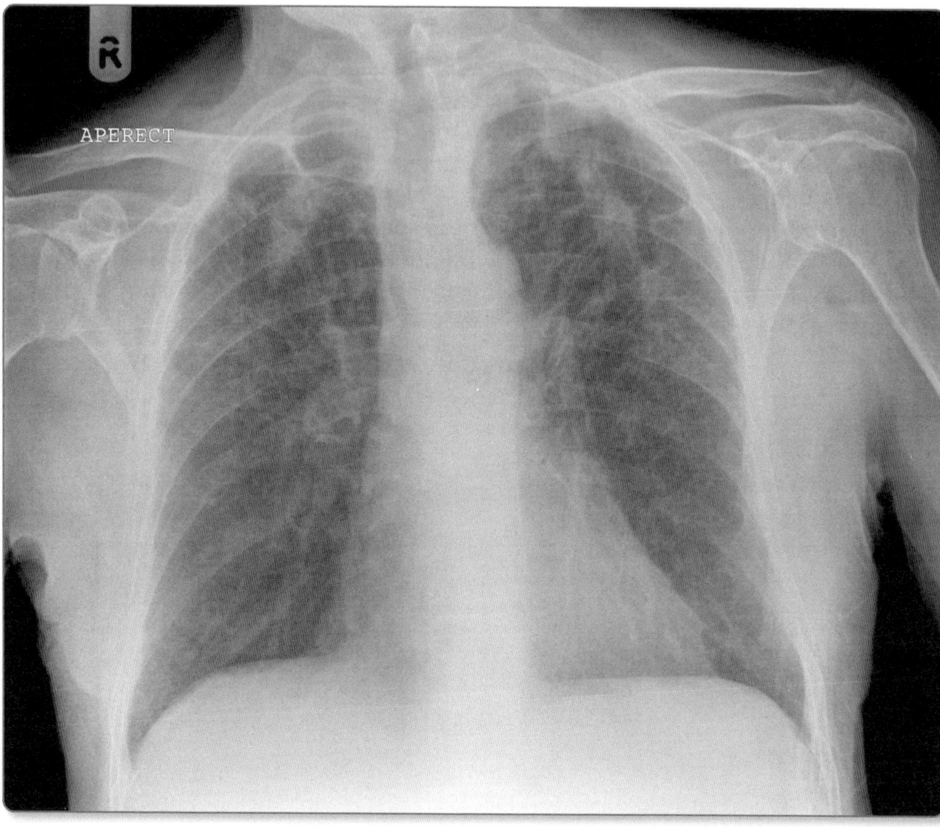

Suggested response

This is an anteroposterior erect chest radiograph of a skeletally mature patient. The first thing to note is that there is bilateral, relatively symmetrical interstitial shadowing, predominantly in the upper and mid zones. There are elongated opacities, each of which measures several centimetres in length, centred in the upper zones bilaterally. These show no evidence of cavitation and are not typical for pulmonary scarring. While the right hilum appears bulky on this film, it should be noted that the patient is rotated to the right side, hence this may be due to rotation. No convincing hilar calcification is identified.

If there is a history of occupational dust exposure, the findings could represent silicosis or coal worker's pneumoconiosis and the mass-like lesions could represent progressive massive fibrosis (PMF) or – less likely, given their symmetry and overall appearance – bilateral tumours. If there is no history of occupational dust exposure then alternative causes of upper zone pulmonary fibrosis should be considered, including tuberculosis and sarcoidosis. In either case, it would be useful to review any available previous imaging to assess for change. Overall, the findings are most in keeping with silicosis with progressive massive fibrosis and a respiratory referral is advised if this has not already occurred.

Diagnosis

An 80-year-old man with silicosis and PMF. Findings stable since a previous radiograph from 6 years earlier.

Tips: Upper zone interstitial lung disease

Key points

Symmetrical upper zone fibrosis suggests a dust-related aetiology (ankylosing spondylitis being a notable exception) due to the proportionally greater ventilation in the upper zones.

If the findings are asymmetrical, then look for well-defined edges to the lung changes with co-existent bony changes. These features would suggest previous radiotherapy.

Hilar nodes with 'eggshell' calcification and upper zone fibrosis are most suggestive of silicosis, although this pattern may also be seen in other conditions such as sarcoidosis. Inactive tuberculosis is not typically associated with hilar lymphadenopathy.

Progressive massive fibrosis is often bilateral and symmetrical with 'sausage-shaped' masses that exhibit slow change. Silicosis is a predisposing factor for tuberculosis, so pulmonary masses may be infective. Remember also that tumours can co-exist and that this risk is increased in silicosis. Always review previous imaging where available to assess for change and have a low threshold for suggesting a CT scan if there are suspicious features or unilateral abnormalities, or if there is no previous imaging.

Silicosis

Occupational exposure to silica, as experienced by miners and ceramic workers, can give rise to silicosis. Simple silicosis is predominantly seen in the upper and posterior lungs with multiple small centrilobular nodules (typically 2–5 mm), a pattern which is indistinguishable from coal worker's pneumoconiosis. Pseudoplaques may be seen if subpleural nodules aggregate. Hilar and mediastinal lymphadenopathy is a common associated feature. Complicated silicosis (or PMF, as in this case) is seen when nodules expand and coalesce into larger irregular opacities, which are usually >1 cm in diameter and located in the posterior and apical segments of the upper lobes. These masses have the potential to cavitate or calcify. Acute silicosis is most commonly seen in sandblasters, who present within 3 years after exposure. Imaging appearances are variable but include ill-defined centrilobular nodules, consolidation and ground glass opacification with septal thickening (i.e. 'crazy paving' on CT).

Case 61

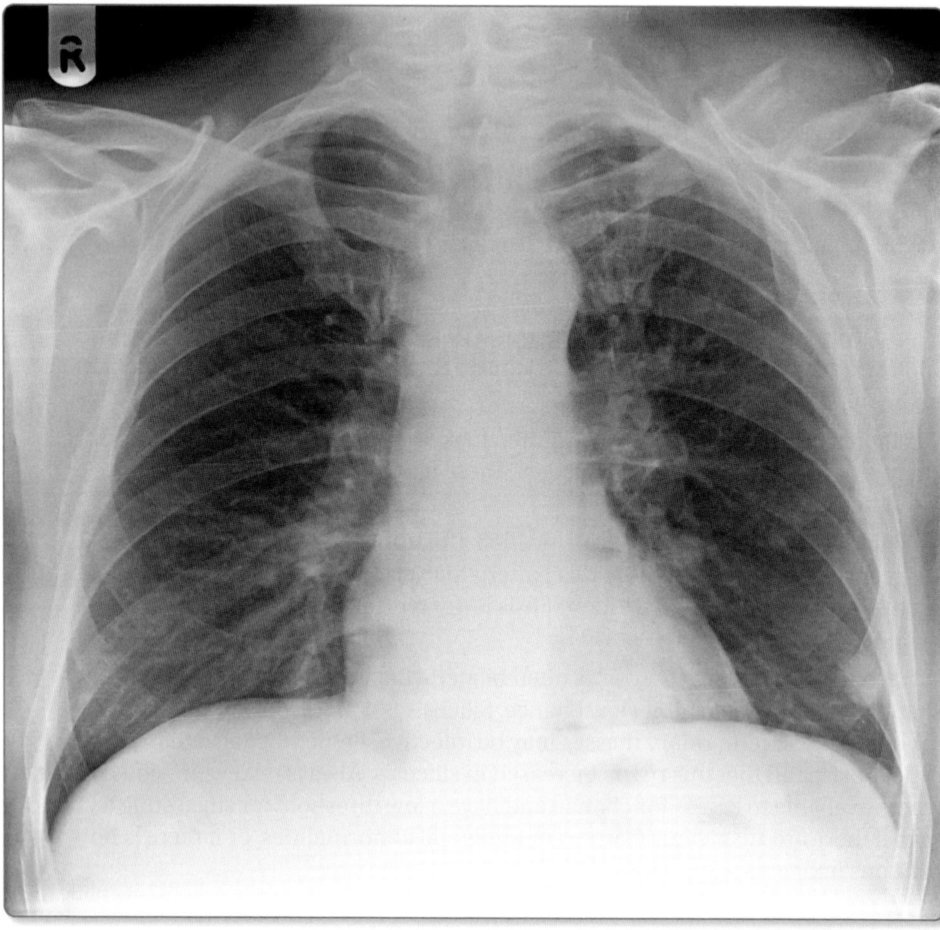

Suggested response

This is a frontal chest radiograph of a skeletally mature patient. Several abnormalities are evident on this radiograph. Firstly, there are multiple nodules projected in the left lung, the largest of which is projected in a retrocardiac location and measures several centimetres in diameter. Some of these nodules appear to exhibit cavitation. The left hilum in particular is rather bulky, with an irregular outline and loss of the normal hilar point. There is also bony destruction of the lateral aspect of the left clavicle, with disruption of the normal fat planes in the left side of the neck and supraclavicular fossa, consistent with there being a soft tissue component to this lesion. No further destructive bony lesions are evident, although there are old right-sided rib fractures. The most likely explanation for this collection of findings is metastatic disease, with pulmonary, left hilar nodal and osteolytic skeletal metastases. The site of the primary lesion is uncertain. Knowledge of the clinical presentation and a review of previous imaging would be helpful, although if this is the initial presentation, a staging of CT scan may be appropriate.

Diagnosis

Metastatic bladder cancer with pulmonary, left hilar nodal and skeletal metastases in an adult male.

Tips: Absence of the distal clavicle

Key points and differential diagnosis

Look for ancillary findings that help to narrow the differential diagnosis. If there are masses elsewhere or further osteolytic lesions, the diagnosis is metastases until proven otherwise. If there are multiple fractures elsewhere, consider previous trauma, pyknodysostosis and hyperparathyroidism. Shoulder abnormalities/prostheses suggest rheumatoid arthritis. Osteosclerosis is seen with metastases, pyknodysostosis and hyperparathyroidism. Soft tissue calcification and surgical clips in the neck (parathyroidectomy) are both seen in hyperparathyroidism.

Lateralisation of the abnormality is important. If bilateral, consider inflammatory conditions (rheumatoid arthritis and other arthritides), hyperparathyroidism, cleidocranial dysostosis and pyknodysostosis. Conditions that are more commonly unilateral include infection, metastatic disease, post-traumatic osteolysis and surgery (usually sharply demarcated).

Osteolytic metastases

Lytic bone metastases are only usually evident radiographically if they measure >1 cm in diameter and have destroyed at least one-third of the bone density. Have a (brief) list of differential diagnoses ready for different patient groups. Breast cancer is the most common cause of osteolytic metastases in women but can also cause sclerotic or mixed metastases (skeletal metastases in bladder cancer have a similarly variable appearance). Bronchogenic carcinoma is the most common cause in men. Other frequent primary sources include colorectal, renal and thyroid cancers (with the latter two being the main differentials for expansile or bubbly bony metastases, often with an osteolytic soft tissue mass). Neuroblastoma is the most frequent cause of osteolytic metastases in children.

Case 62

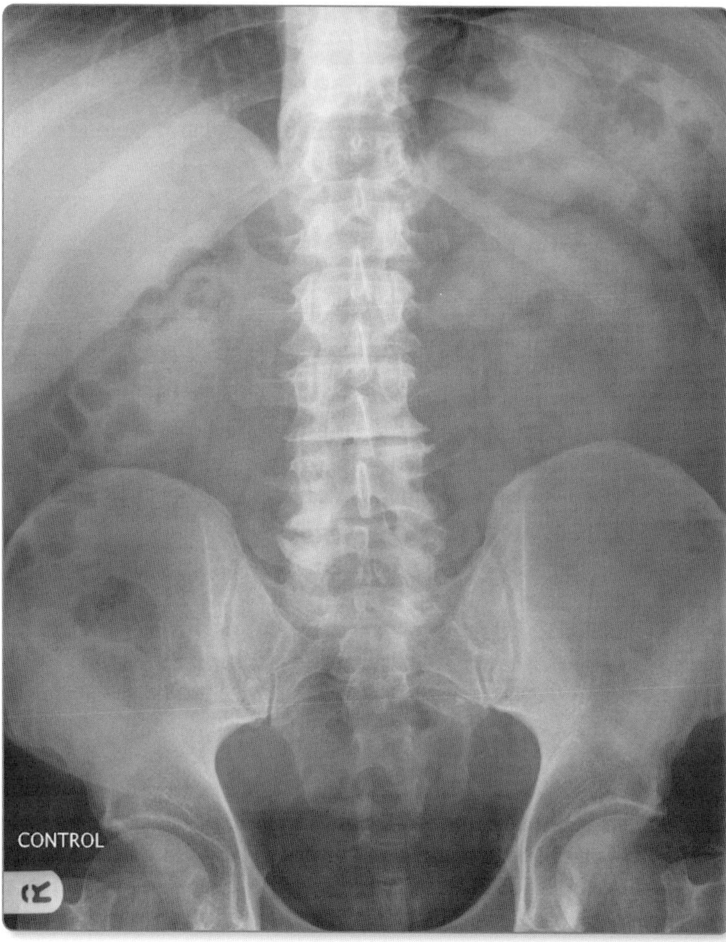

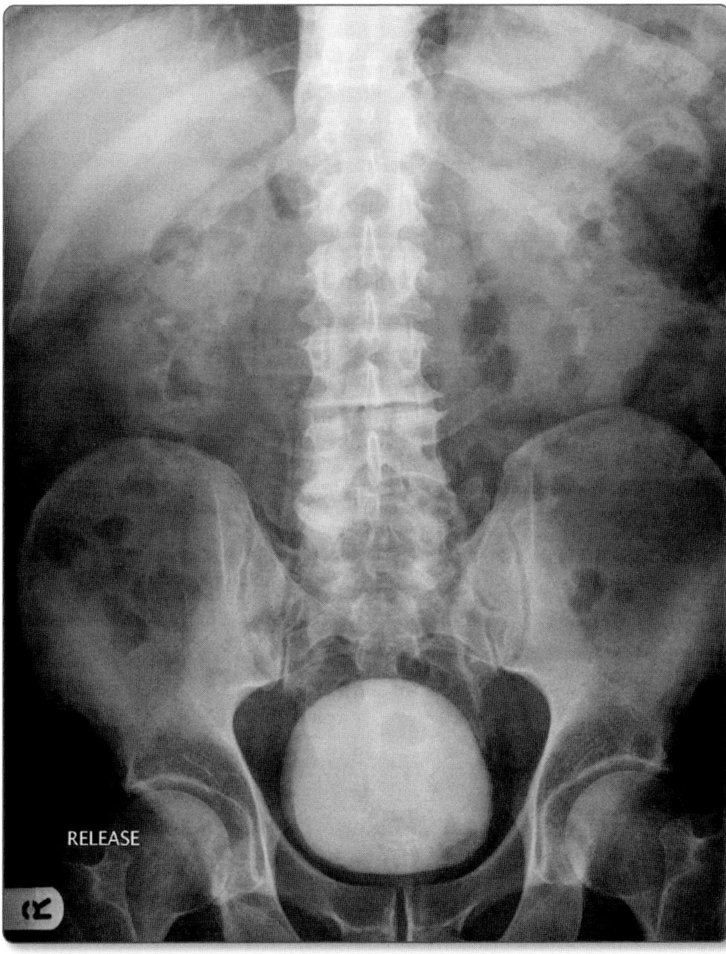

Suggested response

These are films from an intravenous urogram (IVU) series. The postcontrast film is labelled ‘release’, suggesting that the examination has been performed with compression to demonstrate the renal collecting systems and ureters.

I cannot identify any renal tract calcification on the control film. Following contrast administration, the nephrograms are not particularly well seen due to overlying bowel gas. There is a filling defect in the left inferior side of the bladder. Although no definite abnormality is identified in relation to the pelvicalyceal systems or ureters in these images, I would review any other available films in the series in case there is better visualisation of these segments on other films.

Correlation with the clinical history would be helpful but the features on these images are suggestive of a bladder tumour. In my report of the study, I would suggest discussion with the urology multidisciplinary team. The team may proceed to examine the lesion by direct visualisation and biopsy. If bladder tumour is confirmed, then a staging CT scan may be appropriate.

Diagnosis

Transitional cell carcinoma (TCC) causing a filling defect on IVU (see **Figure 1**).

Tips: A finding of a filling defect on IVU

Key points and differential diagnosis

While CT urography has largely supplanted IVU studies they may still feature in examinations. Always keep filling defects in mind whenever you look at a film with contrast in a vessel or viscus, particularly an IVU. Filling defects may be seen due to technical problems (e.g. overlying gas and lack of excretion into that segment), extrinsic compression (e.g. cyst, vessel, extrinsic tumour and fibrosis), intramural causes (e.g. TCC or other tumour and infection) or intraluminal causes (e.g. calculus, clot, sloughed papilla, polyp, debris and air bubble). Most causes of filling defects can be either solitary or multiple (e.g. TCC, polyps and papillae). Bear in mind pyeloureteritis cystica (a rare but classic examination case) as a cause of multiple filling defects (smooth, <3 mm).

Bladder transitional cell carcinoma

More commonly diagnosed by cystoscopy, TCC of the bladder is the most common genitourinary malignancy and is seen far more frequently than upper tract TCC (although the two often co-exist). Occupational history is relevant because exposure to chemicals in a range of industries (typically in dye manufacturing) is a risk factor. Bladder irritation and urinary stasis predispose to TCC, so look for bladder calculi and pay particular attention to bladder diverticula. Chronic bladder wall inflammation due to schistosomiasis may be a particular risk factor in some populations.

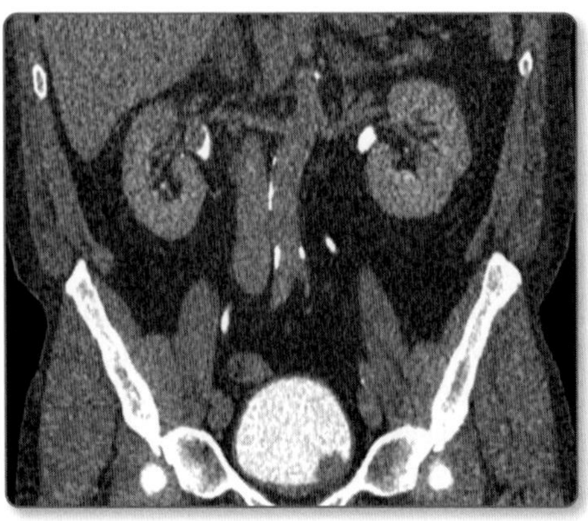

Figure 1 Transitional cell carcinoma causing a filling defect in the bladder on CT urogram. A further apparent defect in the right collecting system was demonstrated to be artefactual on review of the whole study.

Case 63

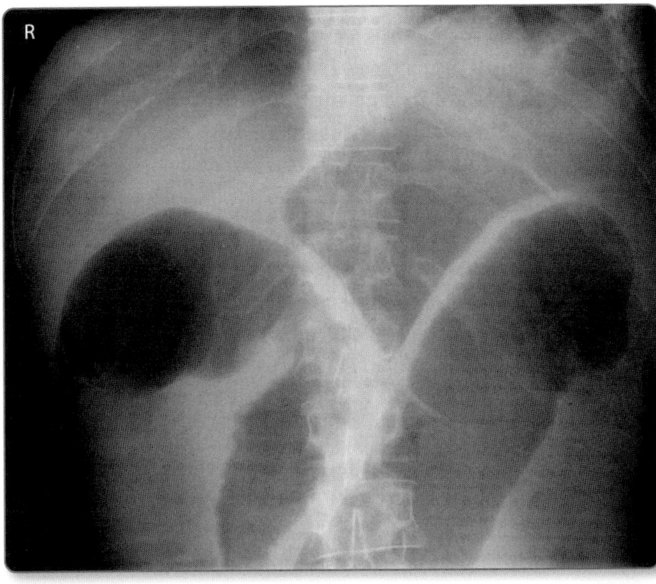

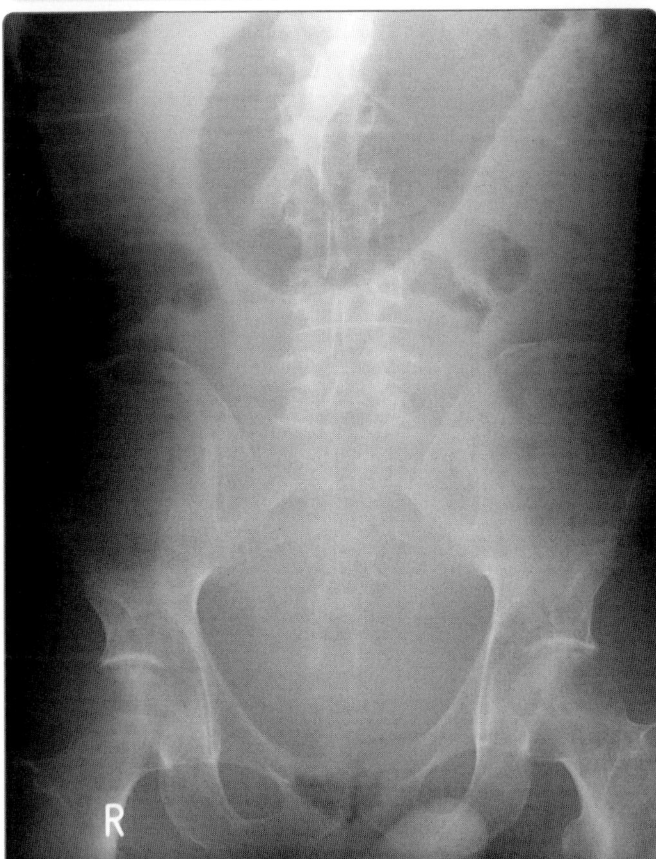

Suggested response

These are two frontal radiographs which together demonstrate the whole abdomen and pelvis of this adult male patient.

The most striking finding is gross distension of the transverse colon with a more normal appearance of the proximal colon. Distally, there is some stool in a normal calibre segment of descending colon. I cannot see the sigmoid colon or rectum and cannot identify any gas in the small bowel. The wall of the transverse colon is thickened suggesting that it is very oedematous.

The left 12th rib is abnormal with an expansile lucent lesion in the mid-portion of the bone. I cannot see a periosteal reaction or any other aggressive feature. There is no clearly defined pattern of matrix within the lesion and overlying bowel makes assessing for 'ground glass' more difficult. I would like to magnify this section of the image to confirm that there are no aggressive features and compare the appearance with any available previous imaging. If the rib lesion is stable and there are no aggressive features, then it is likely to represent an indolent lesion, possibly an enchondroma or fibrous dysplasia.

I am not sure if there is a unifying underlying diagnosis to link the bowel and bony findings, but the large bowel obstruction with mural thickening represents toxic megacolon which is a surgical emergency. The aetiology is likely to be inflammatory, ischaemic or infective and I would discuss the patient with the on-call surgical team as a matter of urgency.

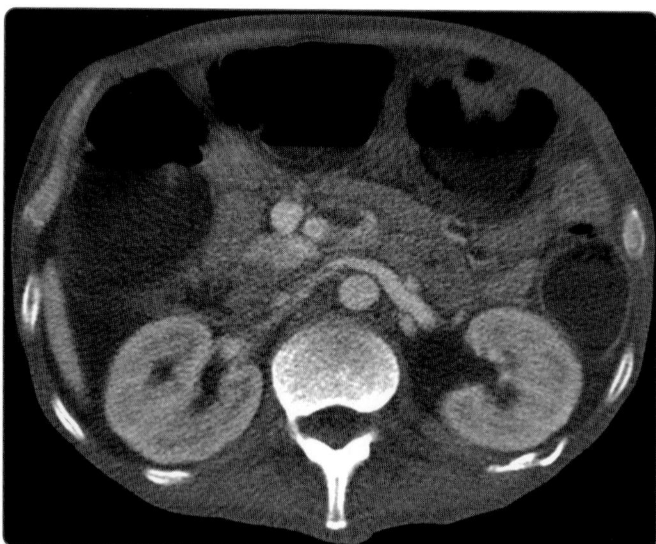

Suggested response

This is an axial image from a contrast-enhanced CT scan of this patient showing multiple small locules of gas in the dependent portion of the colonic wall within what I take to be the distended transverse colon.

If the patient is unwell, perhaps peritonitic, and/or there are inflammatory changes in the peri-enteric/colic fat then this may represent ischaemia. I would search for stenosis/thrombosis in the mesenteric arteries and veins.

If the patient is clinically well then mural or even portal venous gas may be dismissed as an indicator of bowel ischaemia as some patients have stable mural gas for years, although ongoing clinical vigilance is important.

In the acute setting and even if there is no portal venous gas or other affected segments of bowel, I would still be concerned this might represent a surgical emergency and I would immediately contact the senior surgeon responsible for this patient to inform them of my findings and discuss them in the light of the patient's clinical condition.

Diagnosis

Toxic megacolon with intramural gas in an adult male with *Clostridium difficile* colitis. Incidental fibrous dysplasia in left-sided rib.

Tips: Surgical emergencies

Key points

Dilated large bowel has been considered elsewhere in this book (see Case 7), but this case is a good example of a 'surgical emergency'.

It is not necessarily the case that the referring clinician will be aware of the gravity of any diagnosis unless you communicate it to them by telephone. Nonsurgical clinicians and junior surgical trainees may not react with appropriate promptness unless the implications of the diagnosis are spelt out to them. For instance, intramural gas can be a benign appearance. However, given the other findings, it implies infarction of bowel in this case. Furthermore, toxic megacolon has a 20% mortality rate! You must make it clear to the examiners that you will ensure that the diagnosis is conveyed to an appropriate member of clinical staff who will appreciate the importance of the diagnosis and is in a position to act on the findings.

This is discussed further in the introductory text in this book before the cases.

Megacolon

The definition of megacolon varies with some using (differing) absolute measurements of colon as cut-off points. Perhaps a better way of describing it is the presence of dilated large bowel in the absence of mechanical obstruction. Toxic megacolon is seen in inflammatory bowel disease (more commonly in ulcerative colitis than in Crohn's disease), infection, ischaemia and pseudomembranous colitis. Contrast enemas are absolutely contraindicated due to the significant risk of perforation.

Case 64

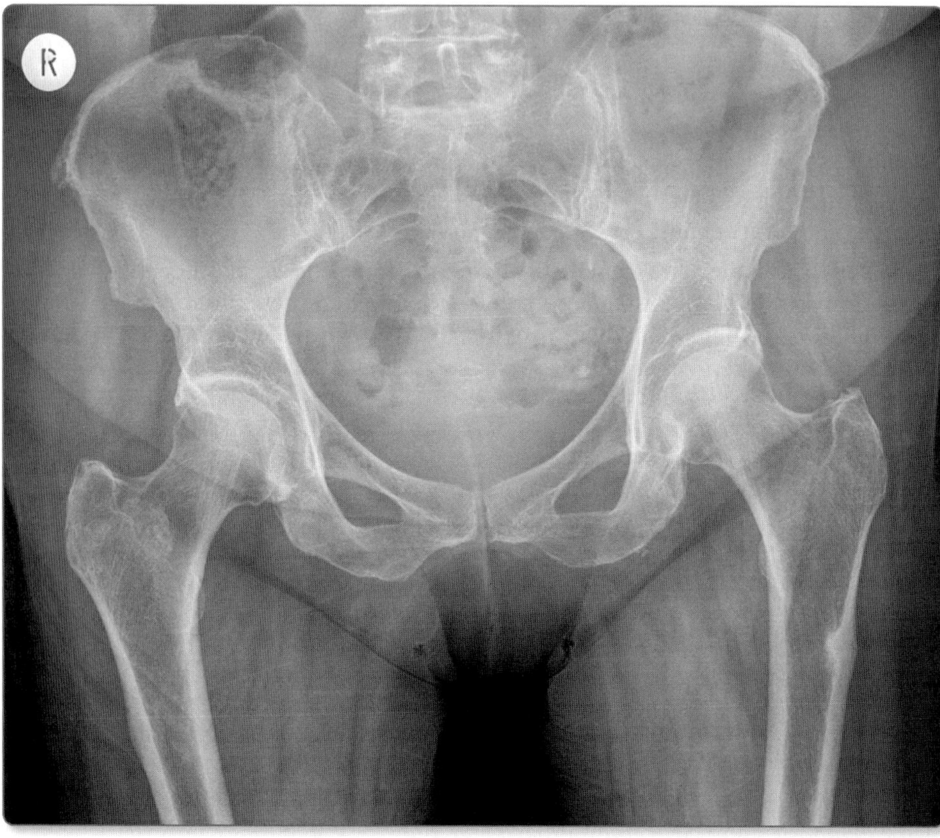

Suggested response

This is an anteroposterior radiograph of the pelvis of an adult female.

In the left proximal femur, there is focal thickening of the lateral cortex with a transverse lucent line running through it, likely to represent a fracture. The medial cortex appears intact. The right femur is also abnormal with focal thickening of the cortex but without any visible fracture line. No underlying destructive lesion is visible on either side.

The appearance could be due to osteomalacia or a stress response but, assuming that the patient is on bisphosphonate therapy, it is more likely to be due to insufficiency fractures associated with bisphosphonate therapy. I would discuss the case with the referring clinician to explore which medications the patient is on, for how long, and if they are symptomatic. I would also suggest an orthopaedic opinion to consider off-loading in order to avoid a completed fracture, or pre-emptive internal fixation.

Diagnosis

Bisphosphonate-associated insufficiency fractures.

Tips: A stress fracture

Key points and differential diagnosis

Stress fractures can be due to insufficiency (normal stresses on abnormal bone, e.g. in osteoporosis, renal osteodystrophy, osteomalacia and Paget's disease; look for other manifestations of metabolic bone disease) or fatigue (abnormal stresses on normal bone, usually seen in athletes or those performing repetitive physical actions).

Sites of insufficiency stress fractures include the spine (osteoporotic wedge compression fracture), pelvis (e.g. acetabulum, pubic rami/parasymphysis and sacrum; the latter may be difficult to identify radiographically due to osteopaenia and overlying bowel gas, but look for the characteristic 'Honda' sign on bone scintigraphy) and femur (usually subcapital and may be very subtle).

Sites of fatigue stress fractures include the spine [e.g. pars interarticularis defects (in the contralateral arm of fast bowlers) and clay shoveller's fracture which involves the spinous process of a lower cervical or upper thoracic vertebra, usually C7], sacrum, upper limb (e.g. hook of hamate and coracoid process of scapula) and lower limb (e.g. second metatarsal and femoral shaft).

Insufficiency fractures

Insufficiency fractures are very common in clinical practice, particularly in elderly patients. Loss of normal bone trabeculae reduces its elastic resistance and predisposes to fracture without the need for abnormal stress (unlike in fatigue stress fractures). Bone scintigraphy and MRI are the imaging modalities of choice.

Case 65

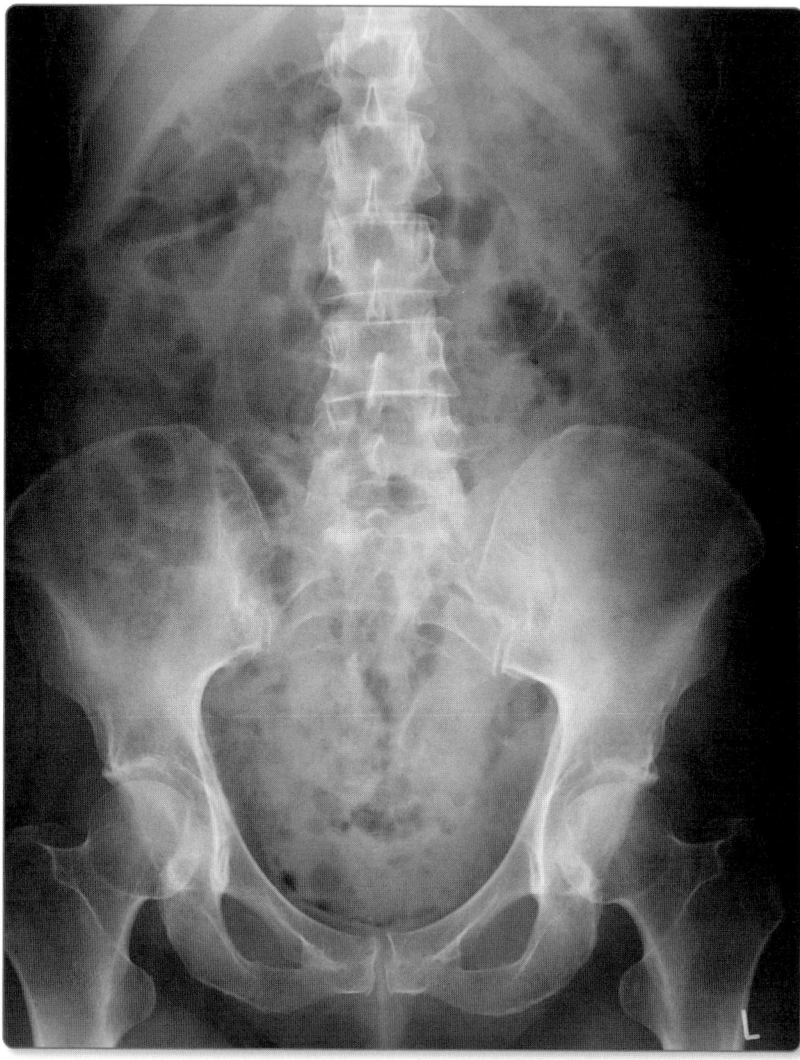

Suggested response

This is an abdominal radiograph of a skeletally mature patient. The bowel gas pattern is unremarkable with no evidence of pneumoperitoneum, but a crescent of gas is evident in the right hemipelvis with further locules of gas in the left hemipelvis. These do not appear to lie within the bowel and are projected along the inferolateral aspects of the urinary bladder, highly suggestive of the presence of gas within the wall of the bladder.

If this patient is unwell, septic and particularly if they are known to have diabetes mellitus, then the appearance is highly suggestive of emphysematous cystitis. I would discuss this case urgently with the referring clinicians. CT scanning may be appropriate to clarify the diagnosis.

Diagnosis

Emphysematous cystitis in an elderly female diabetic patient (see also **Figure 1**).

Tips: Renal tract gas

Key points and differential diagnosis

A CT scan is the optimal medium for evaluation of renal tract gas. It may be visible but difficult to detect on plain film (e.g. due to overlying bowel gas) or ultrasound (obscured by bowel gas or gas in the perinephric space). Hyperechoic gas may also mimic calculi.

Renal gas, if only present in the pelvicalyceal system, may be due to reflux of gas from the bladder (e.g. postcatheterisation) or urinary diversion, or may be infective (i.e. emphysematous pyelitis, in which a dilated pelvicalyceal system is common and which is less severe than emphysematous pyelonephritis). If gas extends into the parenchyma, this is emphysematous pyelonephritis, a urological emergency with a high mortality rate. Streaky parenchymal gas is a poor prognostic sign.

Gas is more often loculated in an abscess, with gas also often seen simultaneously within the pelvicalyceal system.

On plain film, gas projected over the bladder is most likely to lie outside the bladder, e.g. rectal gas. If of bladder origin, it is most likely to be intraluminal gas (e.g. secondary to catheterisation/other instrumentation or enterovesical fistula). Gas in the bladder wall (emphysematous cystitis) may manifest on plain film as a ring of bubbles or streaky lucencies (as in this case) and possibly as an air-fluid level in the bladder itself. Hyperechoic areas in a thickened bladder wall are evident on ultrasound.

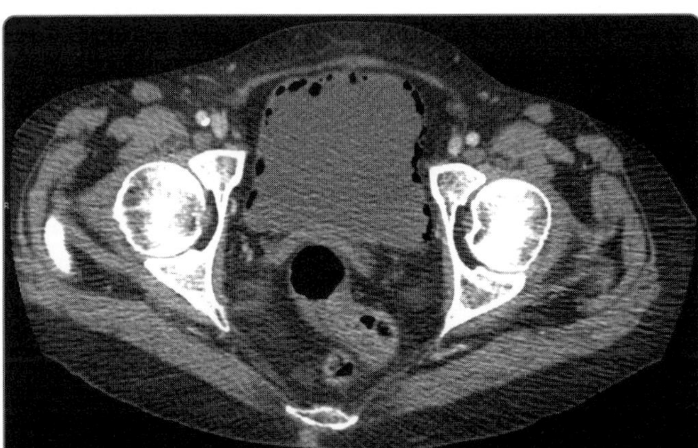

Figure 1 Axial CT from the same patient.

Emphysematous cystitis

Emphysematous cystitis is usually seen in people with diabetes mellitus, most commonly in females. Presentation is variable, ranging from symptoms of urinary tract infection to overt sepsis. It may be associated with the emphysematous pyelonephritis.

It can be difficult to appreciate on plain film, so make sure – particularly if faced with an otherwise unremarkable abdominal radiograph in the viva – that you scrutinise the bladder area carefully. CT is the most sensitive and specific modality for identifying intramural bladder gas.

Case 66

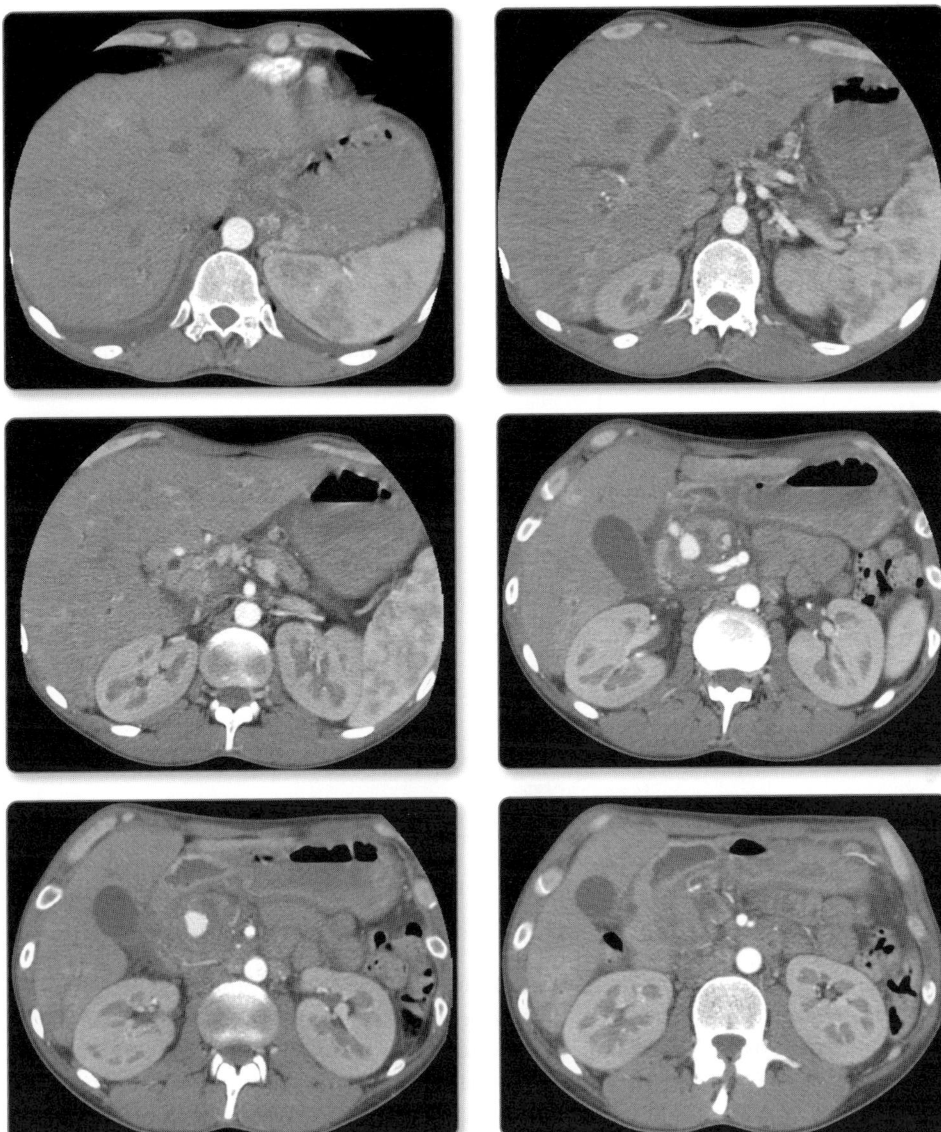

Suggested response

These are arterial phase images from a CT study of the upper abdomen.

There is poor definition of the soft tissue planes around the porta hepatis and pancreatic head and an area of low attenuation in the region of the pancreatic head. In the middle of this region, there is a rounded 2 cm focus of vivid arterial enhancement.

A large artery arises from the superior mesenteric artery and passes to the right towards the liver, close to this region on the fourth image. This is presumably a replaced hepatic artery.

I would routinely review the remainder of the study but cannot see any further abnormality on these images.

If there is a history of pancreatitis, then these findings would make me think of a pseudoaneurysm at the centre of a large pseudocyst. In the absence of a history of pancreatitis, I would consider other causes for an aneurysm or pseudoaneurysm having developed such as an invasive malignancy, vasculopathy, infection and trauma (including recent surgery).

I would correlate the findings with the clinical history and recommend consideration of a catheter angiogram with a view to confirming the diagnosis and potentially treating by endovascular means. In view of the potential urgency of the clinical situation, I would contact the referring clinicians myself and ensure that they were aware of the importance of the findings.

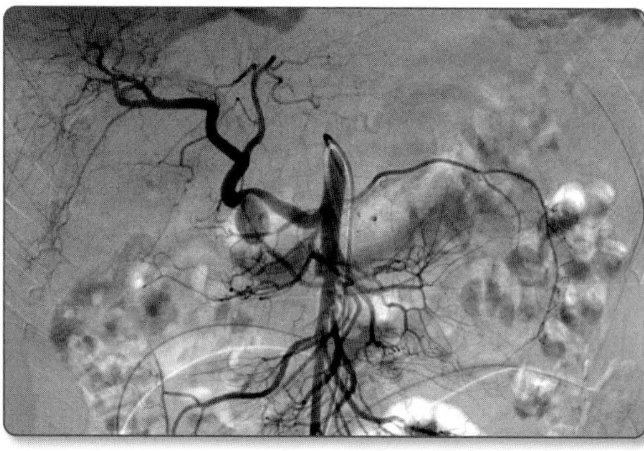

Suggested response

This is an image from a selective angiogram of the superior mesenteric artery which appears to have been performed via a femoral approach, with what appears to be a replaced hepatic artery. There is a 2-cm rounded opacity inferior to and intimately associated with a focal narrowing of the hepatic artery a few centimetres distal to its origin, which I suspect is a pseudoaneurysm. I would confirm the appearance by reviewing the full angiographic series. I would confirm the patient is under the care of an interventional radiologist who may already be considering endovascular therapy. Options would include occlusion of the artery by embolisation or perhaps stent-grafting across the neck of the pseudoaneurysm.

Diagnosis

Pseudoaneurysm from replaced hepatic artery, formed in a pseudocyst, secondary to pancreatitis in an adult male. No cause for pancreatitis visible.

Tips: Pancreatitis

Key points

Firstly, look for the cause of the inflammation, e.g. gallstones and tumour.

Secondly, look for any other conditions associated with the cause. These include cirrhosis resulting from excessive alcohol intake (look for HCC and ascites), cholecystitis or cholangitis (look for gallstones), infiltration of other organs in autoimmune pancreatitis, lung disease in cystic fibrosis and evidence of other injuries in post-traumatic pancreatitis.

Look for any complications of pancreatitis such as pseudocysts, phlegmon, pseudoaneurysms, infection, necrosis or splenic/portal vein thrombosis (avoid overanalysing arterial phase images; CT for pancreatitis is typically performed with three phases including a portal venous phase).

Pancreatitis

Pancreatitis is common both in everyday practice and in examinations and is often associated with multiple findings. There should always be careful examination for vascular findings, making use of all available contrast phases. Some candidates might struggle with the angiographic anatomy in this case, but remember that anatomical knowledge is often also tested as part of radiology viva. Unless you are an interventional radiologist yourself it is probably wise to avoid making bold statements such as 'I would embolise this pseudoaneurysm'; instead, state that you would discuss the case with an interventional radiologist with a view to intervention, which would be perfectly reasonable.

Case 67

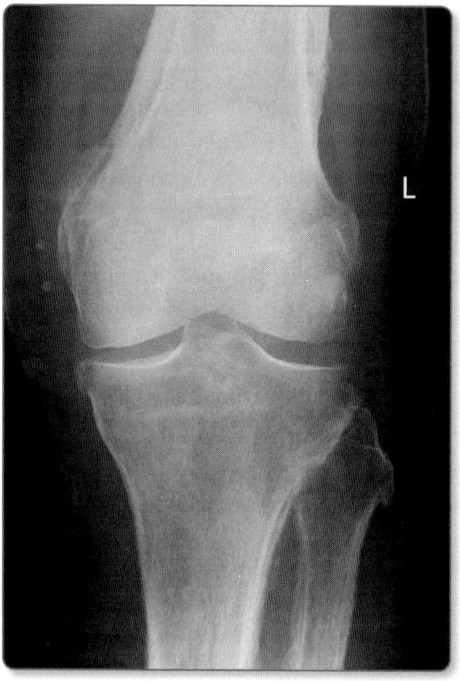

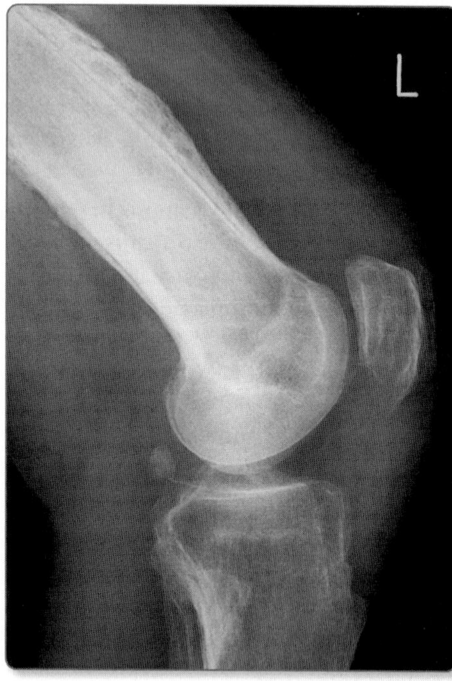

Suggested response

These are anteroposterior and lateral views of the left knee in a skeletally mature patient. There is cortical thickening and mature lamellated periosteal new bone formation involving the diametaphyseal regions of each of the tibia, fibula and femur. The epiphyses are spared. There is a small joint effusion but no fracture or bony destruction. Two rounded calcific densities are projected medial to the medial femoral condyle and, given their lucent centres, are likely to be phleboliths and of doubtful clinical relevance.

If only the left knee is affected, causes such as unilateral vascular insufficiency should be considered, although this could be a rare presentation of hypertrophic osteoarthropathy. If the findings are bilateral, then hypertrophic osteoarthropathy is much more likely.

Pachydermoperiostosis (also known as primary hypertrophic osteoarthropathy) can give similar appearances, but involves the epiphyses that are typically spared in the secondary form. In my usual practice, I would like to review any other available relevant imaging for this patient in conjunction with clinical information, including smoking history. If not already obtained, a chest radiograph should be acquired to assess for thoracic causes of hypertrophic osteoarthropathy, the most important of which is bronchogenic carcinoma. Other causes should also be considered, including inflammatory bowel disease. I would discuss this case with the referring clinician, with further investigations being dependent on the findings on chest radiography.

Diagnosis

Hypertrophic pulmonary osteoarthropathy (HPOA) in a patient presenting with bilateral knee stiffness and subsequently found to have bronchogenic carcinoma.

Tips: Diffuse periosteal reaction

Key points

Consider metabolic conditions (e.g. hypervitaminosis A), primary hypertrophic osteoarthropathy (HOA) and Caffey's disease in young children. Pachydermoperiostosis occurs in children and young adults but rarely affects the over 40s. Secondary HOA (e.g. HPOA) is rare in children.

Distribution is usually very helpful in narrowing the differential. In skeletally mature patients, unilateral periosteal reaction may be due to vascular insufficiency and metastases (usually less diffuse) but rarely HOA. Bilateral periosteal reaction makes pachydermoperiostosis, HOA or vascular insufficiency more likely. HOA typically spares the axial skeleton, instead involving the long bones. HOA is diametaphyseal and spares the epiphyses.

Hypertrophic osteoarthropathy

Hypertrophic osteoarthropathy can be primary (i.e. no underlying condition is found, typically the case with children) or secondary. The case shown here is a typical examination case of secondary HOA (HPOA in this case) with a patient presenting with pain or swelling in the appendicular skeleton and subsequently being found to have a lung tumour. Despite the terms often being used interchangeably, HPOA is only one type of HOA, and bronchogenic carcinoma is far from the most common cause of HOA. Other causative conditions include lymphoma, bronchiectasis and inflammatory bowel disease.

The radiographic findings here are classical of HOA. Bone scintigraphy shows increased uptake along the diametaphyseal cortical margins (see **Figure 1** below, with findings most conspicuous in the lower limbs).

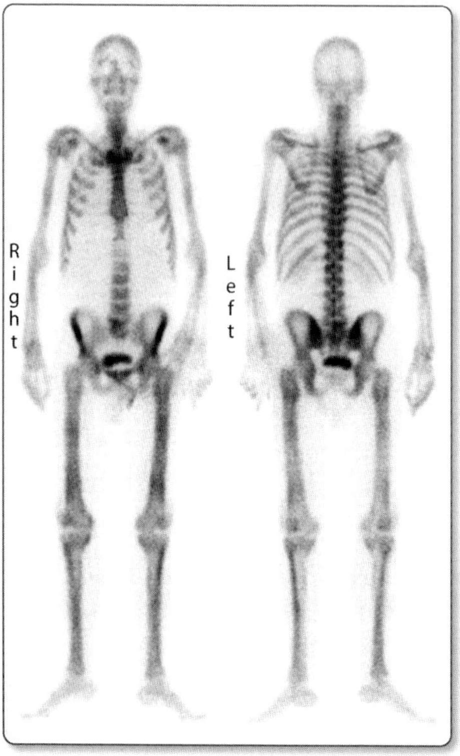

Figure 1 Bone scintigraphy demonstrating increased tracer uptake along the diametaphyseal cortical margins, particularly in the lower limbs. Note that this is a superscan.

Case 68

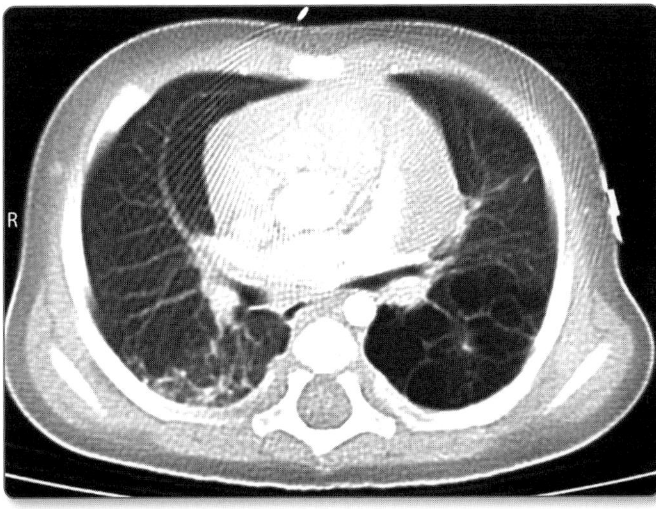

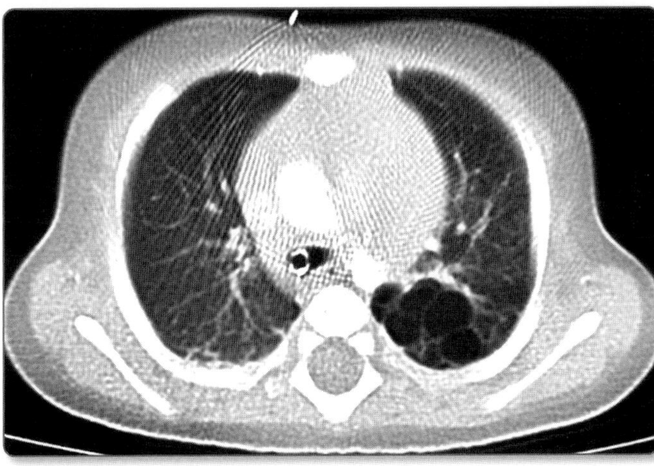

Suggested response

These are selected images from an axial thoracic CT scan viewed on lung windows and the appearance suggests that the patient is a young child.

There is some streak artefact from an external metallic density on the chest wall, but the lungs remain clearly visible. An endotracheal tube is evident, the tip of which is not visualised on these images.

There is an abnormality at the left lung base, with multiple thin-walled contiguous cysts of various sizes. In my usual practice, I would measure these cysts. Nevertheless, several cysts appear to measure >1 cm in diameter. On these images, the abnormality appears to be localised to the left lower lobe. The remaining left lung appears somewhat hypoplastic relative to the right lung, although there is no appreciable mediastinal shift and there is no herniation of the abdominal viscera or fat on these images. There is atelectatic change posteriorly at the right lung base which may be related to the intubation.

The most likely cause of this multicystic abnormality is a left lower lobe congenital cystic adenomatoid malformation, although other differentials including congenital diaphragmatic hernia should be considered. Review of previous imaging and reports (including from antenatal ultrasound) would help to confirm the diagnosis. The child should be evaluated for associated abnormalities including renal and cardiac anomalies.

Diagnosis

Congenital cystic adenomatoid malformation (CCAM) in a 4-month-old infant.

Tips: Paediatric congenital lung disease

Key points

If a focal abnormality is visible, then consider if it is air-filled or solid. CCAM, congenital diaphragmatic hernia (CDH), bronchopulmonary sequestration and congenital lobar emphysema (CLE) may all appear solid at birth. CCAM (type 3) and bronchopulmonary sequestration (extralobar) usually remain solid. CCAM (types 1 and 2), CDH and CLE typically become air-filled as the infant ages. It is also important to remember the effects of superadded infection.

Conditions such as CLE can cause mediastinal deviation *away* from the side of the abnormality. If, however, there is associated pulmonary hypoplasia, then deviation towards the side of the abnormality may be evident. (CCAM and CDH can cause mediastinal deviation either way, depending on the extent of hypoplasia.)

Specifically look for common associated abnormalities such as congenital heart disease, renal dysplasia and vertebral anomalies.

Differential diagnoses

Consider other alternative causes of mediastinal masses in children. An anterior mediastinal mass may represent a Morgagni variant of CDH (remember that MorgAgNi is ANterior). A middle mediastinal mass may be a bronchogenic cyst (this may also be wholly intrapulmonary and may contain air, therefore it is an important differential for type 1 CCAM). Posterior mediastinal masses may also be a Bochdalek variant of CDH (remember that BochdaLEk is Back and LEft in around 80% of cases, although it may also be right-sided or bilateral).

Congenital cystic adenomatoid malformation

Congenital cystic adenomatoid malformation accounts for a quarter of all congenital lung diseases and may be detected antenatally. It has variable imaging appearances, depending on the histological classification. Type 1 is the most common and presents with one or more large cysts. Type 2 (seen in this case) has multiple moderate sized cysts. Type 3 manifests as a confluence of tiny cysts and as such appears solid (hyperechoic relative to the liver) on antenatal ultrasound. It has no lobar or side predominance. A typical plain film would demonstrate a unilateral expansile mass with contralateral mediastinal shift. Pleural effusions and spontaneous pneumothoraces may also be seen.

Case 69

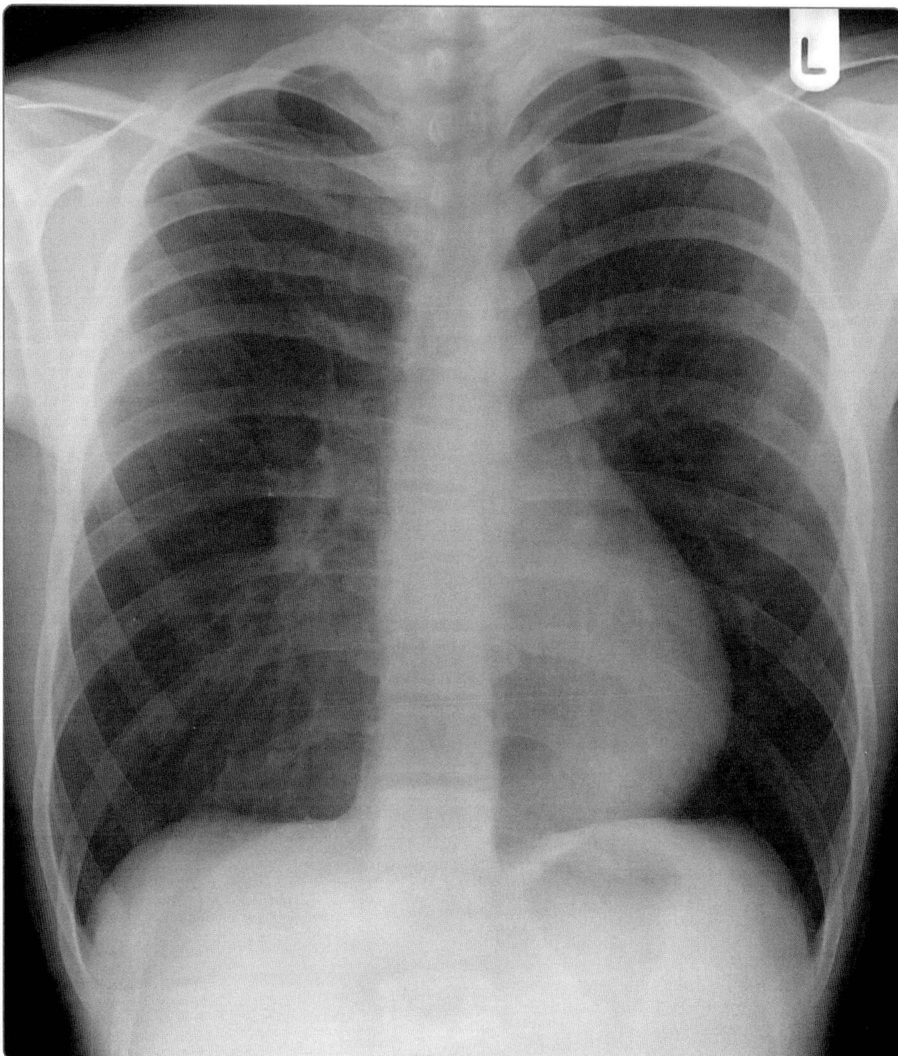

Suggested response

This is a frontal chest radiograph of a skeletally mature patient. There is increased translucency of the left hemithorax which I attribute to rotation to the left. The right heart border is indistinct, with increased opacification medially in the right lower zone. The remaining lungs are clear. The heart itself is displaced to the left but is not significantly enlarged. There is a structural abnormality of the thoracic cage. The posterior ribs are predominantly horizontal with sharp inferior angulation anteriorly.

The findings are consistent with a pectus excavatum deformity. The right 4th rib is also noted to be bifid. The right lower zone opacification is almost certainly a consequence of the pectus deformity rather than middle lobe consolidation, although if there is clinical suspicion or a history of an infective illness then consolidation is a possibility.

Diagnosis

Pectus excavatum in an adolescent male.

Tips: A structural abnormality of the thoracic cage

Key points

Unilateral thoracic cage deformity suggests previous trauma or thoracoplasty. Thoracoplasty is now rarely performed for tuberculosis but has a typical appearance with the upper ribs displaced towards the mediastinum.

If the ribs are angulated, then consider pectus excavatum, in which the ribs are horizontal posteriorly with inferior angulation anteriorly (as in this case, giving the appearance of the number '7'), or barrel chest (usually secondary to chronic obstructive pulmonary disease), in which the lateral part of each rib is elongated and vertically orientated.

Counting the number of ribs may be helpful. 11 pairs may be normal but can also be seen in a number of syndromes including Down's syndrome and cleidocranial dysplasia. 13 pairs are similarly associated with several syndromes including Down's syndrome and VATER syndrome (which is an acronym for vertebral anomalies, anal defects, tracheo-oesophageal fistulae and renal abnormalities).

Abnormally short ribs are associated with a number of congenital conditions in which there are a variety of other bony abnormalities (such as achondroplasia, thanatophoric dwarfism and Jeune's asphyxiating thoracic dysplasia). Respiratory failure makes many of these conditions incompatible with life.

Pectus excavatum

Pectus excavatum (Latin for hollowed chest) is usually an isolated phenomenon. Although often clinically inconsequential, it can cause cardiorespiratory compromise if severe. You may not notice it on first glance, but double checking the ribs on any seemingly normal chest radiograph is a critical review area. Similarly, if the right heart border is indistinct, ensure that there is no pectus excavatum deformity before diagnosing a right middle lobe pneumonia (although clearly the two may co-exist, in which case previous imaging may prove invaluable). The reduced anteroposterior intrathoracic diameter (easily identified on the lateral view) displaces the heart and causes a reduction in cardiac density.

Case 70

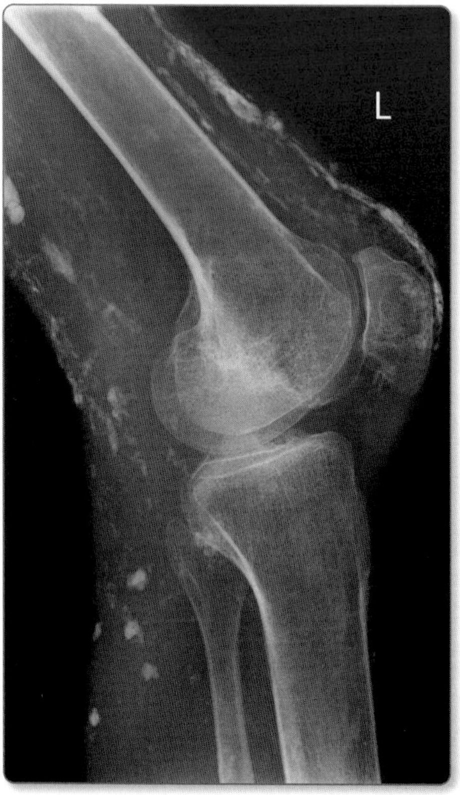

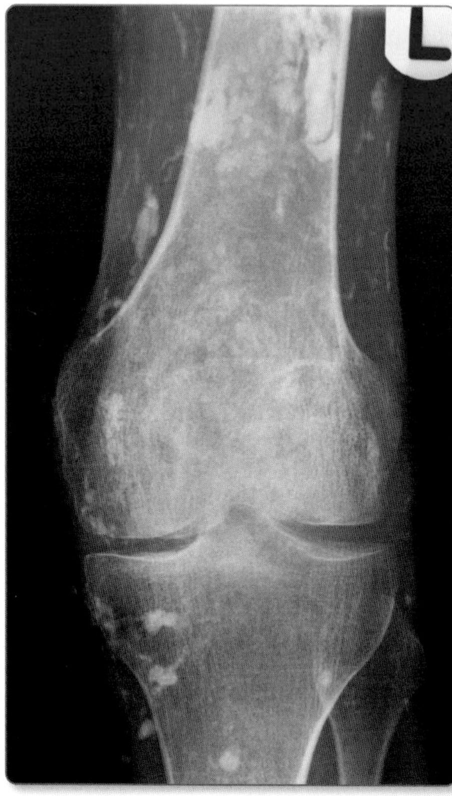

Suggested response

These are frontal and lateral radiographs of the left knee of a skeletally mature patient. The most striking abnormality is the presence of widespread soft tissue calcification, some of which extends in a sheet-like fashion parallel to the long axes of the bones and some of which is in nodular form. Calcifications are predominantly projected in the subcutaneous planes. The underlying bones and knee joint appear normal. There is loss of volume of the soft tissues consistent with skeletal muscle atrophy. Findings are most in keeping with polymyositis or dermatomyositis.

Although the clinical history would be relevant, I cannot identify any fractures on these films and would routinely review any available previous imaging to assess for progression and confirm that the disease is multifocal. If there is known pulmonary disease, this would favour a diagnosis of dermatomyositis.

Diagnosis

Dermatomyositis in an adult female.

Tips: Soft tissue calcification in the extremities

It is good to acknowledge that the differential diagnosis is vast and then make an effort to narrow it down.

Differential diagnosis

There are three main types of soft tissue calcification. The most common is dystrophic calcification, which accounts for >95% of all soft tissue calcifications. This is not associated with metabolic disorders, but occurs in damaged and degenerating tissue and appears as amorphous calcifications of varying sizes (which may eventually ossify). Common examples are calcific tendonitis, phleboliths, atherosclerosis and tissue infarction sites (e.g. myocardial infarction). More unusual causes include osteosarcoma and cysticercosis (rice grain calcifications).

Metastatic calcification manifests as fine specks of calcification in otherwise normal tissues and is often associated with an underlying metabolic disorder such as hyperparathyroidism.

Calcinosis occurs in cutaneous or subcutaneous tissues and is not usually associated with a metabolic disorder, although collagen vascular disorders are a common association. Specific variants include: calcinosis circumscripta associated with scleroderma, which produces sharply marginated/punctate calcifications in the fingers (associated with scleroderma); calcinosis universalis associated with dermatomyositis, producing superficial nodules and plaques and also deeper sheet-like/periarticular calcifications later in the disease process; and tumoural calcinosis, in which multiloculated calcifications appear in or near large joints and which is usually polyarticular.

Distinguishing between calcification and ossification on plain films relies on identification of the trabecular pattern and corticomedullary differentiation of bone during ossification. A feature of ossification on MRI is that a fatty marrow signal may be seen internally on T1-weighted images. Ossification occurs after trauma (in myositis ossificans), in association with bone tumours (e.g. parosteal osteosarcoma) and may also be seen in congenital disorders (e.g. melorheostosis and fibrodysplasia ossificans progressiva).

Dermatomyositis

Dermatomyositis is a multisystem autoimmune disorder which, as the name suggests, predominantly affects the skin and striated muscle. The imaging findings shown here are typical of late-stage dermatomyositis, with muscular atrophy and diffuse confluent sheet-like calcifications **(Figure 1)**. The lower limbs are affected more than the upper limbs. Various pulmonary manifestations may be seen, including pulmonary fibrosis (basal predominance) and a scleroderma-like pattern of multifocal pulmonary infiltrates.

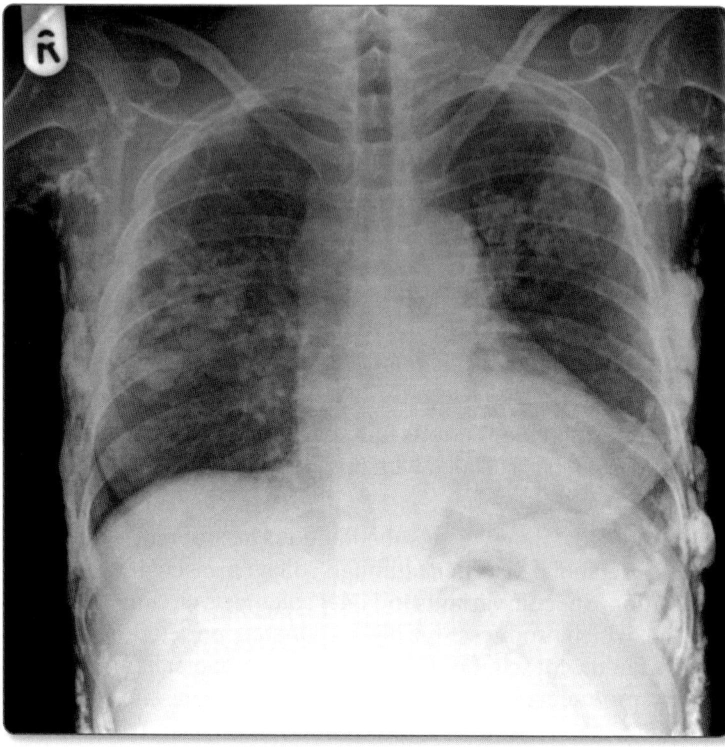

Figure 1 Frontal chest radiograph from this case, also showing extensive soft tissue calcification.

Case 71

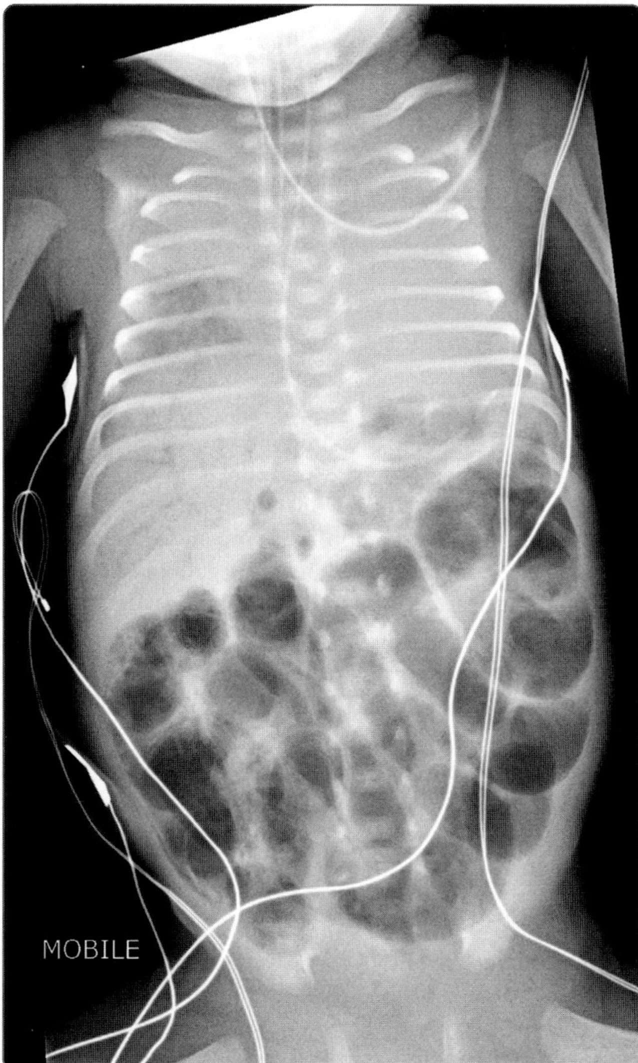

Suggested response

This is a neonatal chest and abdominal radiograph. Judging by the fact that the proximal humeral ossification centres are not yet visualised this is likely to be a neonate, possibly premature.

An endotracheal tube is evident with its tip projected in the region of the carina. There is opacification of the left hemithorax and the right upper and mid zones, likely to reflect endotracheal tube malposition. A nasogastric tube appears to be located appropriately.

There are multiple dilated loops of bowel in the abdomen, some of which in the right flank exhibit features suspicious for the presence of intramural gas. No definite pneumoperitoneum is identified. There are also branching linear gaseous areas projected over the liver, likely to reflect portal venous gas.

The abdominal findings are most in keeping with necrotising enterocolitis.

I would immediately contact the clinicians to ensure that they are aware of the suboptimal endotracheal tube position and also to discuss the abdominal findings.

Diagnosis

Necrotising enterocolitis (NEC) in a 2-week-old infant with malpositioned endotracheal tube.

Tips: Portal venous gas

Key points

There are several features that help to discriminate between portal venous gas and biliary tract gas. Portal venous gas is usually peripheral, in narrow calibre branching structures. It may be associated with gas in the main portal vein and mesenteric veins and/or pneumatosis intestinalis. Pneumobilia is typically more central, in wider calibre branching structures, and may be seen in the gallbladder. In emphysematous cholecystitis (high mortality), gas is seen in the gallbladder lumen and also in the wall.

In children, portal venous gas may be seen in cases of necrotising enterocolitis, congenital disorders (e.g. oesophageal or duodenal atresia), imperforate anus or iatrogenic causes (e.g. corrective bowel surgery or umbilical vein catheterisation). In adults, portal venous gas may be seen in association with any of the '3 Is': *i*nfarcted bowel (e.g. ischaemic or ulcerative colitis), *i*nflammatory disorders (including pancreatitis, diverticulitis and abscess) and *i*atrogenic causes (e.g. colonoscopy or barium enema).

Necrotising enterocolitis

Usually a disease of prematurity, NEC is a serious acquired disease of the neonate with a mortality rate in the order of 20–40%. It usually presents within the 1st or 2nd week of life (slightly later if born very prematurely). Intramural gas gives a 'bubbly' or curvilinear appearance on plain film. Bowel distension is the most common finding in NEC and may be seen prior to the onset of symptoms. Portal venous gas is most commonly seen in neonates following umbilical vein catheterisation, but if evident in NEC it tends to be present in more unwell neonates (although it does not necessarily convey a terminal prognosis and is a much more benign finding than in adults, in whom it is often a sign of imminent demise). Look carefully for evidence of perforation. Small volumes of free gas are often most readily appreciated on a horizontal-beam view, with triangular lucencies anteriorly, between loops of bowel, and/or bubbly/linear gas collections in front of the liver.

If you suggest requesting a horizontal-beam view in a viva, make sure you can interpret one.

Case 72

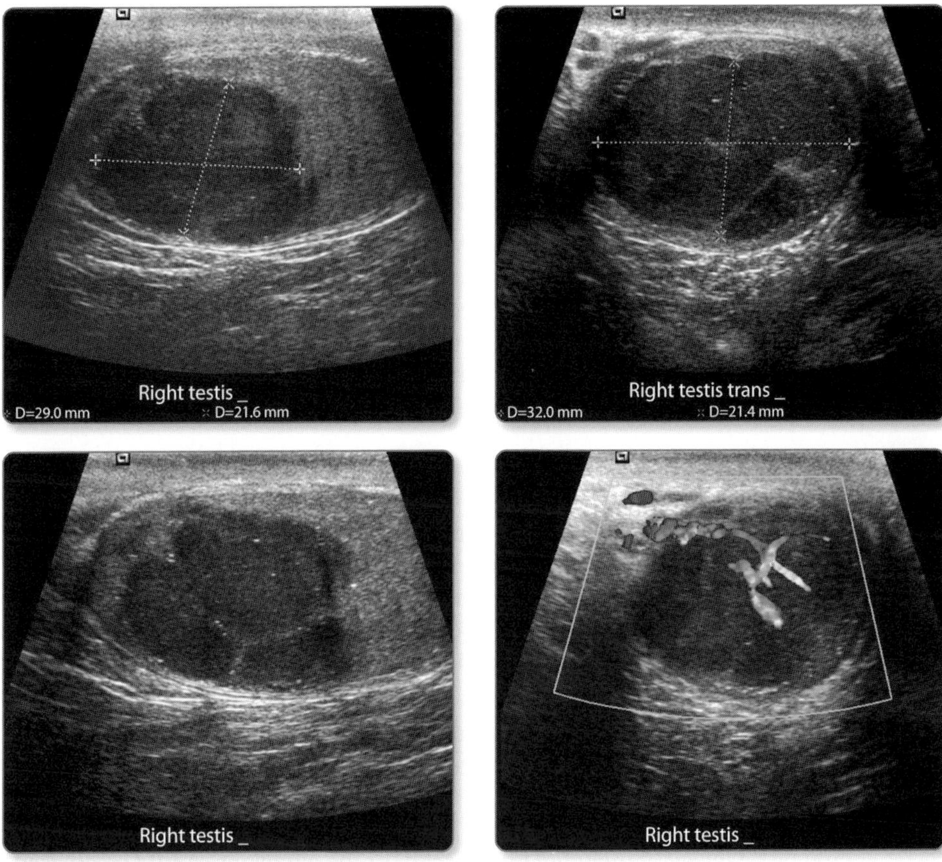

Suggested response

These are selected images from an ultrasound scan of the right testis. There are several contiguous low-reflectivity nodules in the upper pole of the testis, over a total diameter of just over 2 cm, with at least half of the testis being involved. Increased internal colour flow is demonstrated within this area on the colour Doppler image. There are multiple associated tiny hyperechoic foci without convincing posterior acoustic shadowing, consistent with microlithiasis. The tunica albuginea appears intact on these images.

The findings are consistent with a testicular tumour. The testicular volume suggests a post-pubertal male and the most likely differential diagnoses are therefore seminoma, lymphoma and metastases. If I was scanning this patient and identified this abnormality, I would ensure that I evaluated the left testicle and also the abdomen. If this is the first presentation, the patient needs urgent referral to the urologists and a staging CT scan for further evaluation.

Diagnosis

Seminoma in a 30-year-old patient.

Tips: Testicular tumours

Differential diagnosis

Age is the key determinant. In children, teratomas and yolk sac tumours predominate. In young adults, seminomas are most common. In older adults, lymphoma and metastases are both more common than primary germ cell tumours.

Lymphoma and metastases are commonly bilateral, but teratoma and seminoma are almost always unilateral.

On colour flow Doppler examination, larger tumours (>1.5 cm) usually exhibit increased vascularity while smaller tumours (<1.5 cm) usually exhibit reduced vascularity. Many of the common tumour mimics such as haematoma, abscess and infarction are avascular.

Seminoma

Around half of all testicular germ cell tumours are seminomas. They tend to present at a slightly older age (at around 40 years of age) than other primary testicular tumours. The case shown here exhibits typical ultrasonographic findings, with a vascular tumour comprising several confluent hypoechoic nodules without extension beyond the tunica albuginea. Microlithiasis is a common association (follow-up for incidentally detected microlithiasis is controversial).

Remember the pathway of lymphatic drainage from the testes: testicular tumours spread to the para-aortic nodes whereas pathologies involving the scrotum may disseminate to inguinal nodes. Accordingly, if presented with imaging from a male patient which demonstrates para-aortic lymphadenopathy of uncertain aetiology, the testes should be reviewed (if included on the scan) or the clinicians should be advised to ensure that a testicular examination is performed, with a view to ultrasound if required.

Case 73

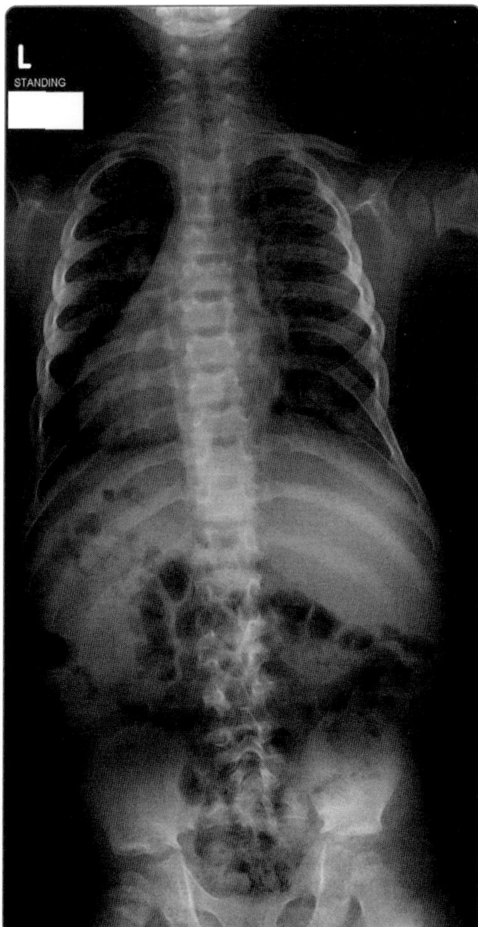

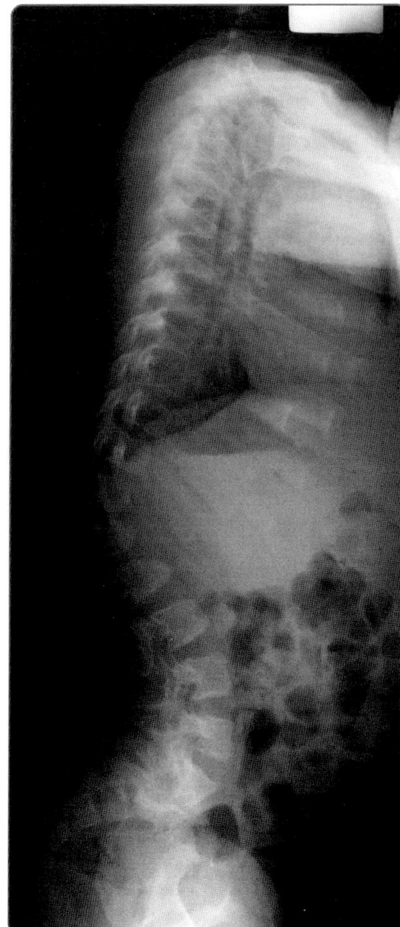

Suggested response

These are frontal standing and lateral views of the whole spine of a skeletally immature patient. Multiple skeletal abnormalities are evident. Focussing initially on the spine, a focal kyphosis centred on the thoracolumbar junction with loss of anterior height and beaking of the upper lumbar vertebrae is visible on the lateral view. The sacral lordosis is exaggerated and there is posterior scalloping of the vertebral bodies. The frontal view shows progressive narrowing of the interpedicular distance in the lumbar spine from cranial to caudal. The pelvis exhibits squaring of the iliac wings with horizontal acetabula and a 'champagne glass' shaped pelvic inlet.

The right proximal humerus shows metaphyseal flaring. Appearances are entirely consistent with a diagnosis of achondroplasia.

Diagnosis

Achondroplasia in a 3-year-old child.

Tips: Posterior vertebral scalloping

Key points

Some degree of posterior vertebral scalloping is a normal finding in over half of the population, but there are several pathological causes for exaggerated posterior vertebral scalloping.

Differential diagnosis

Causes include raised intraspinal pressure secondary to spinal canal tumours, syringomyelia and communicating hydrocephalus. Another cause is dural ectasia (widening of the dural sac) which is associated with Marfan's syndrome, Ehlers–Danlos syndrome and neurofibromatosis (NF) type 1. NF type 1 can also cause localised posterior scalloping as a result of meningocele or 'dumbbell' neurofibroma (intervertebral foramen and flattened pedicle), both of which are usually seen in the lumbar region. The abnormally small spinal canal encountered in achondroplasia and other congenital skeletal disorders such as the mucopolysaccharidoses may also be associated with posterior vertebral scalloping. The soft tissue hypertrophy and bony remodelling associated with acromegaly may lead to diffuse posterior vertebral scalloping.

If anterior vertebral beaking is seen in the central spine, there may be an underlying diagnosis of Morquio's syndrome. If beaking is seen in the lower spine, consider other mucopolysaccharidoses, achondroplasia and Down's syndrome. If there are associated extra-osseous findings, then these effectively exclude diagnoses of achondroplasia and mucopolysaccharidoses (whose manifestations are almost exclusively due to skeletal changes). Aneurysms of the great arteries or lung disease may be seen in Marfan's syndrome and Ehlers–Danlos syndrome, whereas NF type 1 may be associated with subcutaneous neurofibromas, mediastinal masses, bullous or fibrotic lung disease and renal artery stenosis or aneurysms.

Achondroplasia

Achondroplasia is a form of rhizomelic dwarfism. Rhizomelic means proximal limb shortening, a form of short limb disproportionate short stature, as distinct from proportionate short stature or short trunk short stature. Other forms of limb shortening short stature are mesomelic (middle) and acromelic (distal).

Achondroplasia has a range of imaging features of which you should be aware. The classic pelvic and spinal findings are shown in the case above. Look in particular at the configuration of the pelvic bones and for progressive narrowing of the interpedicular distance on the anteroposterior view. Imaging of the skull demonstrates enlargement of the calvaria with frontal bossing and a small foramen magnum, features which are associated with an increased risk of sudden death. Neurological complications are common. Long bones have a 'trumpet' appearance with metaphyseal flaring, which actually reflects the normal metaphyseal width in conjunction with an abnormally shortened diaphysis. 'Trident hand' is pathognomonic, with widening of the distance between the second, third and fourth (shortened) fingers; this feature is usually lost by adulthood.

Case 74

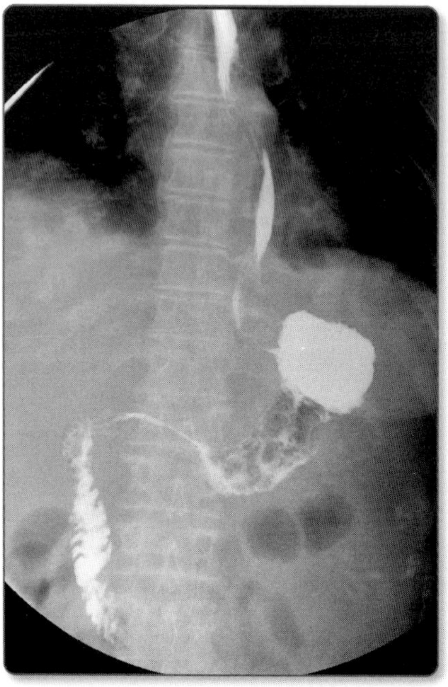

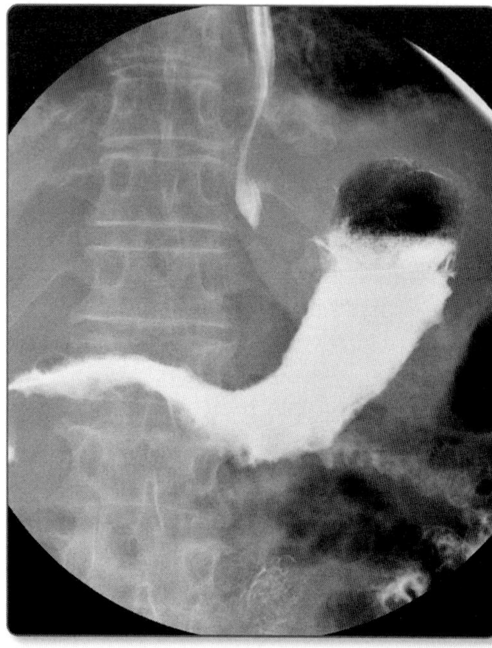

Suggested response

These are two spot views from a contrast meal examination. Contrast is seen to pass through the stomach and into the duodenum. The stomach is partly visualised in double contrast but mostly in single contrast and appears abnormal. Although the fundus distends relatively normally, the lower aspect of the body and the pyloric antrum are significantly narrowed and exhibit mucosal irregularity. In my usual practice, I would review all the images in the study and if this narrowing persisted throughout the examination, then the appearance would be consistent with diffuse wall thickening and stiffening. Inflammatory conditions may cause this linitis plastica appearance, particularly if there is a history of corrosive ingestion or radiotherapy, but the most important differential diagnosis is a diffuse infiltrative neoplastic process.

I would communicate these findings to the referring clinician. If not previously known about, then I would suggest direct visualisation and biopsy of the stomach by endoscopy. Depending on the specific diagnosis, a staging CT scan may be appropriate.

Diagnosis

Elderly female with malignant linitis plastica who presented with weight loss and dysphagia.

Tips: Linitis plastica

Differential diagnosis

Although typically associated with malignancies, there are other causes of linitis plastica.

The neoplasms typically associated with linitis plastica are gastric carcinoma, lymphoma (the stomach is the most common gastrointestinal site) and metastases from breast or lung tumours.

Linitis plastica may also be caused by nonmalignant aetiologies such as chronic inflammation associated with Crohn's disease, eosinophilic gastritis and protracted peptic ulcer disease. Chronic inflammation caused by syphilis or tuberculosis is another unusual cause, along with radiotherapy and corrosive ingestion.

Ancillary findings may suggest a specific diagnosis. Examination of the skeleton may reveal bone metastases, radiotherapy changes (well-demarcated area of sclerosis) or sacroiliitis (associated with Crohn's disease). Perigastric lymphadenopathy is evident in over 75% of patients with gastric carcinoma. Metastases may also be seen in the liver, adrenal glands and ovaries (Krukenberg's tumours occasionally precipitate clinical presentation before the primary lesion manifests).

Malignant linitis plastica

Although often used interchangeably with diffuse malignant infiltration of the stomach, the term *linitis plastica* can be used to refer to any cause of diffuse gastric wall thickening that results in luminal narrowing. Particular subtypes of gastric cancer can cause linitis plastica. As seen in this case, these typically start in the distal stomach (near the antrum) and gradually extend proximally to involve the body and fundus **(Figure 1)**. Around half of cases of gastric lymphoma cause diffuse wall thickening which is usually less rigid than in gastric carcinoma. Breast cancer is the most common extra-gastric primary neoplasm to give rise to metastatic linitis plastica.

Beware of over-diagnosing wall thickening on CT scans in which the stomach is not distended: an empty stomach can appear artificially thick-walled. If the stomach is the target of a study, a negative contrast agent (e.g. water) is typically used to distend it, to enable optimal evaluation, and administration of intravenous hyoscine butylbromide can be considered to paralyse gastric muscle activity.

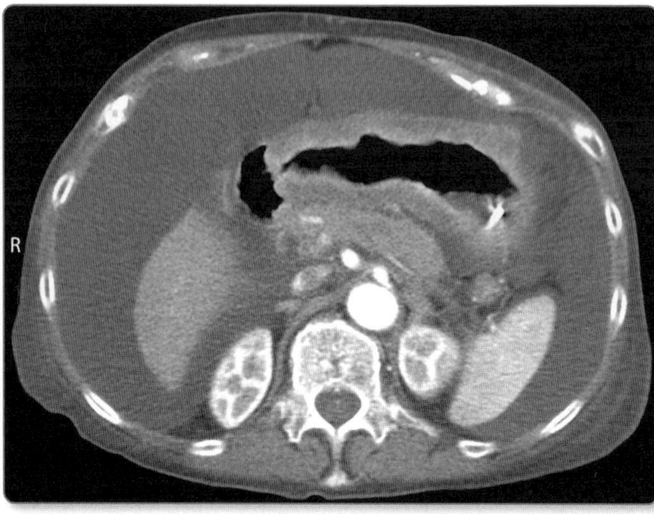

Figure 1 Arterial phase axial CT from this case, showing diffuse stomach wall thickening and large volume ascites.

Case 75

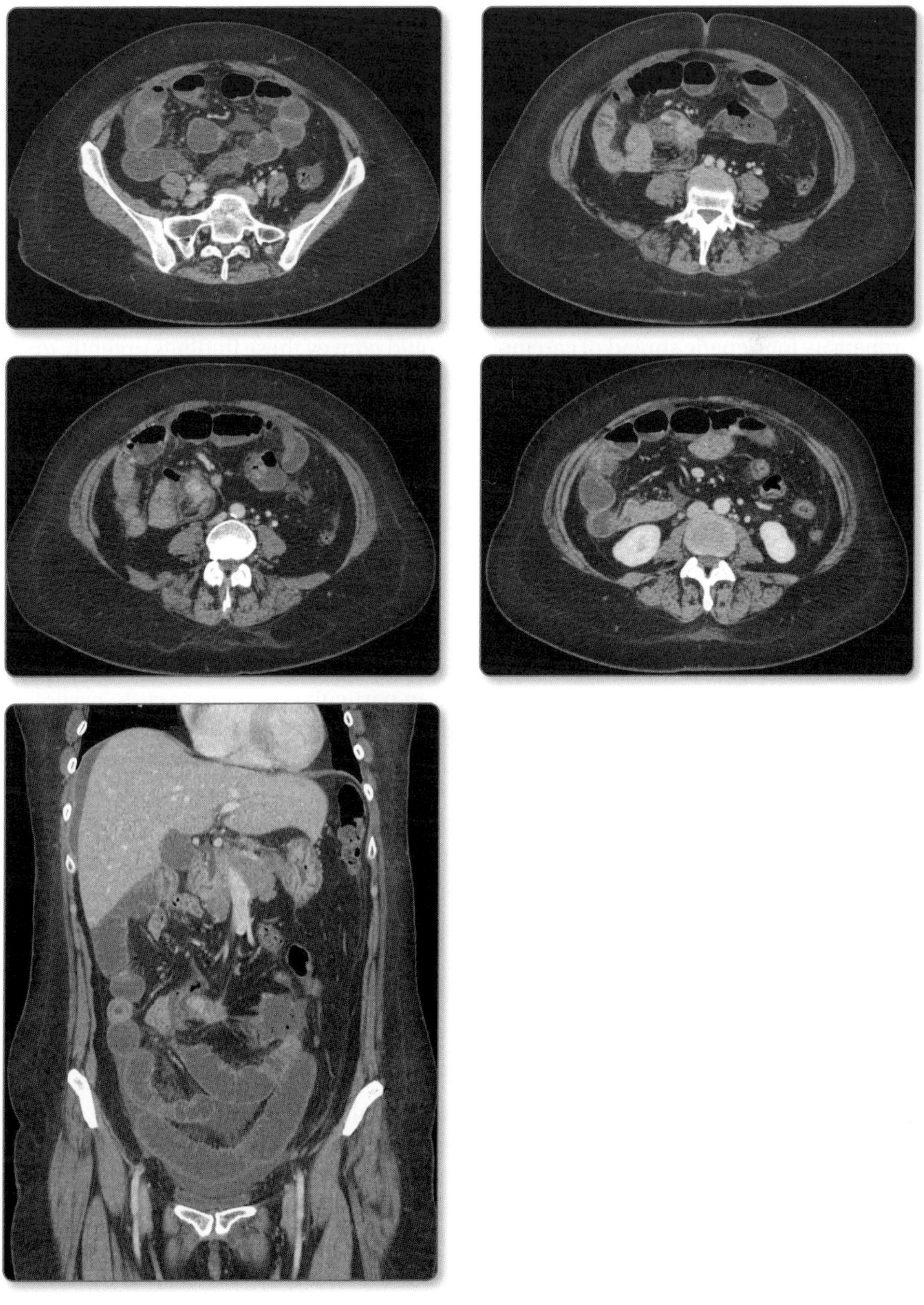

Suggested response

These are selected axial views from a post-contrast CT scan of the abdomen with a further coronally reformatted image. There is a spiculated mass in the mesentery of the mid-abdomen which appears to be in contiguity with a loop of small bowel. It measures several centimetres in diameter and is heterogeneous but predominantly isoattenuating with the liver, most likely due to enhancement. It appears to be causing a desmoplastic/cicatrising/scirrhous reaction.

There are fluid-filled loops of small bowel, some of which are dilated, which are likely to reflect a degree of obstruction, and some local small bowel loops exhibit wall thickening. There is a small volume of ascites.

This appearance almost certainly represents a neuroendocrine tumour of carcinoid type. What is seen of the liver is unremarkable, although in my usual practice I would review all images on this scan, paying particular attention to the liver given the propensity for hepatic spread of carcinoid. I would convey these findings urgently to the referring clinicians, highlighting the partial small bowel obstruction.

Diagnosis

Adult female with a small bowel carcinoid tumour causing a desmoplastic reaction with partial small bowel obstruction.

Tips: Mesenteric masses

Key points

Mesenteric masses are most commonly cystic, in particular mesenteric cysts, cystic lymphangiomas or pseudomyxoma peritonei.

Solid mesenteric masses are usually tumours. Primary mesenteric malignant masses are less common than metastases or benign masses. Malignant tumours are usually centred at the root of the mesentery whereas benign tumours are more peripheral. Colonic and ovarian primary malignancies are the most common source of mesenteric metastases so evaluate these organs carefully.

Carcinoid tumour is likely if there is a stellate (spoke-wheel, scirrhous) pattern on CT and/or stippled internal calcification. The differential diagnosis for a scirrhous mesenteric mass is sclerosing mesenteritis (very rare).

Carcinoid tumour

Carcinoid is the most common appendiceal and small bowel primary tumour. Only a minority of patients present with characteristic carcinoid syndrome (caused by tumoural hormonal activity, usually in the presence of liver metastases). Carcinoid tumours of the appendix or stomach rarely metastasise, but small bowel carcinoid tumours commonly spread to lymph nodes, liver, bone or peritoneum.

Various imaging appearances might be encountered in the viva scenario. The CT appearances shown in the case above are classical, with a radiating spoke-wheel pattern. Contrast follow-through examinations might show angulated loops of small bowel with a resulting obstruction, a submucosal mass or separation of bowel loops by metastases. There is often increased tracer uptake in I^{123} MIGB (iodine-123 metaiodobenzylguanidine) scintigraphy. Carcinoid tumours are typically hypervascular on angiography and may give a 'sunburst' appearance. Note that carcinoid liver metastases are characteristically hyperarterialised and consequently may be overlooked on portal venous phase acquisitions. CT scans to assess for liver metastases should therefore include an arterial phase acquisition.

Case 76

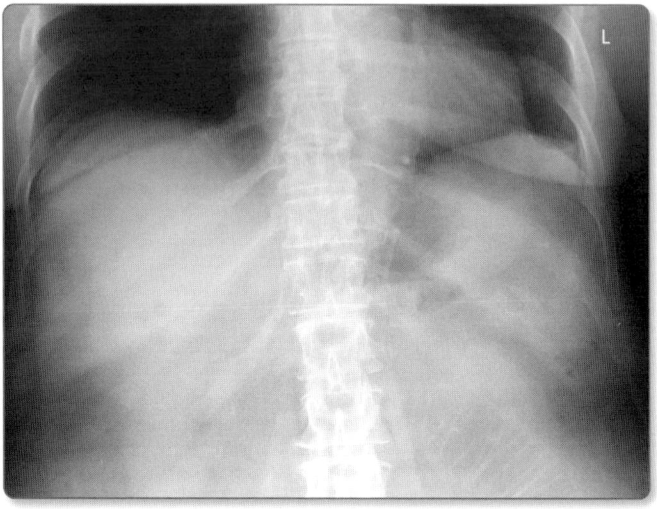

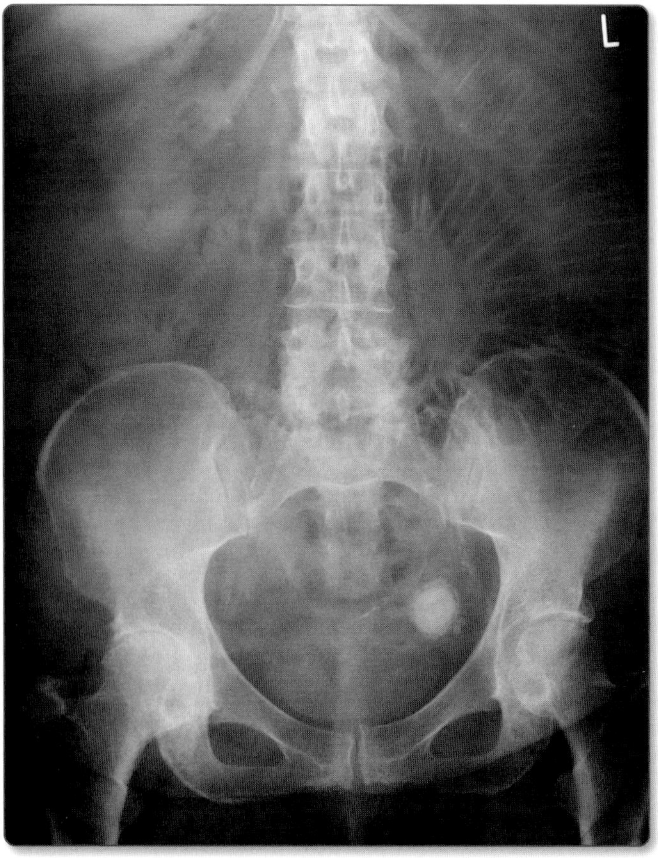

Suggested response

This is a pair of abdominal radiographs covering the upper and lower abdomen of an adult patient.

There are dilated loops of small bowel on the left side of the abdomen. No dilated loops are seen on the right side. In the left low pelvis, there is a large densely calcified ovoid radio-opaque structure with a lamellated appearance, suggestive of a calcified gallstone. Adjacent to this large calculus are a number of smaller, round, calcified opacities which appear to be pelvic phleboliths. I am unsure whether gaseous foci projected over the inferior edge of the liver lie within bowel or the gallbladder, but appearances are not typical for gas in the bile ducts.

The appearance is that of gallstone ileus. There is no Rigler's sign or other feature of free gas, but if perforation is a clinical concern then an erect chest radiograph could be performed for clarification. If I encountered this film at work, I would contact the referring clinicians immediately myself to convey the diagnosis.

Diagnosis

Gallstone ileus without perforation.

Tips: Gallstone ileus

Key points

Keep in mind the triad of small bowel obstruction, a large calculus (which may be lamellated) projected over the abdomen and gas in the biliary tree, but remember that often only two of the three are present.

If the small bowel obstruction is chronic then the dilated bowel loops may have filled with fluid, in which case they will not be visible. Remember to specifically comment on whether there is evidence of perforation. If you do not want to suggest doing a CT scan immediately, then you can conclude by showing you know something about the management – suggest an urgent discussion with the on-call surgeon in which any need for further imaging can be considered.

See also Case 7 and Case 12 for further discussion of large and small bowel obstruction.

Gallstone ileus

The cause of gallstone ileus is chronic cholecystitis. The inflamed gallbladder wall adheres to the proximal duodenum (or rarely the colon) and a fistula forms through which gallstones may pass into the bowel lumen **(Figure 1)**. Giant gallstones may cause small bowel obstruction. Not all cases of gallstone ileus will require assessment with CT, but CT may be appropriate if it is necessary to confirm the diagnosis, help operative planning or determine whether conservative management is a possibility.

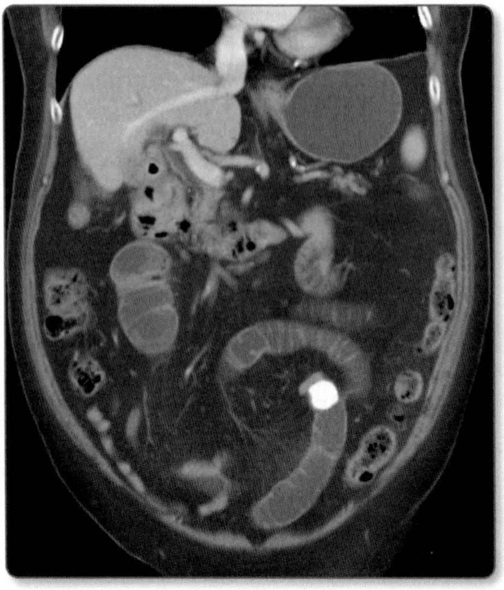

Figure 1 Coronal CT scan image showing the obstructing gallstone in a small bowel loop in the left lower quadrant. The image also demonstrates inflammatory changes around the gallbladder and upper duodenum, with gas evident in the gallbladder. This is the site of the fistula between the gallbladder and the bowel which allowed the large gallstone to enter the bowel lumen.

Case 77

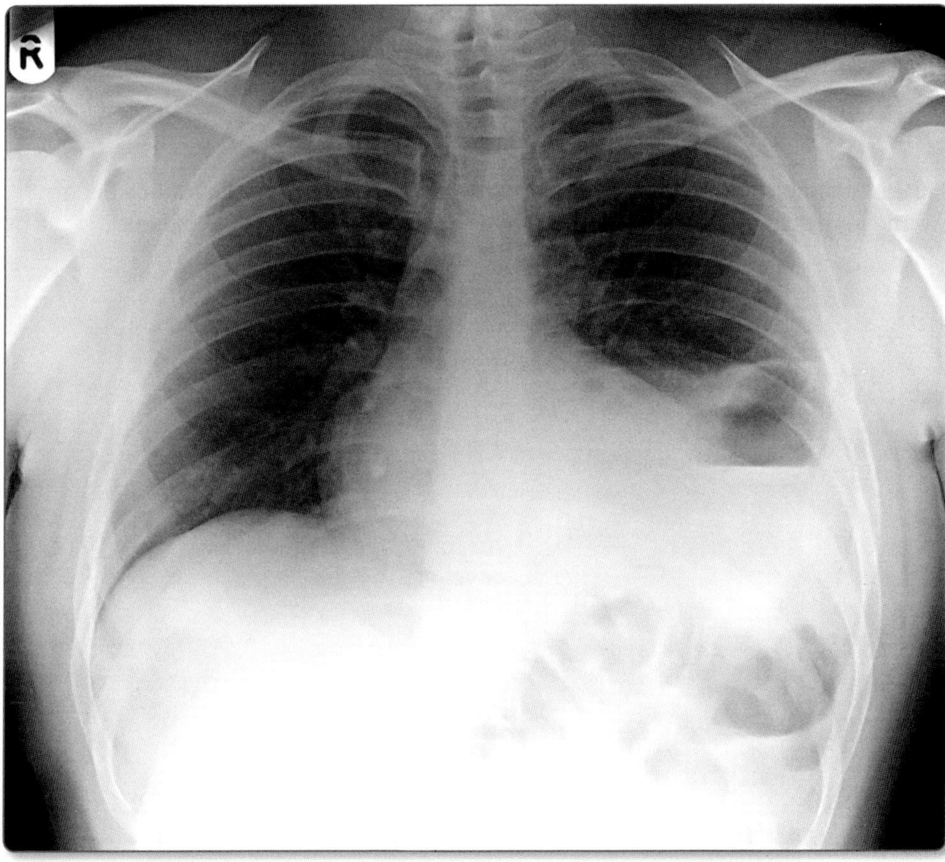

Suggested response

This is a frontal chest radiograph of a skeletally mature patient. There is an abnormality at the left lung base. The left hemidiaphragm is neither clearly visualised in its usual location nor is the air bubble of the gastric fundus, although a loop of bowel is evident in the left upper quadrant of the abdomen. There is an air-fluid level at the left base and the left heart border is partly obscured. The left upper and mid zones appear normal with no evidence of pneumothorax or rib fractures. The right lung is also normal. The nonvisualisation of the gastric fundus and left hemidiaphragm in their normal locations suggests either a left-sided diaphragmatic hernia or rupture.

The overall clinical picture is important in this case. If there has been a history of trauma I would be concerned about diaphragmatic rupture, although the lack of ancillary features of recent trauma on this radiograph makes me suspect the findings may be more long-standing. Review of available previous imaging may help to confirm this. Further possibilities include air-fluid levels within a left lower zone cavitating lung lesion or hydropneumothorax, although these do not explain the nonvisualised gastric bubble. I would discuss the case with the referring clinician and plan management and imaging in the light of a more detailed clinical history. Cross-sectional imaging may make a useful contribution to further define the abnormality.

Diagnosis

Left hemidiaphragmatic hernia in an adult male occurring following trauma (stab wound to the chest) several years earlier (see **Figure 1** from the same patient).

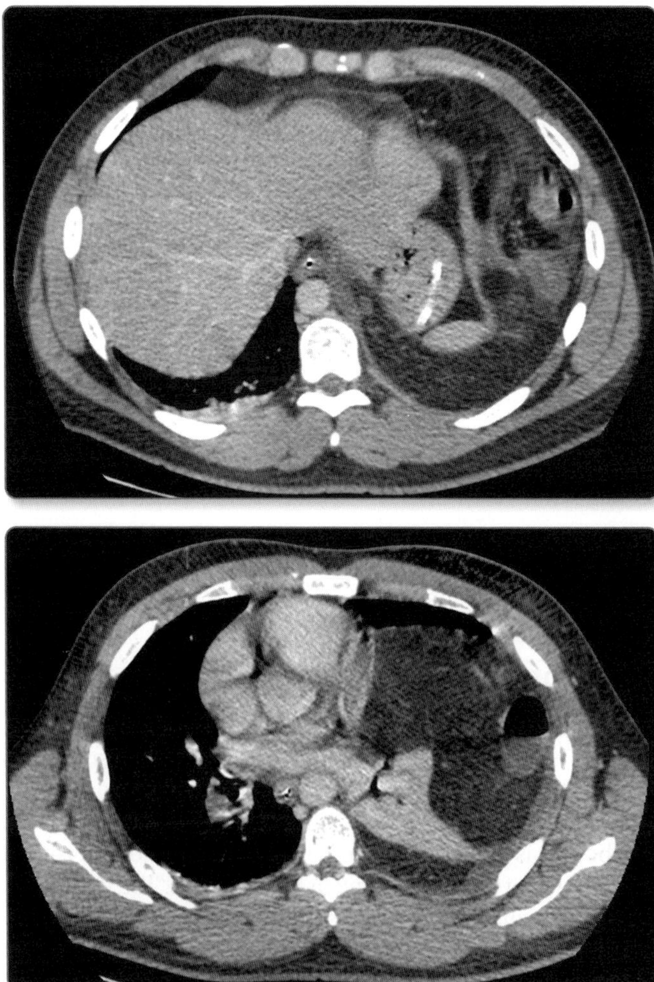

Figure 1 Axial CT images from the same patient.

Tips: Suspected diaphragmatic hernia

Key points

When evaluating the diaphragm, it is important to consider the possibility of an eventration (where the diaphragm is weakened but intact and the abdominal contents are displaced superiorly), which is usually right-sided with a lobulated contour.

Traumatic diaphragmatic rupture is usually left-sided, may be secondary to blunt or penetrating trauma and may present months or years after the traumatic event.

Congenital diaphragmatic herniae give variable imaging appearances, dependent on the type (e.g. Bochdalek and Morgagni), and usually present in children. They are more commonly left-sided and associated anomalies are not uncommon.

Bochdalek herniae are more common, tend to present in babies and the majority are left-sided with a posterolateral defect (BochdaLEk are Back and Left). Morgagni herniae tend to present in older children and the majority are right-sided with an anteromedial (cardiophrenic angle) defect (morgAgNi is Anterior).

Differential diagnosis

Consider other causes of a raised 'hemidiaphragm' such as a subpulmonic effusion (where the 'dome' moves laterally towards the costophrenic angle; this is not a true hemidiaphragm elevation), loss of lung volume, phrenic nerve palsy or intra-abdominal abnormalities (e.g. colonic interposition and subphrenic abscess).

Traumatic diaphragmatic hernia

Symptoms may manifest years after the traumatic insult (whether a blunt or penetrating injury). The imaging findings in this case are typical, with nonvisualisation of the left hemidiaphragm (right side affected in around 10% of cases) and herniation of abdominal contents (most commonly stomach, colon and small bowel) into the thorax. If a nasogastric tube is present, it has a characteristic 'U' bend since the gastro-oesophageal junction remains normally sited. Strangulation is reported far more often in traumatic diaphragmatic herniae than in other types of diaphragmatic hernia. On CT scanning, it is most readily appreciated on sagittal and coronal images.

Case 78

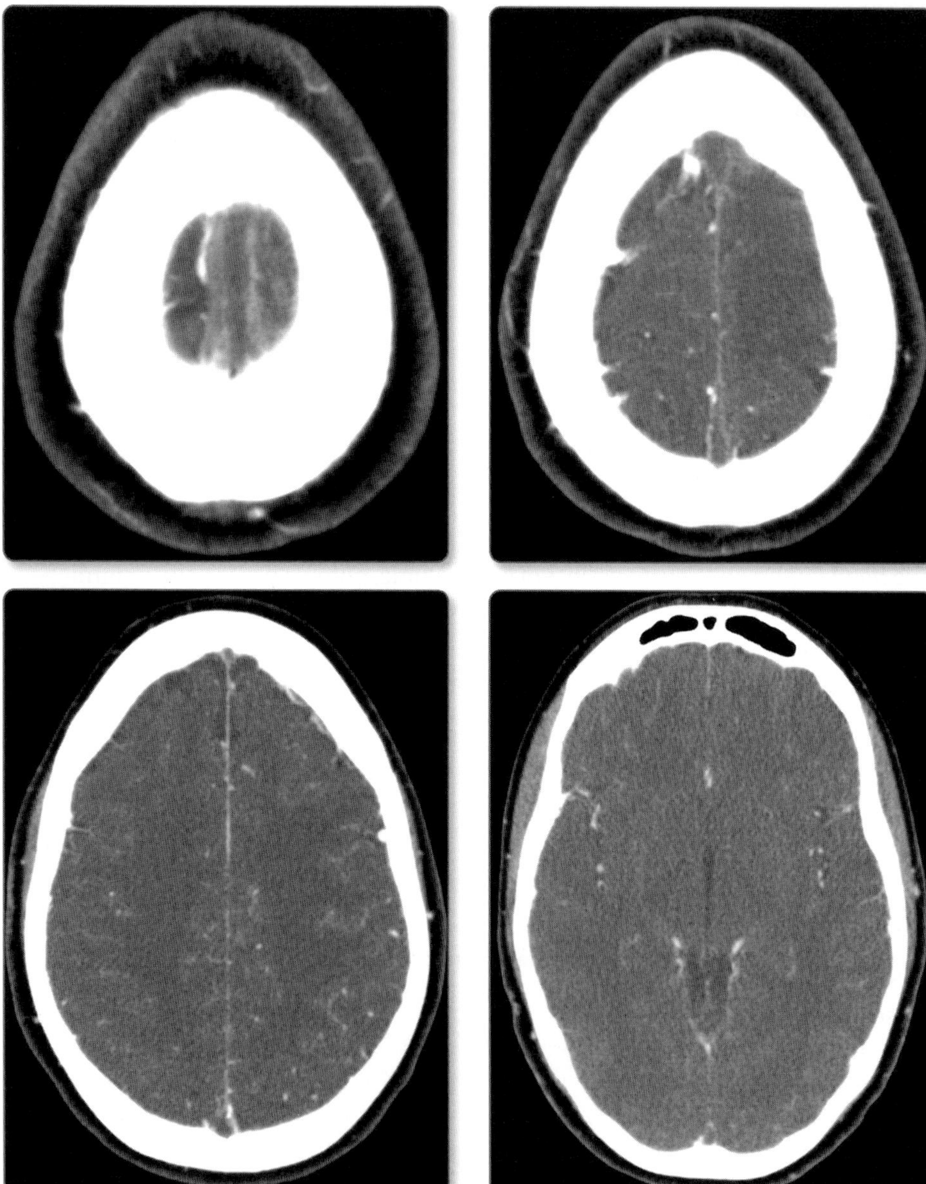

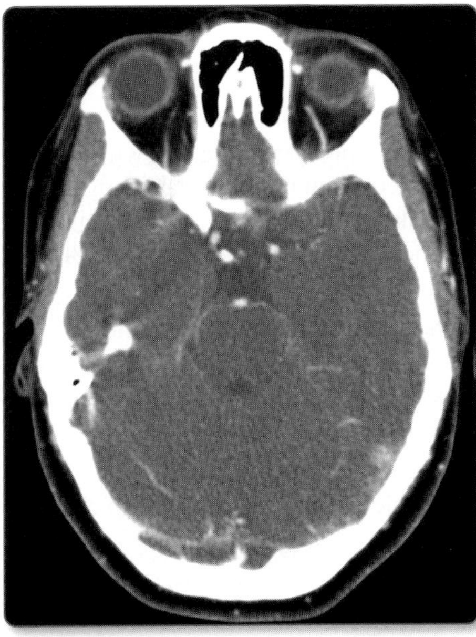

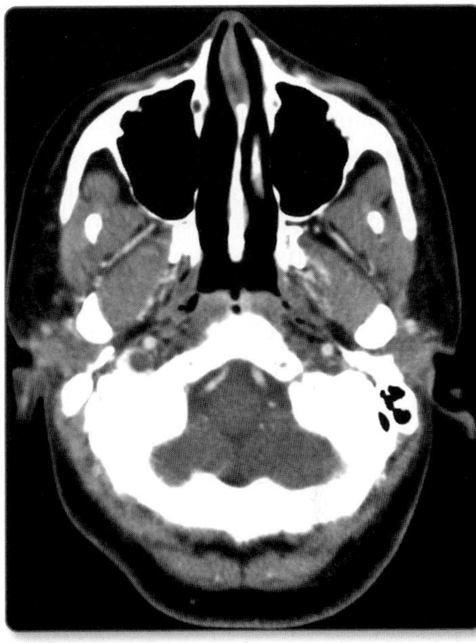

Suggested response

These are selected axial images from a postcontrast CT brain study which appears to have been windowed to evaluate the intracranial vasculature. None of the dural venous sinuses, including the transverse and sigmoid sinuses, appear to be opacified. The 'reverse delta' sign is evident in the superior sagittal sinus. Filling defects are also evident in both internal jugular veins. A high-attenuation crescent of contrast is evident around the filling defect in the right internal jugular vein implying that the contrast phase is truly venous and is optimised for evaluation of the venous sinuses. The most likely explanation for the nonopacification of the venous sinuses is extensive thrombosis.

An area of low attenuation in the left frontal lobe is suggestive of an infarct, although I would routinely review the whole study on brain windows in addition to these selected images. What is seen of the intracranial arterial system is unremarkable, although again I would routinely review all available imaging. If this is the initial diagnostic examination, I would discuss this case with the referring clinicians urgently.

Diagnosis

Extensive dural sinus thrombosis in an adult patient presenting with headache and neurological symptoms following a viral infection.

Tips: Defects in the dural venous sinuses

Key points

On unenhanced CT, look for hyperattenuation in the dural venous sinuses, although false positives may occur with a raised haematocrit in polycythaemia and with reduced brain density (young children). A clue to this is that the attenuation of all blood, including arterial, will be increased. Also look for the 'cord' sign, resulting from thrombosed veins, and venous infarcts, which do not follow the arterial territories and are often haemorrhagic. Also specifically look at the paranasal sinuses.

On enhanced CT, consider if the filling defects are focal or widespread and check for any abnormal enhancement that could be responsible for dural sinus thrombosis, such as subdural empyema or intracranial abscess. Consider if the focal filling defects could be due to large arachnoid granulations, which tend to be rounded.

On MRI, any signal change in thrombosis varies with the age of the blood. Hypointense T2 signal in chronic thrombus may mimic normal signal void and chronic thrombus may enhance as it becomes organised.

Anatomically small/absent sinuses can mimic dural sinus thrombosis on MRI or CT venography.

The bone contour may be helpful as if there is a diminutive impression on the skull, this tends to imply a constitutionally small sinus rather than a thrombosis. Conversely, with a large impression on the bone, a nonopacified sinus is more likely to be due to thrombus.

Dural sinus thrombosis

Dural sinus thrombosis may be clinically unsuspected and carries a high mortality rate, despite being potentially treatable. Both the clinical presentation and the radiographic findings can be very subtle, hence dural venous sinuses should form a critical review area on imaging of the brain. It often occurs spontaneously, but secondary causes include coagulation disorders, dehydration, trauma and sepsis (intracranial and otherwise). The latter two groups in particular may have ancillary findings on CT scanning which should be sought carefully.

There is a range of findings on imaging, but on CT scans the combination of the 'delta sign' (hyperattenuation of the superior sagittal/straight sinuses) and 'reverse delta sign' (filling defect on venography surrounded by a triangle of enhancement) are strongly suggestive.

Case 79

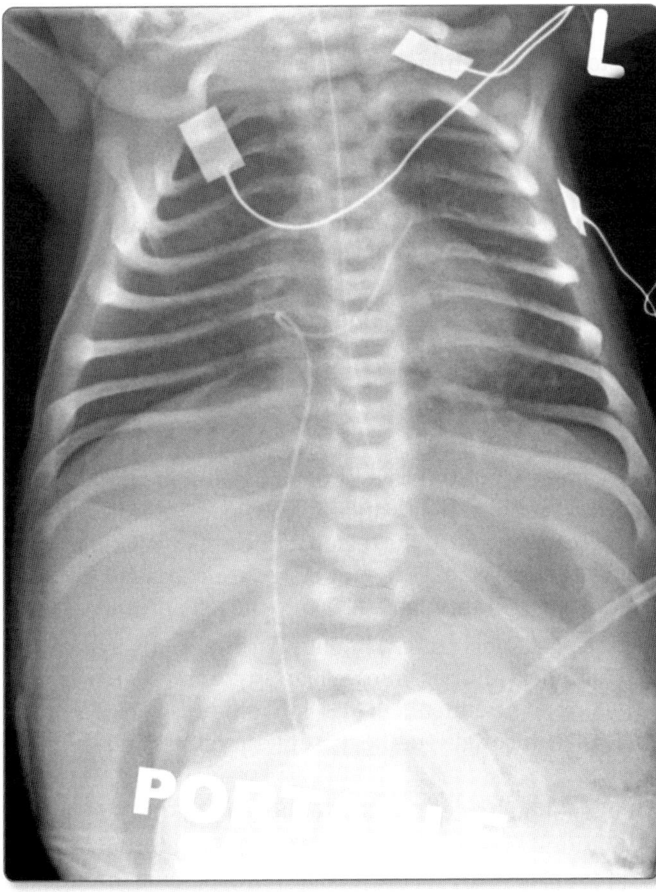

Suggested response

This is a supine chest and abdominal radiograph of an infant. There are cardiac monitoring leads and a nasogastric tube is in an apparently satisfactory position. A further line, presumably vascular and most likely a long-line or peripherally inserted central catheter (PICC), is seen to pass superiorly from below the inferior extent of this film along the anticipated course of the inferior vena cava (IVC). It appears to kink in the right atrium, with the tip crossing the midline to be projected over the left atrium. This could be explained by inadvertent passage of the venous line through a patent foramen ovale (PFO).

The cardiothymic contour is within normal limits. There is minor parahilar haziness, which is a rather nonspecific finding in a supine radiograph in a patient of this age. Further tubing is projected over the lower abdomen which I think is most likely to be outside the patient.

I would discuss this patient with the referring clinicians as the venous line should be retracted to minimise the risk of cardiac complications.

Diagnosis

Peripherally inserted central catheter passing through a PFO into the left atrium in a 4-day-old infant.

Tips: Paediatric lines and tubes

There are important considerations when reviewing lines and tubes placed in paediatric patients (particularly neonates). Accurate line placement can be more difficult than in adults due to their smaller size, altered anatomy or a range of different pathologies. Be aware of not only incorrectly sited lines and tubes but also abnormal positions which indicate an underlying pathology or anatomical variant.

Key points

Umbilical venous catheters (UVCs) pass through the umbilicus and course superiorly via the umbilical vein, left portal vein, ductus venosus, middle/left hepatic vein and IVC. The tip should be projected in the region of the upper IVC/inferior cavoatrial junction. An unusual course of an UVC may be seen, e.g. passing laterally in the liver (portal venous placement) or through a PFO into the left atrium.

Umbilical arterial catheters (UACs) initially pass inferiorly in the pelvis through one of the paired umbilical arteries, into an iliac artery and then pass superiorly into the aorta. The tip can be either high (T6–T10) or low (L3–L5). Intermediate tip positions could involve the origins of the mesenteric vessels and should generally be repositioned.

Long lines/PICCs should have their tips in the inferior SVC (for upper limb placement) or superior IVC (for lower limb placement). Look out for lines coiling back on themselves, flipping up (e.g. into the jugular vein), passing through a PFO into the left atrium or passing through the tricuspid valve into the right ventricle.

A nasogastric tube coiled in the proximal aerodigestive tract in a neonate should raise suspicions of oesophageal atresia (look for the gastric bubble). In left-sided congenital diaphragmatic hernia, the tip of the tube may be projected in the left hemithorax.

For endotracheal tubes, the shorter but variable length of the trachea in young children makes accurate placement more difficult. Look for inadvertent bronchial passage or oesophageal intubation, in which gaseous distension of the oesophagus, stomach and bowel may be seen.

Patent foramen ovale

Strictly speaking, patency of the foramen ovale is a normal finding in neonates and as such is not 'pathological' in the case shown above, but merely an indicator of an unsatisfactorily sited PICC line. Reversal of atrial pressure gradients at birth (with left exceeding right) is usually sufficient to physiologically seal this interatrial communication. A PFO is diagnosed when this communication persists after the age of 1 year. It is typically asymptomatic but has been implicated in migraines and in decompression illness in subaqua divers and is an important cause of stroke in younger patients due to passage of a paradoxical embolus.

Case 80

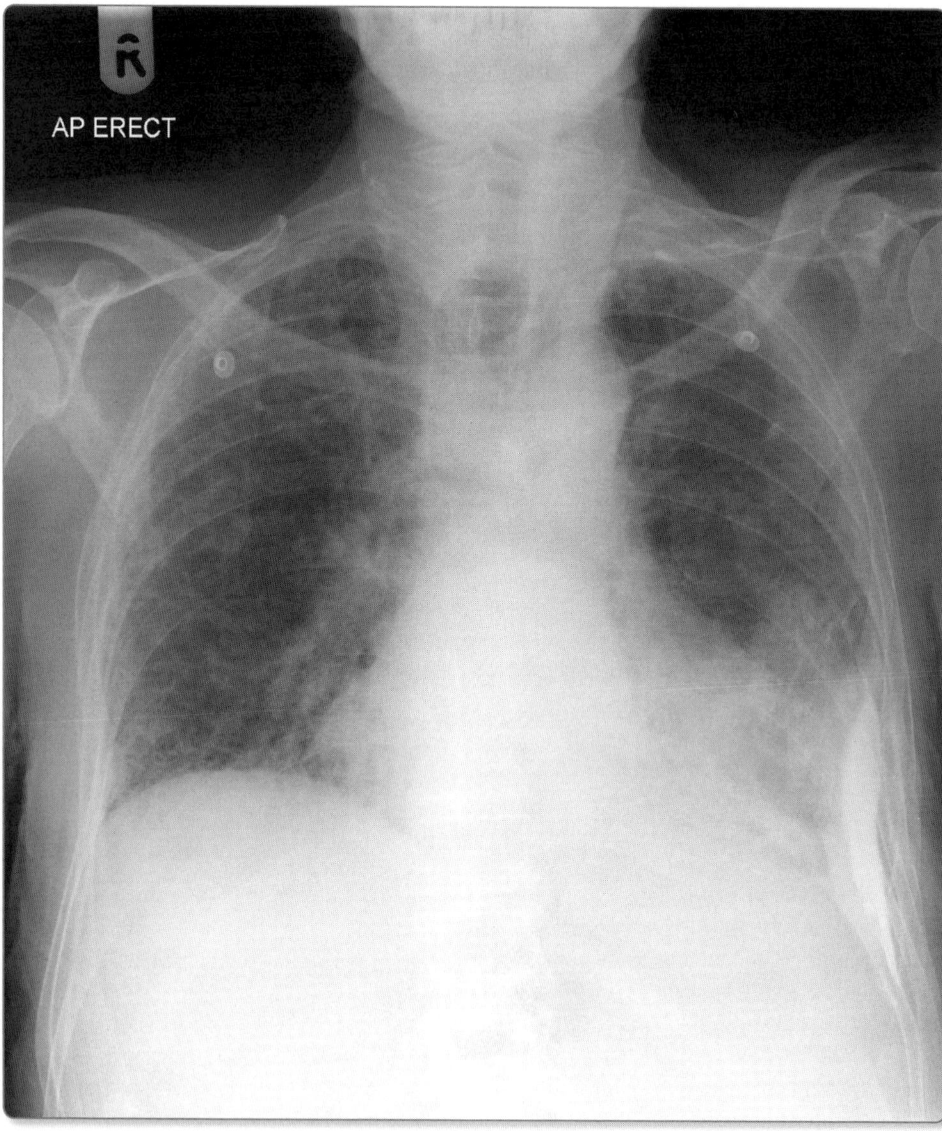

Suggested response

This is a rotated anteroposterior erect chest radiograph of a skeletally mature patient. There is loss of volume of both lungs. An area of dense calcification is projected peripherally within the left hemithorax, extending from level of the 6th to 10th ribs laterally. The superior aspect of a relatively well-defined opacity is projected medial to this. The appearance is most in keeping with calcified pleural plaque disease. There are also increased interstitial markings bilaterally, predominantly at the bases and most conspicuous on the right. These are in keeping with fibrotic lung disease with basal predominance. Although there is a broad differential for this, if there is an appropriate occupational history and in light of the pleural plaques, then the most likely diagnosis is pulmonary asbestosis. Review of any available relevant previous imaging would be useful to assess for change or, if this is the first presentation, respiratory referral and high-resolution chest CT is advisable in the first instance.

Diagnosis

An 81-year-old with pulmonary asbestosis.

Tips: Lower zone interstitial lung disease

Key points and differential diagnosis

If relatively symmetrical, lower zone fibrosis tends not to be inhalational (asbestosis is the important exception to this) and usual interstitial pneumonia (UIP) is by far the most common cause. If asymmetrical, consider radiotherapy, chronic aspiration and lymphangitis carcinomatosa (unilateral if secondary to bronchogenic carcinoma, otherwise bilateral).

Look for ancillary findings that suggest a particular diagnosis. For instance, oesophageal dilatation (seen in scleroderma and chronic aspiration), pulmonary mass or mastectomy (lymphangitis carcinomatosa), pleural plaques (asbestosis), soft tissue calcification (dermatomyositis), shoulder joint or cervical spine abnormalities (rheumatoid arthritis) and hilar/mediastinal nodes (various causes but make asbestosis less likely).

Pulmonary asbestosis

Exposure to asbestos (often occupational, e.g. in textile manufacturing or shipbuilding) can give rise to a spectrum of conditions, including malignant mesothelioma and pleural plaque disease. The term 'asbestosis' specifically refers to the chronic fibrotic interstitial lung disease that occurs secondary to asbestos exposure. There may be a latent period of 20+ years. Interstitial fibrosis is most marked in subpleural regions and is seen in the posterior lung bases, hence high-resolution CT should be performed with the patient lying prone to facilitate differentiation from physiological dependent changes. Note that the presence of calcified pleural plaques **(Figure 1)** does not indicate a diagnosis of asbestosis (which is parenchymal) but merely suggests a history of asbestos exposure. Asbestos exposure is associated with five chest conditions: transient pleural effusion, pleural plaques, asbestosis, lung cancer, and mesothelioma. In many jurisdictions it is treated as an occupational disease where compensation may be payable and additional scrutiny after death, such as referral to the coroner in the UK, is required even if that occurs due to unrelated factors.

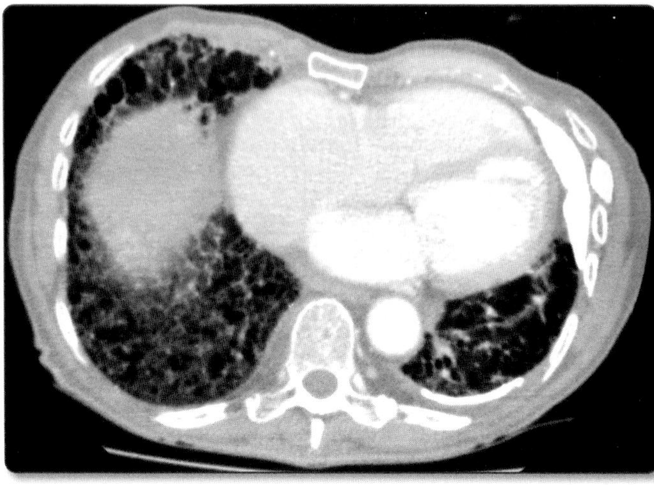

Figure 1 Axial CT image on lung windows from this case, showing right basal pulmonary fibrosis with left basal pleural plaques.

Case 81

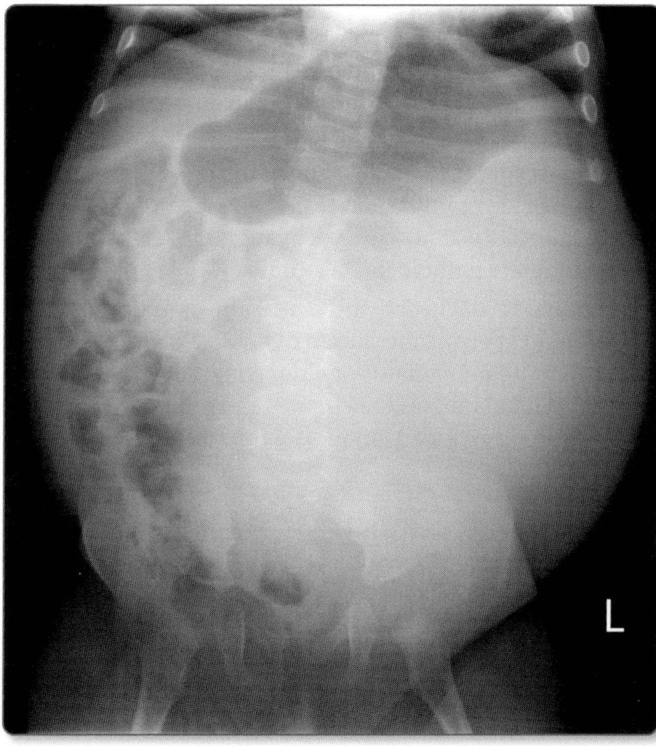

Suggested response

This is an abdominal radiograph of a skeletally immature patient and the stage of bone development suggests a child within the first year of life. There is abdominal distension. Gas is evident in the stomach and rectum which appear to be normally sited. Aside from these, nondistended bowel loops are almost entirely confined to the right flank, with appearances suggestive of displacement by a large left-sided mass. No abnormal calcification is identified. There are no further pertinent findings. Whilst review of available previous imaging would be relevant if available, the most likely causes of a left-sided abdominal mass of this size in a young child are either of renal origin, such as Wilms' tumour or hydronephrosis, or adrenal origin, namely neuroblastoma. I would discuss this case urgently with the paediatric team. If this is the initial presentation, an ultrasound scan should be performed in the first instance for further evaluation.

Diagnosis

Left-sided hydronephrosis in a 3-month-old infant (see also **Figure 1** from this case).

Tips: A paediatric abdominal mass

Key points and differential diagnosis

Look for displacement of bowel loops. They will be displaced laterally in flank pathology (as seen here), superiorly in pelvic pathology (e.g. hydrometrocolpos) and inferomedially in hepatic or splenic pathologies (e.g. hepatoblastoma). Look also for calcification, which is seen in hepatoblastoma and in 50% of neuroblastomas but in only 10% of Wilms' tumours.

It is important to consider the lateralisation of the mass. Renal/adrenal pathologies could manifest on either side or both sides (e.g. Wilms' tumour is bilateral in 5% of cases, polycystic kidneys are almost always bilateral). A left-sided mass makes appendiceal or hepatobiliary pathologies very unlikely.

The age of the patient is vital in arriving at a diagnosis (a useful reference is that the capital femoral epiphyses typically start to ossify at 2–8 months). Tumours are far less common in neonates than in infants or older children. Hydronephrosis is the most common cause of abdominal masses in neonates and multicystic dysplastic kidney is the second most common (Wilms' tumour is more common than this after the age of 1 year).

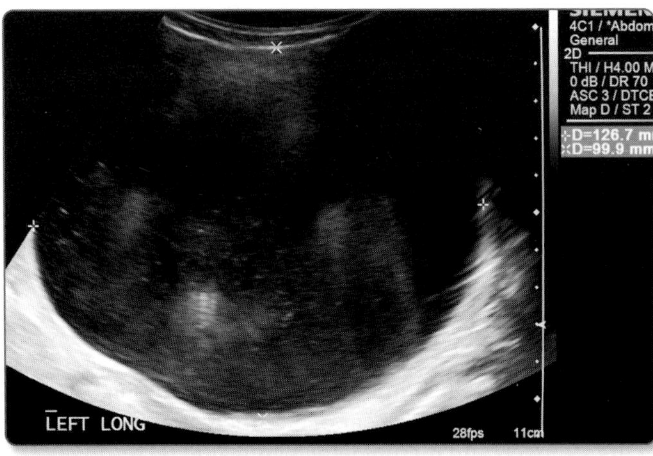

Figure 1 Ultrasound image from this case showing a grossly hydronephrotic left kidney.

Paediatric hydronephrosis

Hydronephrosis accounts for around one-quarter of all abdominal masses in neonates and is usually congenital. Pelviureteric junction obstruction (see also Case 24) is the most common cause.

Posterior urethral valves can present in male patients of any age but most commonly manifest in the first year of life. In such cases, there is vesicoureteric reflux (predominantly left-sided) with dilatation of the posterior urethra.

The presence of a duplex system predisposes to hydronephrosis of the upper moiety as a result of the ectopic upper moiety ureter obstructing at the insertion site secondary to stenosis or ureterocoele. The upper moiety ureter usually inserts inferomedially to the lower moiety ureter, as predicted by the Weigert–Meyer rule. The lower moiety ureter is prone to reflux.

Prune–belly syndrome is an 'Aunt Minnie' case, with a triad consisting of hypoplastic abdominal wall musculature, markedly dilated ureters (particularly in their lower thirds, with or without hydronephrosis) in the absence of obstruction and bilateral cryptorchidism. Varying degrees of renal dysplasia are seen and the bladder is characteristically dilated and elongated. Pulmonary hypoplasia is a common consequence.

Case 82

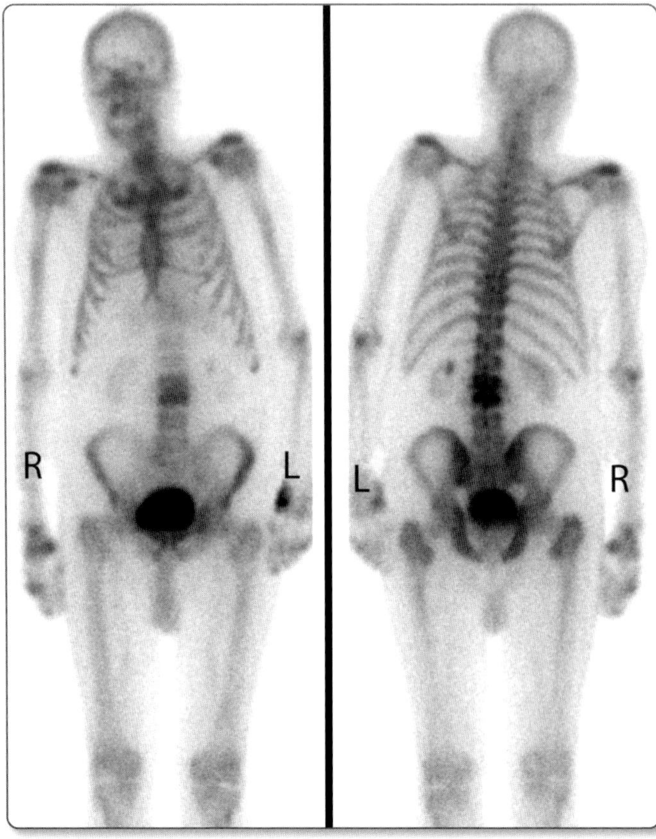

Suggested response

These are two views (anterior and posterior) from a radionuclide bone scan. The most striking abnormality is increased tracer uptake in the L3 and to a lesser degree L2 vertebrae. Uptake in the axial skeleton is otherwise within normal limits, allowing for features typical of degenerative disease. Increased tracer uptake in the left wrist most likely corresponds with the radioisotope injection site.

If this patient had a known primary malignancy, the bone scan findings could represent skeletal metastases. Alternatively, if the patient presents with a history of back pain and pyrexia of unknown origin or bacteraemia, then the findings are more likely to represent discitis. The findings could also be degenerative in origin, but this is less likely given the extent of vertebral body involvement. Review of any available relevant previous imaging would be helpful but, depending on the clinical picture, this patient is likely to require further imaging with MRI.

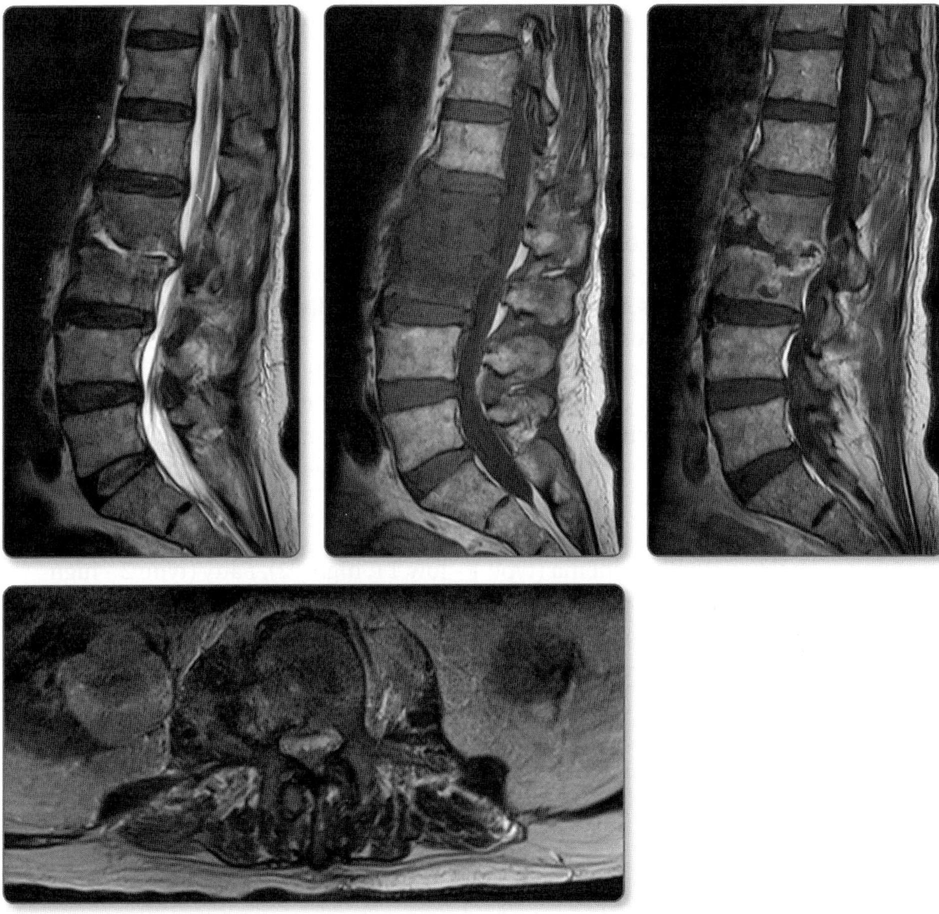

Suggested response

These are selected images from MRI of the lumbar spine with sagittal T2, T1, and T1 postcontrast imaging and axial T2 imaging. There is a cleft of fluid signal in the narrowed L2/L3 intervertebral disc space, with protrusion of disc material posteriorly into the spinal canal at this level. The L2 and L3 vertebrae are of heterogeneous but mostly low signal on T1 imaging compared with adjacent vertebrae, and there is avid enhancement following contrast administration. Axial T2 imaging demonstrates high signal in the adjacent psoas major muscles, most conspicuous on the left where there appears to be a focal collection. Incompletely visualised renal cysts are also evident.

The findings are most in keeping with discitis with psoas abscess formation. Appearances on sagittal imaging are concerning as they suggest cauda equina compression. I would therefore want to evaluate the remainder of the MRI scan to clarify the presence of nerve root involvement and also to evaluate the extent of abscess formation. I would discuss this case urgently with the referring clinicians and recommend immediate consultation with the spinal surgical team.

Diagnosis

L2/L3 discitis in an elderly male presenting with back pain.

Tips: Vertebral endplate changes

Key findings and differential diagnosis

Discitis and metastases can be differentiated as follows. Metastases may involve contiguous or noncontiguous vertebrae at any level but rarely involve the disc space, with the vertebral endplates remaining intact. Pyogenic discitis usually affects the lumbar spine and is rarely seen above T9 (except in intravenous drug users), with vertebral endplate destruction occurring (sclerosis and then bony fusion occur in later stages). Tuberculous discitis can, however, mimic metastases. This most commonly affects the thoracic spine and subligamentous spread can cause multiple noncontiguous vertebrae to be affected. Endplates/disc spaces are often apparently unaffected until a late stage.

Modic endplate changes are an important differential diagnosis for discitis. Remember MOFS – *M*odic: *O*edema (type 1 – low T1, high T2), *F*atty (type 2 – high T1 and T2) and *S*clerosis (type 3 – low T1 and T2). Modic type 1 changes can initially appear similar to discitis. However, the endplates remain intact, there is low or normal T2 signal in the disc space and paraspinal abscesses are not a feature.

Other relevant findings in discitis include relative preservation of posterior elements in the face of endplate destruction (the latter being characteristic of pyogenic discitis but not usually a feature of tuberculous discitis) and psoas abscesses (far more common in tuberculous discitis than pyogenic discitis).

Discitis

Discitis has a bimodal age distribution, with peaks in childhood and at around 50 years of age. In children, infection develops in the intervertebral disc itself due to its inherent vascularity. In adults, the disc lacks a blood supply, hence infection spreads from one vertebra to another via the disc. Nuclear medicine studies typically show diffuse uptake early in the disease with more focal uptake later on, but are of little use in assessing for postoperative discitis as they poorly differentiate between postoperative inflammation and discitis. MRI is more sensitive and specific. Plain film manifestations of discitis (e.g. loss of crispness of endplates and reduced disc space height) are often absent until a few weeks after the onset of symptoms. The appearance of early discitis overlaps with other diseases including common degenerative changes, and specialist advice and interval follow-up can be invaluable.

Case 83

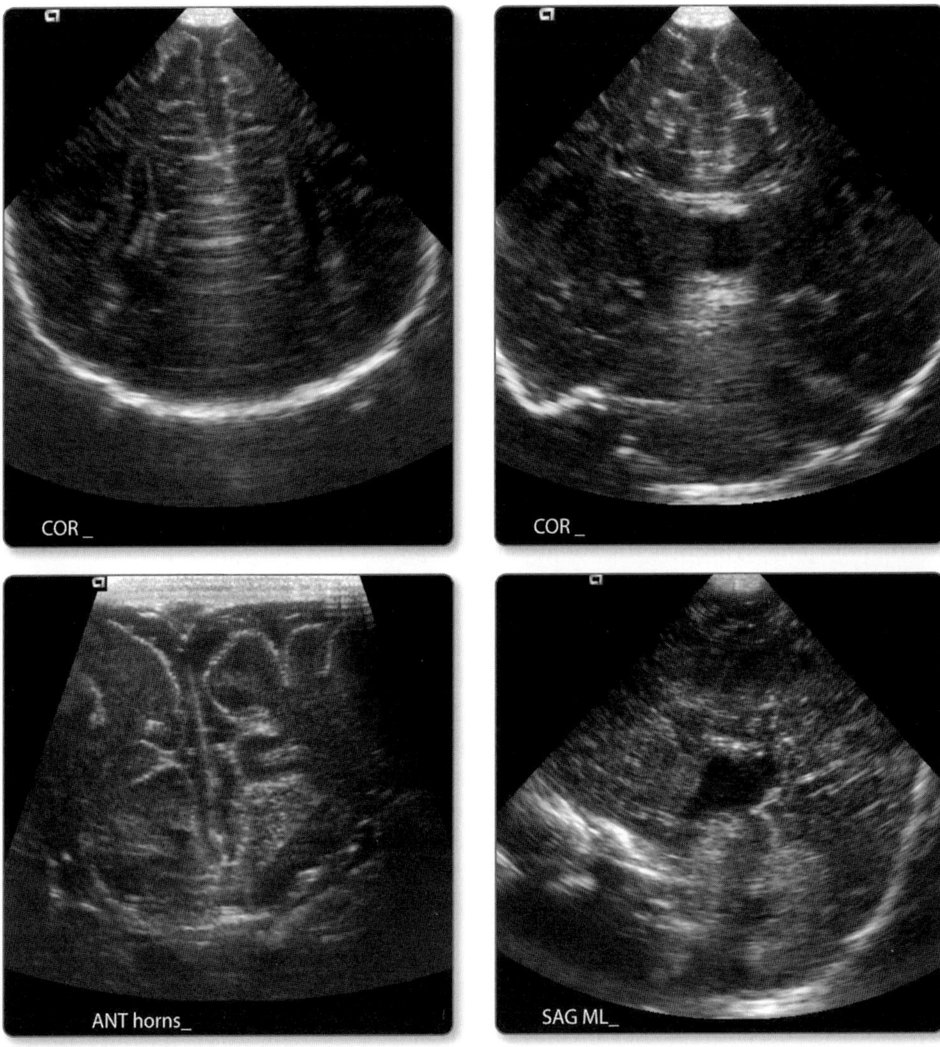

Suggested response

These are selected coronal and sagittal images from a cranial ultrasound scan, obtained by scanning through the fontanelle of a baby. The nondilated lateral ventricles are seen to be parallel but spaced widely apart, with a 'bat-wing' appearance on the coronal images and without a visible corpus callosum. The corpus callosum is again not identified on what I take to be a midline sagittal image (lower right image), and there is an abnormal pattern of gyri radiating from the 3rd ventricle. The visible extra-axial spaces appear normal and symmetrical. No further abnormalities are identified, although in my normal practice I would review the remaining images from the ultrasound scan. These findings are consistent at least with significant dysgenesis and possibly agenesis of the corpus callosum. I would want to discuss this case with the referring clinicians and further imaging with MRI may be appropriate to clarify the extent of the anomaly and to look for any associated abnormalities.

Diagnosis

Agenesis of the corpus callosum in a 2-month-old infant.

Tips: Paediatric cranial ultrasound

Paediatric cranial ultrasound scanning is highly specialised and in general examiners will not expect detailed knowledge of specialist techniques but will want to test anatomic knowledge and transferrable skills. You should at least have a reasonable understanding of the anatomy, of ultrasound and of the more common abnormalities.

Key points

Look for the presence or absence of normal structures (e.g. the corpus callosum is absent here). Look at the extra-axial spaces for findings such as subdural haematoma and hygroma. The subarachnoid space is normally <3.3 mm but widens in atrophy or macrocephaly. Look for masses and hydrocephalus. Ask yourself, 'Is the posterior fossa normal or are there features of Dandy–Walker spectrum?' Look at the resistive indices on Doppler imaging (normal range 0.6–0.9) which may be reduced (e.g. in hypoxic ischaemic brain injury) or elevated (e.g. in patent ductus arteriosus).

Look specifically for evidence of germinal matrix haemorrhage, scrutinise the caudothalamic groove (ensure you know where this is!) and look for blood in the groove/ventricles, hydrocephalus and cystic change (porencephalic cysts may form). Look also for evidence of periventricular leukomalacia such as hyperreflectivity adjacent to the ventricles and formation of cysts of varying sizes (depending on the grade). This can be differentiated from haemorrhage by the absence of mass effect.

Dysgenesis of the corpus callosum

Dysgenesis of the corpus callosum may be partial or, as seen in this case, complete (agenesis). It is commonly associated with other central nervous system abnormalities including midline lipomas, Chiari type II malformation, hydrocephalus and Dandy–Walker malformation, so carefully scrutinise the images for these associated findings. Corpus callosum dysgenesis may be detected antenatally.

In agenesis, cranial ultrasound reveals absence of the corpus callosum and septum pellucidum. A characteristic 'bat-wing' appearance is seen on coronal imaging, with widely separated parallel lateral ventricles. The third ventricle sits high and the occipital horns of the lateral ventricles are dilated. A 'sunburst' pattern of gyri is seen on sagittal imaging, with absence of the cingulate sulcus and radiation of the medial hemispheric sulci towards the third ventricle. If dysgenesis is partial, the genu (the first part of the corpus callosum to develop in utero) is invariably present.

Case 84

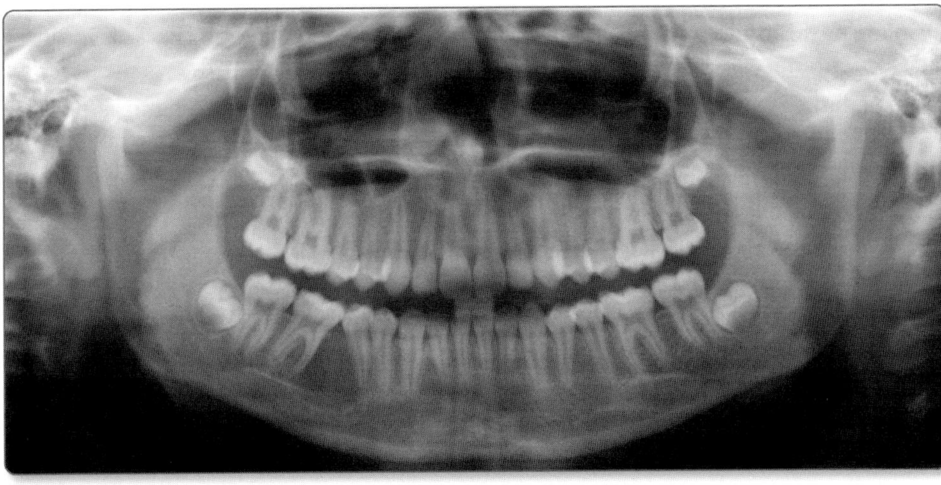

Suggested response

This is an orthopantomogram, probably of an adolescent as the wisdom teeth have not yet erupted. A well-defined rounded unilocular cystic lesion measuring around 2–3 cm in diameter is projected in the body of the right hemimandible between the roots of the lower right 5th and 6th teeth, which are displaced to either side of the lesion. There is a narrow zone of transition between the lesion and the body of the mandible, with a thin sclerotic rim inferiorly. There is no appreciable root resorption. No further lesions are demonstrated. The most likely differential diagnoses for a unilocular cyst in this location, in the presence of erupted teeth, are odontogenic keratocyst (OKC) and ameloblastoma.

Diagnosis

Odontogenic keratocyst in a 13-year-old girl.

Tips: A cystic lesion of the mandible

A number of mandibular masses are specific to the jaws and are often related to dentition. In general, however, such abnormalities should be described using the same terminology as bony lesions elsewhere in the body (see Cases 2 and 6), i.e. zone of transition, cortical destruction/expansion, multiplicity, periosteal reaction, internal matrix and location.

Key points and differential diagnosis

There are special considerations to be made when considering the location (including the relationship to the teeth). Is the lesion found at the apex of a tooth (radicular cyst, the most common mandibular cyst)? Does it involve an impacted/unerupted tooth [dentigerous cyst, ameloblastoma and OKC (typically 3rd molar)]? Does it lie anterior to first or second molars (giant cell granuloma and brown tumour)? Does it lie in the most vascular part of the mandible, the posterior body/angle (e.g. metastases)? Does it lie in the posterior body/ramus [ameloblastoma, OKC (unless it forms part of Gorlin–Goltz syndrome, which has multiple OKCs with no site predilection)]?

Locularity is another useful means of narrowing the differential diagnosis. Radicular and dentigerous cysts are unilocular. Brown tumours and giant cell granulomas are multilocular. Ameloblastomas (cystic and solid types) and OKCs may be either unilocular or multilocular.

Odontogenic keratocyst

Odontogenic keratocyst imaging appearances are variable, with a unilocular or multilocular lesion that is well-corticated, expansile and may cause cortical thinning as well as displacement of teeth and root resorption. It has a high recurrence rate following curettage as a consequence of daughter cysts outside the primary lesion. Multiple OKCs are a feature of Gorlin–Goltz syndrome, along with multiple cutaneous basal cell carcinomas and skeletal abnormalities (e.g. scoliosis, Sprengel's deformity of the shoulder).

Case 85

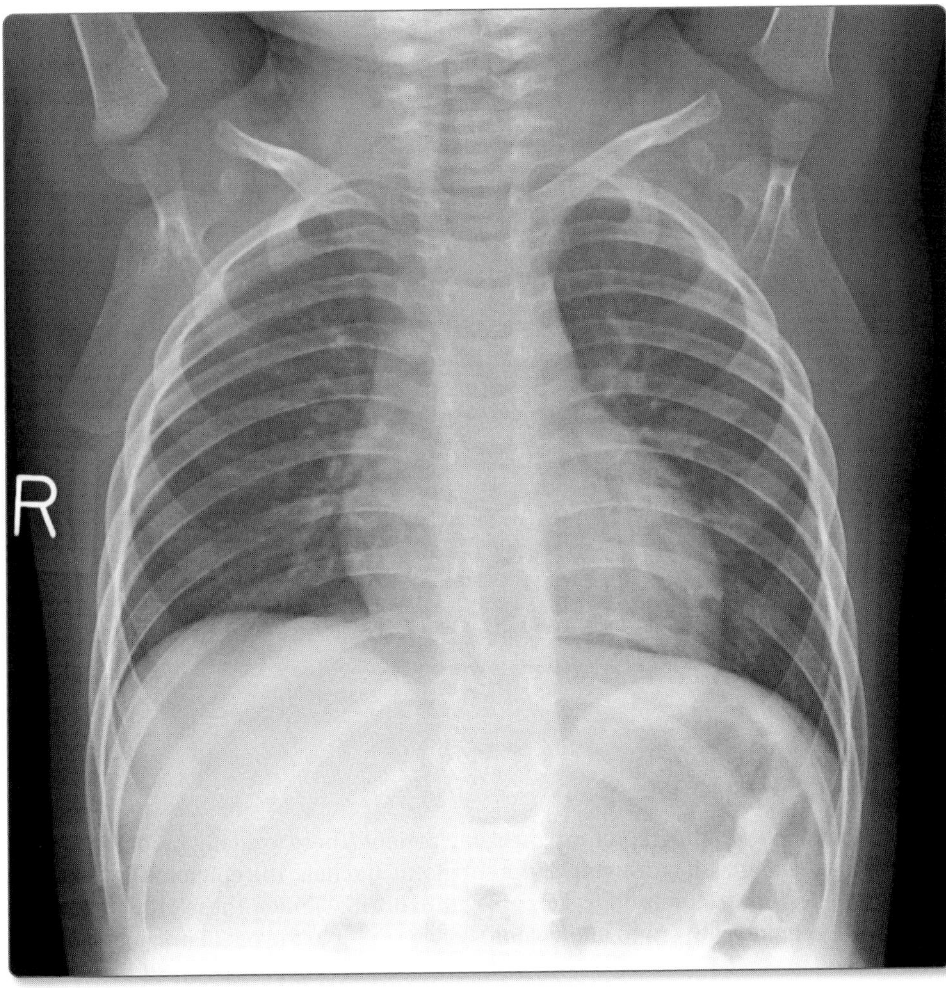

Suggested response

This is a frontal chest radiograph of a young child. The first thing to note is the presence of a 'steeple sign,' in keeping with narrowing of the trachea. There is also bilateral central peribronchial thickening and parahilar infiltrate. The lung volumes are preserved. There are no further pertinent findings. If there is a history of viral illness, then the most likely explanation for these appearances is croup, although epiglottitis cannot be excluded. The appearance could also result from other causes, such as ingestion of a caustic substance.

I would urgently discuss this case with the paediatric team.

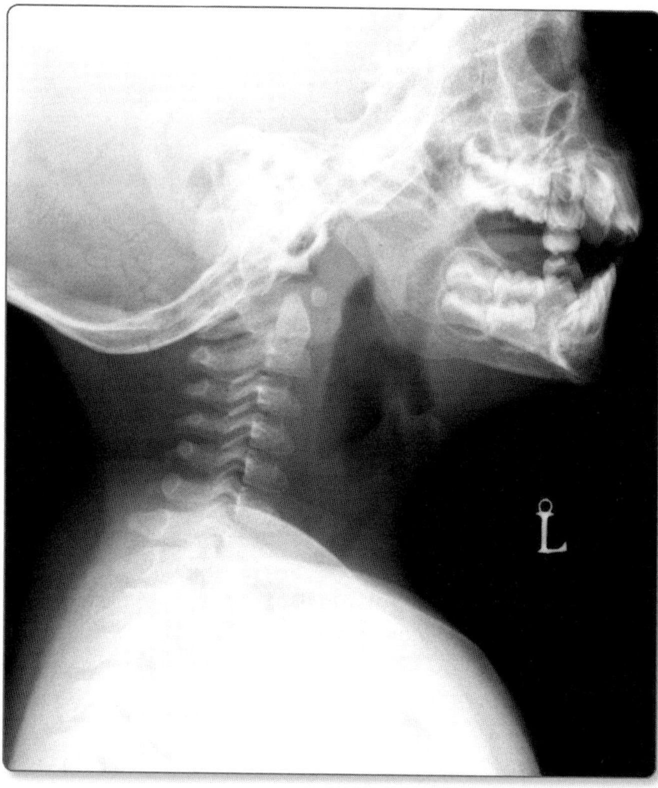

Suggested response

This is a lateral neck radiograph from the same patient. There is dilatation of the hypopharynx along with narrowing of the subglottic trachea. The epiglottis is unremarkable. Prevertebral soft tissues are within normal limits. These findings are most in keeping with croup and I would convey them to the paediatric team immediately.

Diagnosis

Caustic substance intake in an 18-month-old child causing a croup-like pattern of laryngotracheobronchitis.

Tips: Paediatric upper airways disease

Key points

Retropharyngeal abscesses usually present before 1 year of age and croup before 3 years of age. Epiglottitis usually affects those over 3 years old and peaks in incidence at the age of 6 years. The age distribution, however, is changing due to immunisation against *Haemophilus influenzae* and it is increasingly a disease of adults. The terminology is also evolving with 'supraglottitis' coming into use to reflect more varied pathogens and anatomical involvement.

On the lateral neck radiograph, look at the prevertebral soft tissues and assess for thickening (i.e. more than three-quarters of the anteroposterior diameter of a vertebral body, which may indicate an abscess or a haematoma) or gas within the tissues (indicating trauma or an abscess). Also specifically look for foreign bodies.

In epiglottitis, the aryepiglottic folds appear enlarged and thickened: 'thumb-like'. The trachea may be narrowed in epiglottitis, croup, and trauma, or for a number of congenital reasons (including a vascular ring), so look for any abrupt change in its calibre. Finally, inspect the adenoidal/tonsillar tissue for swelling.

Croup

Croup (acute laryngotracheobronchitis) is usually of viral aetiology, although a similar pattern of upper airway disease can be seen following aspiration of caustic substances, as in this case. A characteristic 'steeple' sign is seen on frontal radiographs, with an upturned 'V' replacing the normal shouldering of the air column. This highlights the importance of considering the trachea as a review area on chest radiographs. Findings on the lateral neck radiograph, including tracheal narrowing and hypopharyngeal dilatation, are nonspecific. The primary reason for performing lateral views is to exclude life-threatening epiglottitis, which often requires urgent intubation (unlike croup, which typically runs an indolent course). Radiographs for suspected epiglottitis should be acquired with the child in the erect position to reduce the risk of suffocation, and the mouth and oropharynx should not be examined unless suitably skilled and experienced doctors with advanced paediatric airway management skills (senior paediatric anaesthetists and ENT surgeons) are physically present.

Case 86

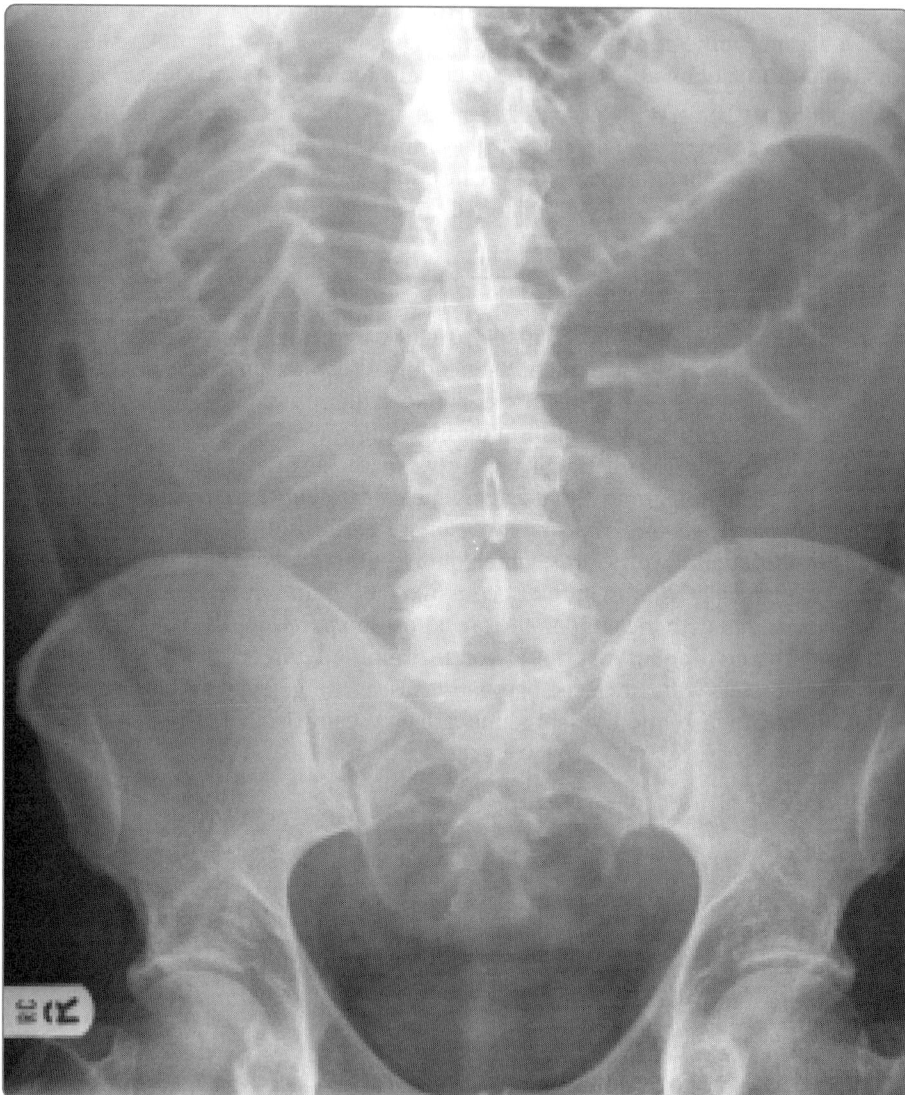

Suggested response

This is an abdominal radiograph of a skeletally mature patient. There are multiple gas-filled distended loops of bowel in the central abdomen with minimal gas visible within the colon, consistent with small bowel obstruction. The bones are unremarkable.

There are no features to suggest a perforation, but if this were a clinical concern, I would advise that an erect chest radiograph be performed to rule it out.

Review of any available previous relevant imaging would be useful to determine whether there has been previous abdominal imaging, for instance. However, I would immediately discuss the findings with the on-call surgical team and discuss whether any further imaging would be useful in the work-up of this patient.

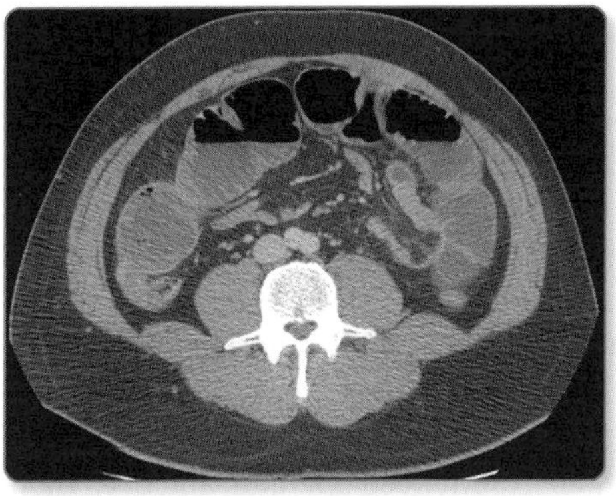

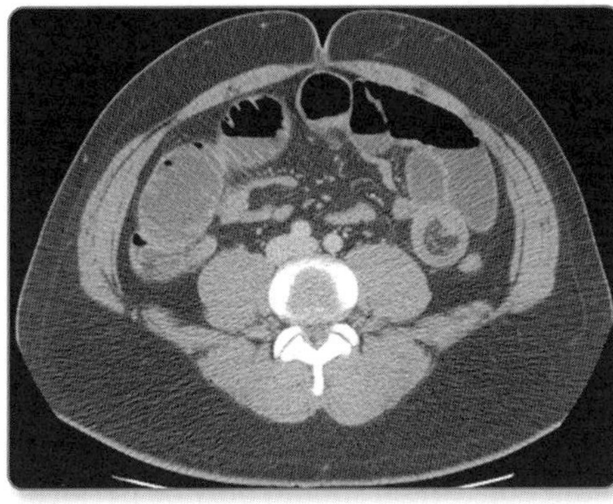

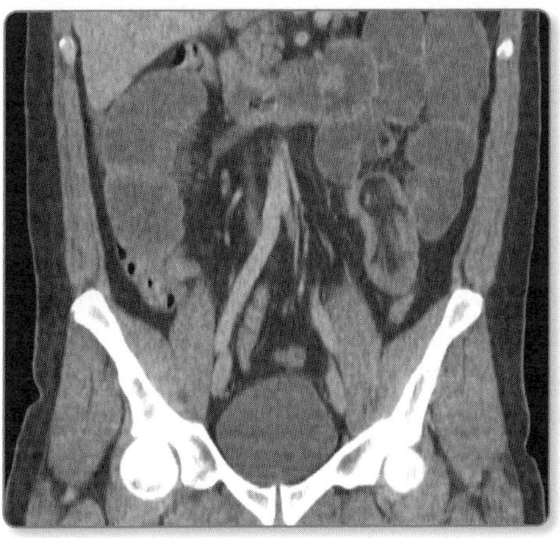

Suggested response

These are selected images from a contrast-enhanced CT study that confirms the finding of small bowel obstruction and demonstrates multiple fluid-filled loops in addition to the gas-filled loops that were visible on the plain film. In the left side of the abdomen, just above the pelvic brim, there is a target appearance with the impression of a segment of mesentery extending to form an intussusceptum. I suspect that the cause of this patient's obstruction is an intussusception.

In an adult patient, there is usually a lead point in an intussusception, and in the small bowel this is most likely to be a benign tumour, although I cannot identify a specific lesion on these images. The patient appears to have high-grade small bowel obstruction and I would urgently discuss the case with the on-call surgical team as it is quite likely that operative intervention will be necessary.

Diagnosis

Ileo-ileal intussusception causing small bowel obstruction secondary to an inflammatory fibroid polyp.

Tips: Intussusception

Key points

Intussusception is the most common cause of acquired bowel obstruction in children and is usually ileocolic. The vast majority are idiopathic (90%+); nevertheless, look for primary causes such as Meckel's diverticulum, polyps (for instance, in association with Peutz–Jeghers syndrome), intramural haematoma or a mesenteric cyst.

Ultrasound is usually the best first test in children. On transverse images look for the 'target' or 'doughnut' sign, and on longitudinal images look for the 'pseudokidney' sign.

Intussusceptions may be treated by hydrostatic (barium) or pneumatic (air) reduction, which should only be performed by an experienced operator, and even then only with surgical expertise immediately on hand. Look for the impression of a mass being progressively displaced by the column of air/barium and be alert for perforation, which is a complication of the procedure that would necessitate urgent surgery.

In adults there is usually a lead point (80–90%), with a neoplastic cause in 65% of cases. Transient incidental intussusceptions are quite commonly seen on CT scans, but intussusception causing obstruction is relatively rare. They are most commonly ileo-ileal (i.e. small bowel affected more than large bowel) and the differential for the lead point varies according to its position in the bowel. In the small bowel, benign tumours, Meckel's diverticulum and malignant tumours (including metastasis and lymphoma) should be considered, with malignant tumours, lymphoma, polyps and surgical anastomoses being the most common causes in the large bowel.

Intussusception

In intussusceptions, a proximal segment of the gastrointestinal tract (the intussusceptum) invaginates into an adjacent segment (the intussuscipiens), possibly at the site of a pathological lead point (more commonly in adults than children). There is no abnormality on plain film in one-quarter of cases, although a soft tissue mass is often seen, particularly in the right upper quadrant. In children, intussusceptions have recently decreased in incidence for reasons that are not well understood but are thought to relate to increased vaccination.

Case 87

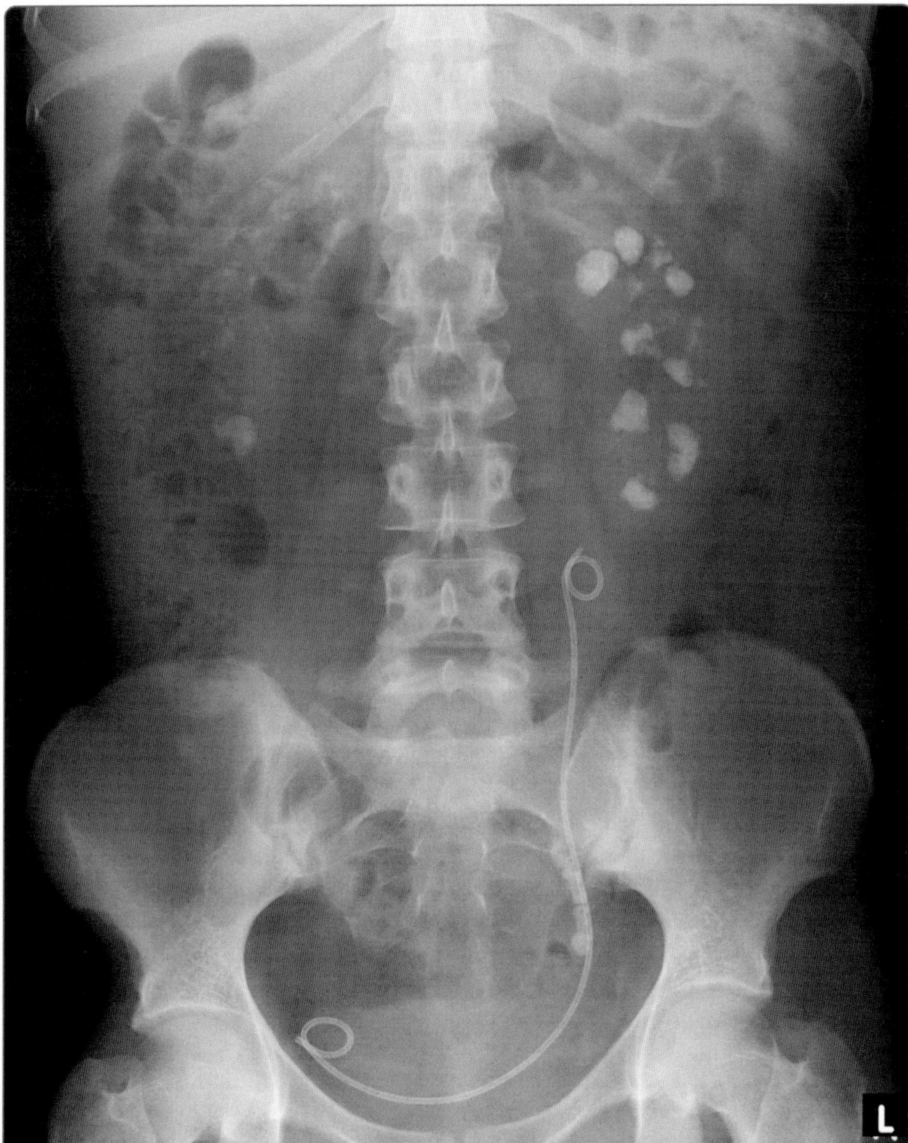

Suggested response

This is an abdominal radiograph of a skeletally mature patient. There are dense calcifications projected over both renal outlines, most conspicuous on the left. Although the renal outlines are partly obscured by bowel gas on both sides, the distribution of calcifications suggests a medullary distribution. The kidneys appear to be of at least normal size. A plastic stent is noted with its proximal aspect projected over the mid left ureter and its distal aspect projected over the bladder, consistent with a migrated left ureteric stent. A row of calcifications projected in the distal left ureter alongside the stent is likely to represent steinstrasse ('stone street') calculi.

The findings are most in keeping with medullary nephrocalcinosis with associated ureteric calculi and complicated by migration of a left ureteric stent. The most likely causes include medullary sponge kidney and metabolic disturbances such as hyperparathyroidism, although no ancillary features of hyperparathyroidism are evident on this radiograph. Given the ureteric stent migration, I would discuss this case with the urologists and, if not previously known about, would offer to perform an ultrasound to assess for hydronephrosis.

Diagnosis

Adult female with medullary sponge kidney and migrated left ureteric stent with steinstrasse calculi in left ureter.

Tips: Bilateral renal tract calcifications

Key points

Decide if the calcification is medullary or cortical.

Medullary calcification is far more common (approximately 95% of cases) than cortical calcification. Calcifications form in the renal pyramids and predispose to calculus formation. The kidneys are usually of normal size (but may be large in medullary sponge kidney). Calcification is commonly caused by a metabolic disturbance such as hyperparathyroidism or renal tubular acidosis. Therefore, look for ancillary features of these diseases including bony changes, vascular calcification and pancreatic calcification (hyperparathyroidism) and osteomalacia/rickets (renal tubular acidosis). Most dystrophic causes are unilateral, such as infection, but renal papillary necrosis is often bilateral.

With cortical nephrocalcinosis the kidneys are often small and there is classically a 'tramline' appearance to the calcification, but it may appear punctate with calcifications between viable and non-viable renal tissue. Cortical nephrocalcinosis is a late sign of acute cortical necrosis which is often associated with complicated obstetric cases.

Calculi are more likely to be bilateral if there is an underlying metabolic cause (e.g. hyperparathyroidism).

Medullary sponge kidney

In a medullary sponge kidney, there is abnormal dilatation of the renal collecting tubules with cystic cavity formation, predisposing to calculus formation and giving a 'bunch of grapes' appearance. As such, it is technically not a true cause of medullary nephrocalcinosis, although you should include it in your differential diagnosis given the imaging similarities. It is usually bilateral but can affect a single kidney or part of one kidney. Cystic cavities may be evident in the medulla. A striated nephrogram may be seen on intravenous urography, due to contrast within ectatic ducts. Associations include Caroli's disease and Beckwith–Wiedemann syndrome. Treatment is rarely required unless there are complications of calculus disease such as hydronephrosis, as happened in this case.

Case 88

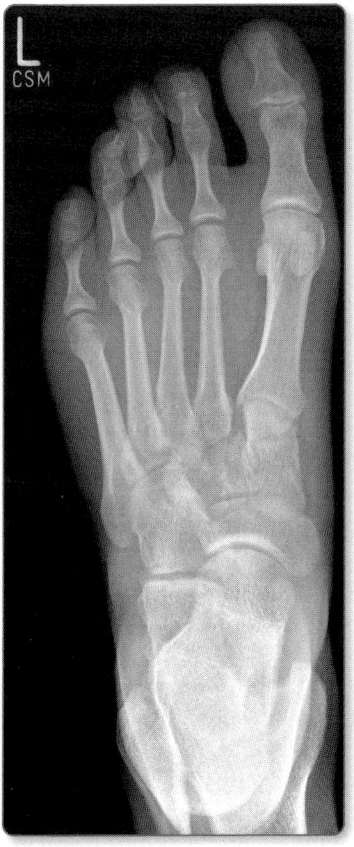

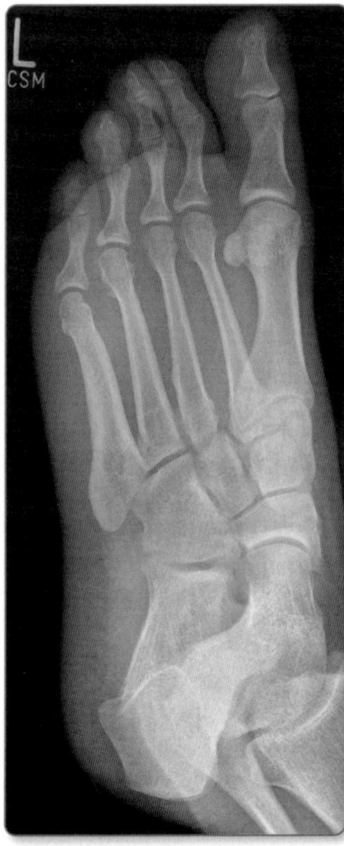

Suggested response

These are dorsoplantar (DP) and oblique views of the left foot in a skeletally mature patient.

The alignment at the Lisfranc joint is abnormal, with lateral subluxation of the base of the third metatarsal compared to the medial border of the lateral cuneiform on the oblique film, and also malalignment between the medial borders of the second metatarsal and the middle cuneiform on the DP view.

The appearance is consistent with an injury involving the Lisfranc joint, which is likely to be unstable. In addition, on the DP view a lucent line extends proximally from the distal surface of the middle cuneiform in the sagittal plane, which in the current context is very suspicious for a fracture.

I would urgently report the films and would ensure that referring clinicians were aware of the injury and that the patient was under the care of an appropriate orthopaedic surgeon. Further imaging may be necessary to guide management.

Diagnosis

Lisfranc fracture/dislocation.

Tips: Foot and ankle trauma

Key points

Injuries are often subtle, so look round the cortical margins of each and every bone. As well as being hard to identify, fractures may also be very complex, so CT is frequently helpful to exclude a fracture (if clinical suspicion is high) or to further evaluate complex injuries.

When reviewing the radiograph, check the alignment along the Lisfranc articulations and specifically look for a fracture at the base of the fifth metatarsal (an unfused apophysis lies parallel to the long axis of bone whereas a fracture line runs perpendicular to it). Also inspect the calcaneum for Bohler's angle (a normal angle is >30°; if the angle is <30° then a fall from a height should be suspected and imaging of the hip and spine may be advisable), an anterior process fracture or a tarsal coalition (not a traumatic injury but a cause of foot pain). Calcaneonavicular coalitions ('anteater sign') are more common than talocalcaneal coalitions ('continuous C sign'). Also check for osteochondral defects, particularly at the talar dome, and beware of distal fibular fractures on foot radiographs.

Lisfranc injuries

The midfoot and forefoot articulate at the Lisfranc joint, which comprises five tarsometatarsal joints. The Lisfranc ligament runs between the lateral margin of the medial cuneiform and medial/plantar aspect of the base of the second metatarsal. Injury to the ligament may or may not be associated with a fracture but should nevertheless be given full recognition due to the significant risk of long-term disability if missed. On a DP view, the medial borders of the second metatarsal and middle cuneiform should normally be in alignment. On a medial oblique view, the medial borders of the cuboid and fourth metatarsal should usually be aligned. Loss of these features together with an increased distance (>2 mm) between the bases of the first and second metatarsals strongly suggests a Lisfranc injury.

Case 89

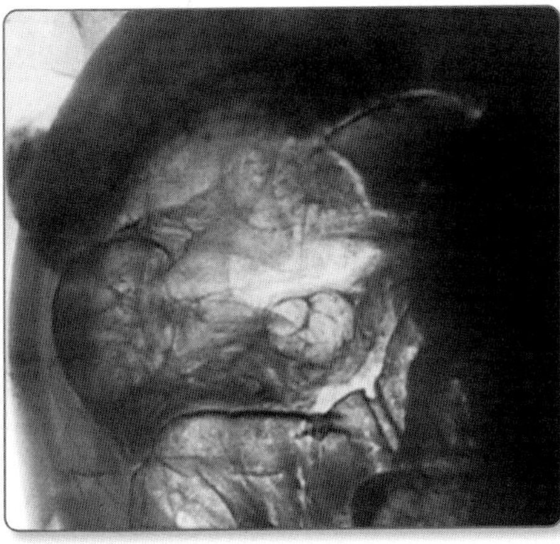

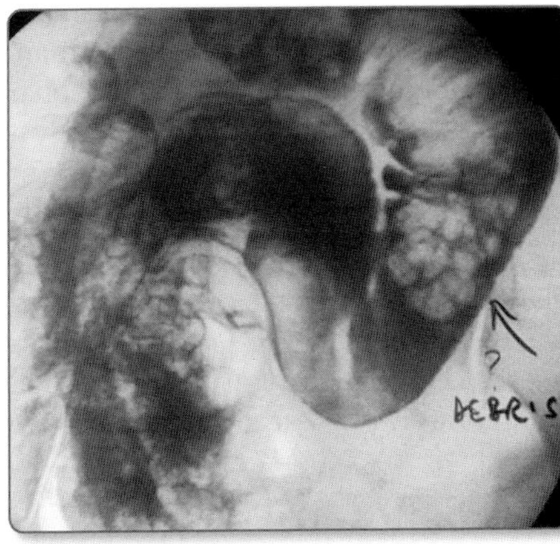

Suggested response

This is a pair of spot images from a barium follow-through examination. The images both demonstrate filling defects of about 1–2 cm across. The lesions both have a multinodular surface appearance. The larger lesion is in the terminal ileum and I note that it is labelled 'query debris.' However, the compact cauliflower-like appearance would be unusual for food debris in the distal small bowel, which is typically in the liquid phase, and this patient appears to have multiple small bowel polyps.

Multiple polyps in the small bowel may be adenomas, hyperplastic polyps, haemangiomas or hamartomas. Hyperplastic polyps may be detected incidentally during upper gastrointestinal endoscopy and are rarely symptomatic. Multiple haemangiomas, hamartomas or adenomas may be associated with obstructive symptoms or gastrointestinal bleeding. If the patient has a past history or family history of colonic polyps, then the lesions may be multiple adenomas associated with a hereditary polyposis syndrome such as familial adenomatous polyposis. If clinical inspection reveals multiple pigmented lesions around the lips and in the mouth, then the lesions may be hamartomas associated with Peutz–Jeghers syndrome. A definitive diagnosis can often be secured by careful history taking and clinical examination, although a biopsy is sometimes necessary to confirm the diagnosis. Therefore, I would discuss this case with the gastroenterology team.

Diagnosis

Multiple small bowel polyps associated with Peutz–Jeghers syndrome.

Tips: Bowel polyps

Key points

Colonic polyps are more likely to be malignant than small bowel polyps. The larger a polyp, the more likely it is to be malignant [particularly adenomas or gastrointestinal stromal tumours (GIST)]. A solitary polyp is more likely to be a lipoma or GIST, whereas multiple polyps are more likely to be haemangiomas, hamartomas or hyperplastic polyps. Adenomas may be solitary or multiple. Ancillary features of malignancy include lymphadenopathy, liver metastases and bone metastases.

Management depends upon the clinical manifestations as well as the specific diagnosis. Resection may be appropriate for symptomatic benign polyps causing bowel obstruction or bleeding, or polyps that are malignant, of high malignant potential or of uncertain malignant status. This may depend on the patient's overall clinical condition, ease of resection and polyp size.

Gastrointestinal polyposis

Polyps may be an incidental diagnosis in patients being investigated for nonspecific abdominal symptoms. Obstruction and gastrointestinal bleeding (which may be chronic and present as iron-deficiency anaemia) may occur. In symptomatic patients, diagnosis of colonic polyps is relatively straightforward as the colon is readily accessible. However, small bowel polyps **(Figure 1)** may be difficult to identify and diagnose, especially if a definitive diagnosis cannot be made on clinical grounds, and biopsy or surgical resection should be contemplated.

Polyposis syndromes include familial adenomatous polyposis (including subtypes Gardner's and Turcot's syndromes) and Peutz–Jeghers syndrome. There are many others, but they are all rare.

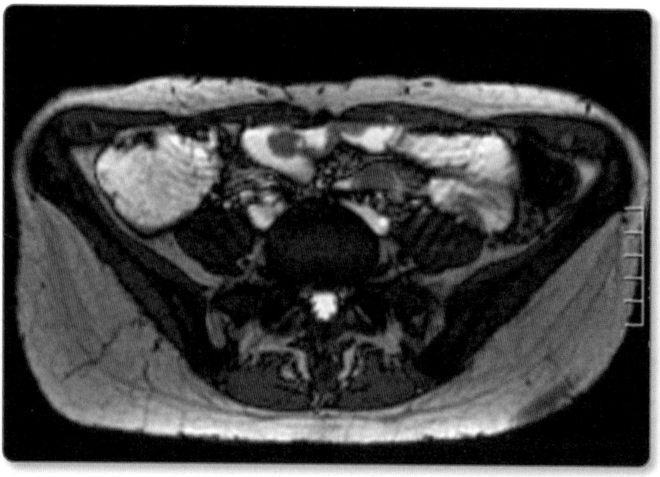

Figure 1 T2-weighted MRI with oral preparation fluid demonstrates a large pedunculated small bowel polyp with a long stalk.

Peutz–Jeghers syndrome is an autosomal dominantly inherited condition in which there are multiple hamartomatous polyps in the small bowel and which may also involve the stomach or colon. The hamartomas are not premalignant but there is an increased risk of gastric, duodenal and ovarian carcinoma. The hamartomas may bleed and may form the lead point of an intussusception. The syndrome is usually associated with pigmentation of the buccal membrane and perioral skin, which often crosses the vermillion border of the lips. These features, in conjunction with the family history, often allow a clinical diagnosis to be made.

Case 90

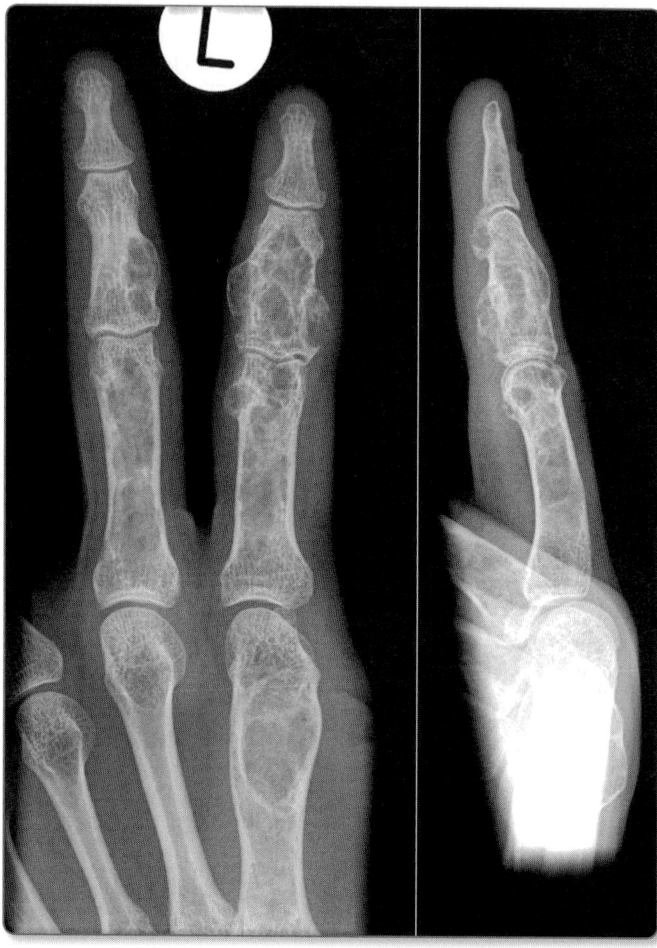

Suggested response

These are dorsoplantar (DP) views of the left index and middle fingers and a lateral view of one finger, probably the index.

Multiple lucent lesions are visible in the middle and proximal phalanges and also the index finger metacarpal. They appear nonaggressive and there is no periosteal reaction. All of the lesions are expansile to some degree, most are eccentric and, other than on the proximal volar radial border of the middle phalanx of the index finger, they are well-defined. At the aforementioned border, there is a defect in the cortex and, although there is no soft tissue swelling, I suspect that there may be a minimally displaced fracture. No phleboliths are identified in the soft tissues.

The lesions are all typical of enchondromas and the patient almost certainly has Ollier's disease. The patient may have suffered recent trauma, but I would like to correlate this with the history and clinical findings.

Diagnosis

Ollier's disease with possible fracture following trauma.

Tips: Enchondromas

Review Cases 2 and 6 for general tips on dealing with bone lesions.

Key points

Enchondromas may occur in any bone and are the most common benign lucent lesion in the phalanges. They are usually solitary, may be expansile and usually contain chondroid matrix, except in the phalanges where they may be entirely lucent. They are not associated with a periosteal reaction, unless there has been a fracture or other pathology. The risk of malignant degeneration is unclear, but the likelihood of malignant transformation is higher in the long bones than in the extremities. It may be impossible to discriminate between low-grade chondrosarcoma and enchondroma.

Differential diagnosis

If multiple enchondromas are identified, the differential lies between Ollier's disease and Maffucci's syndrome. These possibilities are differentiated by the presence of soft tissue haemangiomas which can be found in Maffucci's syndrome (phleboliths may be identified).

Ollier's disease (multiple enchondromatosis)

Noninherited and characterised by multiple enchondromas, this disease usually affects the small tubular bones of the hands and feet in particular. The risk of malignant degeneration is controversial but probably approaches 25% of patients (who each may have many lesions).

Maffucci's syndrome

This is also characterised by multiple enchondromas, but they are associated with soft tissue haemangiomas in which multiple phleboliths are often visible. Maffucci's syndrome is also nonhereditary, but there is a considerably increased rate of malignant degeneration of the enchondromas; some authors suggest that this occurs in nearly all patients.

Case 91

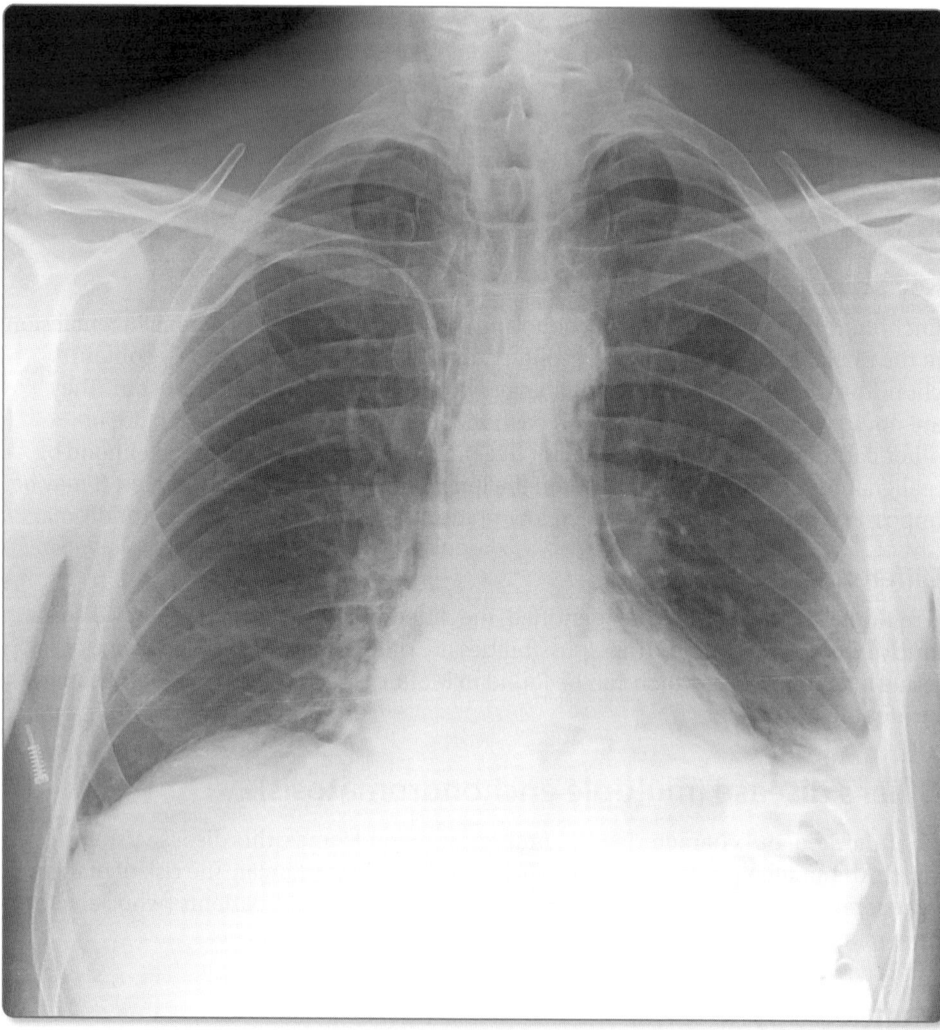

Suggested response

This is a frontal chest radiograph of a skeletally mature patient. There is a right subclavian venous catheter, the tip of which is projected in a satisfactory position in the lower superior vena cava. There is pneumomediastinum with gas outlining the left heart border and descending aorta. There is loss of definition of the left hemidiaphragm laterally with streaky shadowing at the left base. Inferior to this, contrast-filled bowel is noted to be outlined by gas laterally, consistent with pneumoperitoneum. No gas is evident in the soft tissues of the neck and there is no pneumothorax. Concomitant pneumomediastinum and pneumoperitoneum could be due to free gas tracking superiorly from the abdomen or inferiorly from the mediastinum. The fact that contrast is present within the bowel suggests that there has been a recent gastrointestinal contrast examination. One unifying explanation for these appearances might be that there has been a contrast swallow examination to assess for oesophageal perforation. If these findings were not suspected on the referral, I would discuss them urgently with the referring clinicians.

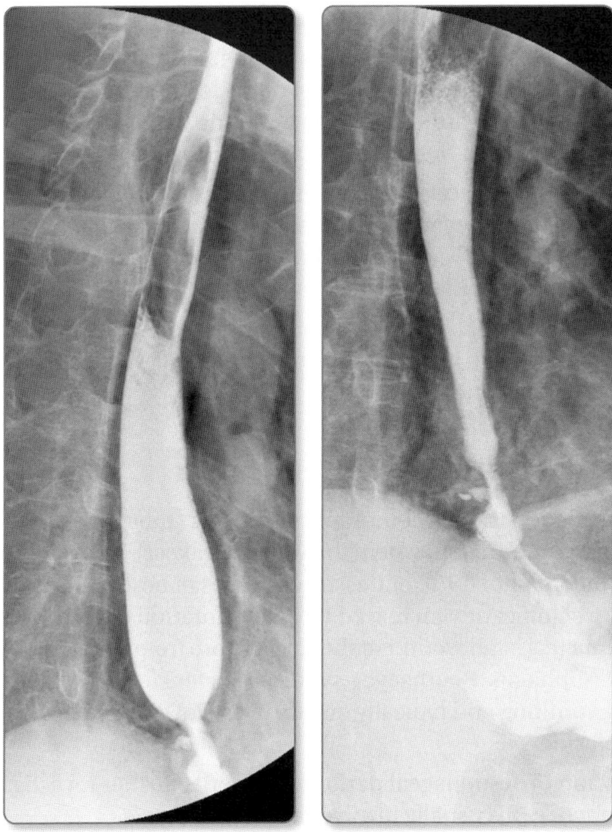

Suggested response

These are two images from a contrast swallow examination. Pneumomediastinum is again evident. There is contrast extravasation from the right side of the distal oesophagus. The oesophagus is narrowed at the site of extravasation. If this area did not open on any image from the examination then a stricture would be most likely, although it is also possible that this area was in spasm when these images were acquired. The findings are those of oesophageal perforation. This may be iatrogenic, for instance as a result of endoscopy which may have been performed to dilate an oesophageal stricture. Alternately, the perforation may be spontaneous (Boerhaave's syndrome). I would urgently discuss these findings with the surgical team.

Diagnosis

Oesophageal perforation secondary to endoscopy with pneumomediastinum and subsequent pneumoperitoneum.

Tips: Pneumomediastinum

Key points

Pneumomediastinum is often accompanied by pneumothorax, pneumoperitoneum, pneumoretroperitoneum or subcutaneous emphysema, so search for each of these. Radiological signs related to pneumomediastinum include the continuous diaphragm sign, 'V' sign (gas outlining the medial aspect of the left hemidiaphragm and left lower mediastinal border), tubular artery sign (gas outlining major mediastinal vessels) and 'sail' sign (where the thymus is outlined by gas in children).

Ancillary signs may suggest a specific aetiology. Look for central venous catheterisation, evidence of recent thoracic surgery (look for hilar clips, rib resection), dilated oesophagus (possible recent endoscopic stricture dilatation) and barotrauma related to intubation and ventilation.

Remember that a faint 'false positive' pneumomediastinum appearance may be produced by the Mach effect, in which the linear edges of a radiodense mediastinum and radiolucent lung abut one another.

Oesophageal perforation

Oesophageal perforation is most commonly iatrogenic (most often in the region of the pharyngo-oesophageal junction, where the wall is weakest). The risk from a 'standard' endoscopy is in the order of 0.1%. Endoscopy in cases of oesophageal dilatation, however, carries a significantly increased risk of perforation (approximately 2%). Penetrating trauma (e.g. stab wound to the neck) more frequently involves the upper than the lower oesophagus. Boerhaave's syndrome refers to oesophageal rupture that occurs following vomiting and typically occurs in the lower third of the oesophagus, usually on the left side.

A high suspicion of oesophageal perforation merits further investigation, in contemporary practice this usually involves a CT scan.

Case 92

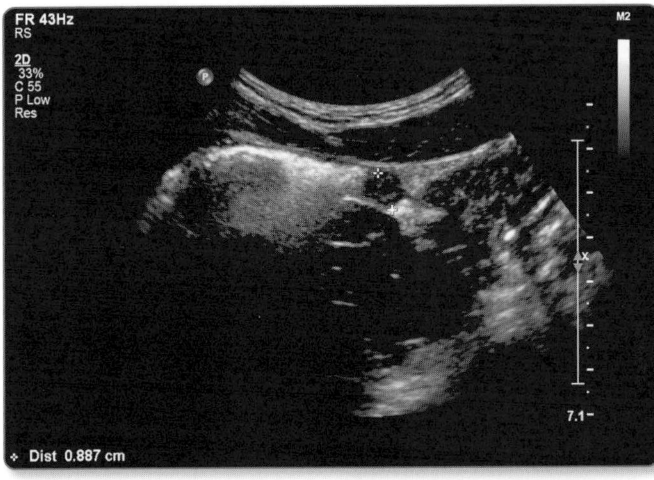

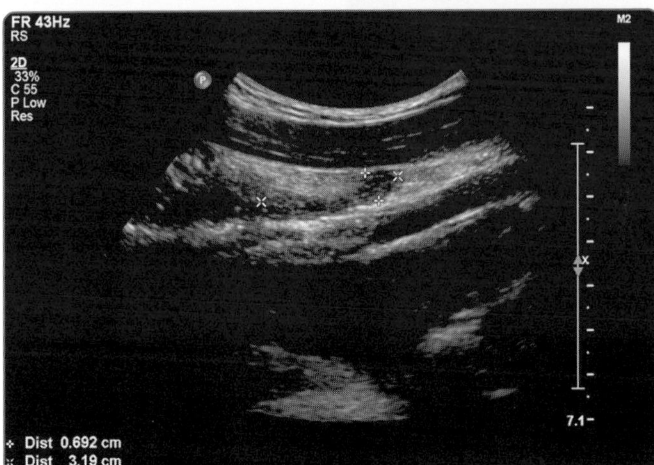

Suggested response

These are two ultrasound images taken with a curvilinear probe showing a tubular structure which has been measured to be approximately 9 mm in diameter. It is surrounded by high-reflectivity fat and lies approximately 2 cm deep to the skin. Knowledge of the region of the body being imaged would be helpful and I would like to correlate the findings with the clinical history and examination, but I suspect that this represents an inflamed appendix. In the first instance, I would continue the study with a high-frequency linear probe.

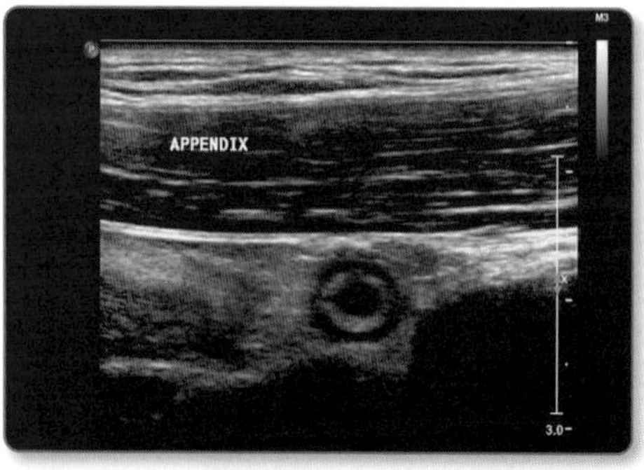

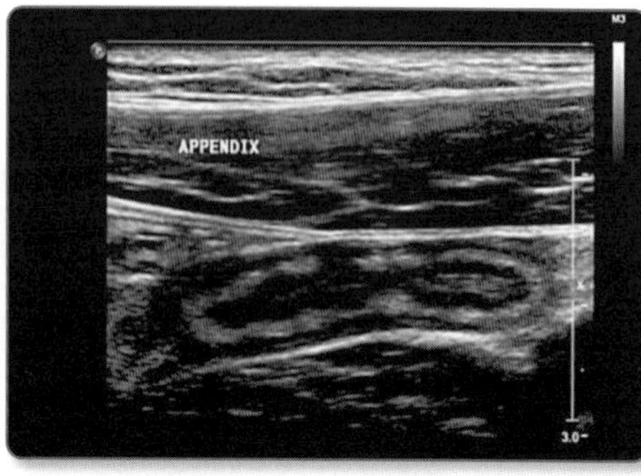

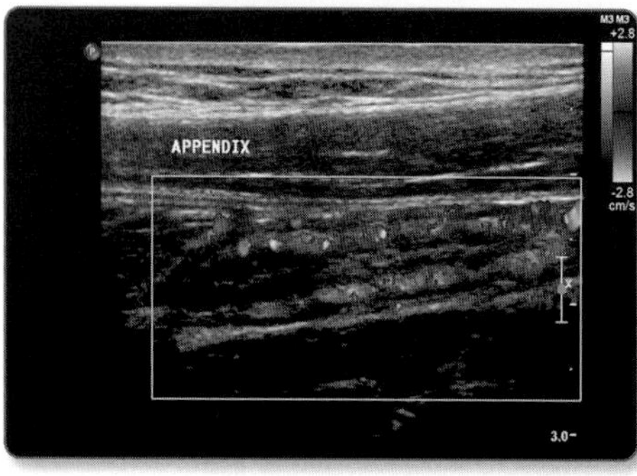

Suggested response

These images are labelled 'appendix' and confirm that the abnormality is a blind-ending, tubular structure with florid hypervascularity in keeping with acute appendicitis. I would urgently discuss the patient with the on-call surgical team and explain my findings to them.

Diagnosis

Appendicitis on ultrasound.

Tips: Ultrasound images that you do not initially recognise

You may encounter a study of any part of the body – even the eyeball. Use every clue you can when scrutinising an examination. Consider any history you are given and try to use any technical information that is recorded to help you. Consider the type of probe, whether a particular preset or scale has been used and whether there are any colour or power Doppler images. Look for any annotations for further clues, including side marking and orientation of image (e.g. axial, longitudinal, medial, lateral, etc.).

If you remain unsure, then try to identify any structure you recognise and talk about that. If something has been measured then mention it, even if only in passing. If you can see a possible abnormality, then describe it and say how you would proceed. For instance, state that you might look with a different probe or Doppler, etc. as appropriate.

Remember that the examiners are not trying to deliberately catch you out. If you cannot fathom what body part is being examined, despite running through a logical system, then say so. In your usual practice, either you would personally be performing the examination or would be told what you were reviewing the imaging for. Guessing which body part is represented is not necessary or desirable, so it is far better to seek clarification.

Imaging appendicitis

Examiners will commonly probe around how and when to image a common condition, and appendicitis is a prime example of this. There may be no absolutely 'correct' answer but have some idea of which test to use and when, and the reasoning behind the decision. Things to consider are when to operate and when to scan, whether to use ultrasound, MRI or CT, and whether age or gender should be a determining factor.

Case 93

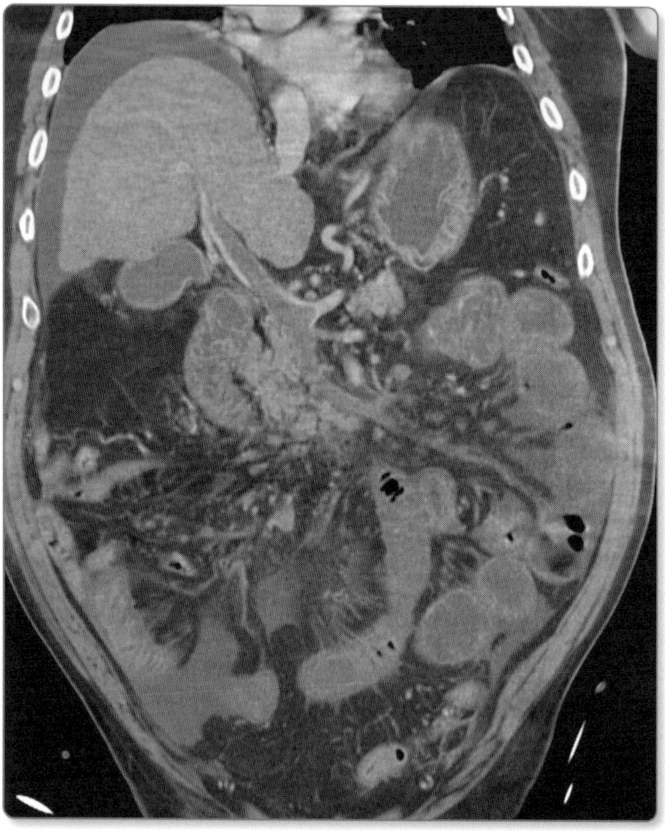

Suggested response

This is a coronally reformatted CT image of the abdomen, presumably acquired in the portal venous phase, demonstrating several abnormalities. There is free fluid around the liver and between some of the mesenteric folds. The small bowel loops appear abnormal, with wall thickening in some areas and patchy interrupted mucosal enhancement evident in the proximal jejunal loops. In this region, there are a couple of small foci of gas which may lie in the bowel wall, although I would routinely review the whole scan to confirm or refute this possibility. The mesentery is diffusely abnormal, with generalised haziness and prominent engorged vasa recta vessels in the central abdomen. There is a 'sausage-like' filling defect in the portal vein that extends inferiorly into the superior mesenteric vein. This is most likely to represent thrombus. I do not see any gas in the portal vein. I also note large serpiginous vessels between the liver and the stomach that are most likely to be varices. The liver itself appears small and the contour of the lateral edge is slightly irregular, suggesting macronodular cirrhosis.

This patient appears to have portal vein thrombosis complicating cirrhosis with portal hypertension. This is associated with venous ischaemia and possible infarction of the small bowel. There is no free intraperitoneal gas on this image, but I would review the whole study thoroughly to identify any features to suggest perforation of the bowel. If I encountered this scan at work, I would contact the referring clinicians immediately myself to convey the diagnosis.

Diagnosis

Portal vein thrombosis with small bowel ischaemia.

Tips: Bowel ischaemia

Key points

Arterial ischaemia is far more common than venous ischaemia. The cause may be thromboembolism, possibly originating from the heart if there has been a recent myocardial infarction or if the patient has atrial fibrillation, or thrombosis in situ at the site of preexisting atherosclerotic disease.

Look for filling defects or abrupt occlusions of the mesenteric vessels, particularly the superior mesenteric artery. Specifically consider if there has been a perforation, which could indicate bowel wall infarction. In the absence of perforation, it is not possible to determine with absolute confidence whether the bowel wall is infarcted. Even the presence of intramural gas does not necessarily indicate infarction. If there is no free gas, the best you can do is to say that there are features that indicate severe ischaemia, possibly infarction, but that complete breakdown of the bowel wall has not been identified.

Conclude by demonstrating that you know that this is a surgical emergency, that surgical exploration may be undertaken depending on a variety of factors (including index of suspicion for infarction and the overall clinical condition of the patient) and that you would discuss the patient urgently with the on-call surgeon.

Portal vein thrombosis

Portal vein thrombosis is usually a complication of a prothrombotic state of any cause, for instance cirrhosis, intra-abdominal infection, inflammation (usually pancreatitis) or compression (for instance, due to cholangiocarcinoma). The diagnosis may be made on Doppler ultrasound or cross-sectional imaging. The aims of treatment are to address the underlying condition, to control portal hypertension and to target the thrombosis itself. It is usual to assess the patency of the portal vein before attempting a transjugular intrahepatic portosystemic shunt (TIPSS), although portal vein thrombosis is not necessarily an absolute contraindication to this procedure.

Budd–Chiari syndrome (thrombosis of the hepatic veins) is associated with portal venous thrombosis in approximately one-quarter of cases.

Case 94

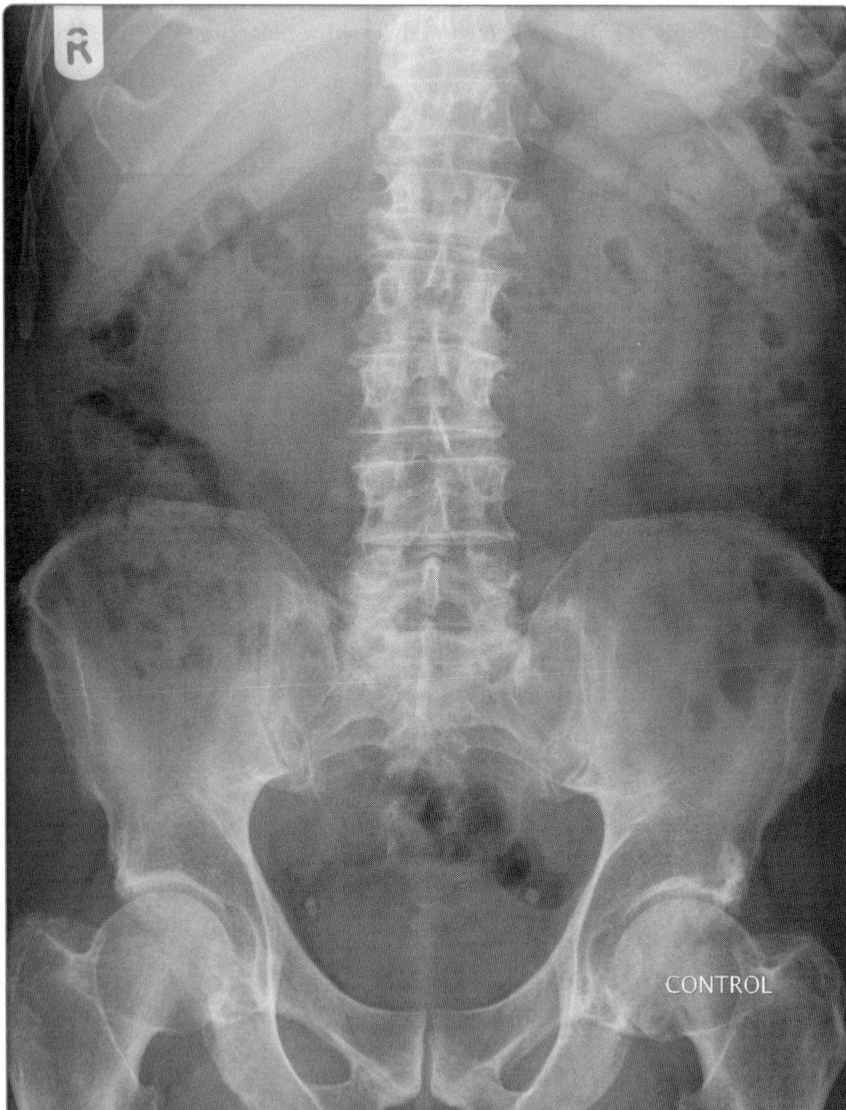

Suggested response

This is an abdominal radiograph of a skeletally mature patient. Degenerative disease in the hips and lumbar spine implies that this is an older adult. The first thing to note is that the presumed renal outlines are projected inferomedially to their usual anatomical locations and their long axes are medially orientated. Whilst the superior poles are relatively well visualised, the inferior poles are not clearly identified and there is an impression of the lower poles extending toward the midline inferiorly at the level of the L4 vertebra. This appearance is therefore likely to represent a horseshoe kidney. At least two irregular calcific densities are projected over the renal outline on the left at the level of L3 and are likely to represent calculi within the horseshoe kidney. Well-defined calcific densities in the pelvis are most likely to represent phleboliths. The bowel gas pattern is unremarkable and there are no more pertinent findings.

As this radiograph is marked 'control', I presume that it is the first film in an intravenous urogram series. I would routinely examine the remaining radiographs to assess for corresponding filling defects or renal tract obstruction.

Diagnosis

Adult patient with horseshoe kidney with calculi in the left 'lower pole'.

Tips: Foci of discrete renal tract calcification

Key points

About 90% of renal tract calculi are radio-opaque, but how visible they are depends on their constituents. Struvite and calcium-based stones are usually visible on plain film but uric acid stones are usually not visible. Any form of calculi can form staghorn calculi but these are most commonly struvite calculi.

CT can visualise almost all of those calculi not evident on plain film, the exceptions including those rare calculi induced by indinavir or atazanavir. If clinical features suggest calculi then look for ancillary features such as hydronephrosis and perinephric/periureteral stranding (which suggest an obstructing calculus) and consider whether it would be helpful to perform excretory phase urography.

In the kidney, calculi are the most common cause of renal calcification. Metabolic disorders (e.g. hyperparathyroidism) and structural abnormalities (e.g. horseshoe kidney and polycystic kidneys) predispose to calculi, so look for other manifestations of these pathologies.

If there is a typical calcification projected along the anticipated course of the ureter, then it is more likely to be a calculus than anything else. The main differential for calcification within the pelvis is phleboliths, which lie outside the ureter and often have a lucent centre with the 'comet tail' sign (i.e. a tail of soft tissue, in continuity with the calcification, which represents the gonadal vein). If you are unsure about the location of the calcification, then excretory phase urography would delineate the course of the ureter and may be helpful.

Bladder calculi may have passed from the upper tract or have formed in the bladder itself. Primary bladder calculi are most commonly caused by stasis due to bladder outflow obstruction (look for a large prostatic indentation), although they also often form in bladder diverticula.

Calculi may also lie in the urethra having passed from the upper urinary tract.

Do not forget other causes of calcification that can be mistaken for renal tract calculi on plain film. Within the renal tract a foreign body (e.g. calcified catheter balloon), calcified tumour (transitional cell carcinoma or squamous cell carcinoma), tuberculous abscess or renal artery aneurysm may give this appearance. Outside the renal tract, there is a longer differential list including mesenteric lymph nodes, gallstones, pancreatic calcification, vascular calcification, phleboliths and prostatic calcification.

Horseshoe kidney

Horseshoe kidney is the most common renal fusion anomaly, with the left and right kidneys being united at their lower pole by a parenchymal or fibrous bridge that crosses the midline at the level of L4/L5. The long axes of each kidney (normally laterally orientated) instead point medially, and the renal pelvises and (multiple) ureters emerge anteriorly. Horseshoe kidneys are often an incidental finding but predispose to hydronephrosis (secondary to pelviureteric junction obstruction as a result of the high insertion of the ureter into the renal pelvis), vesicoureteric reflux, infection, calculi (as seen in this case) and tumours (in particular transitional cell carcinoma).

Case 95

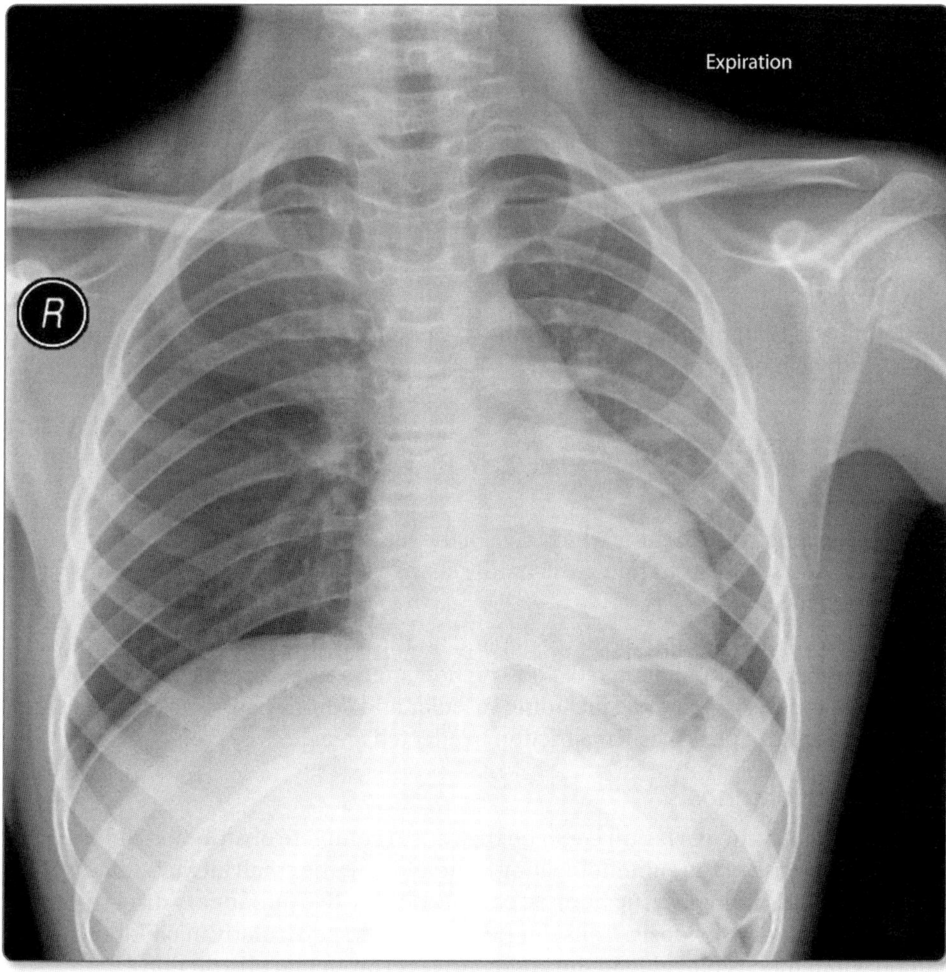

Suggested response

This is an erect frontal chest radiograph of a skeletally immature patient taken in expiration.

There is an area of increased transradiancy and volume within the right lung which involves the whole of the lower zone with a sharply defined upper border which I take to be the displaced horizontal fissure.

The left lung and right upper lobe are of uniform density, which is normal for an expiratory radiograph. The mediastinal contour and the thoracic wall are normal.

It would be useful to compare the appearance with a radiograph taken on inspiration, if one is available, but I think the findings represent air trapping in the right middle and lower lobes.

This suggests partial obstruction of the bronchus intermedius. Correlation with the clinical history would be helpful, but the most likely causes are an aspirated foreign body or mucous plugging. I cannot see any other features of airways disease and would favour a radiolucent foreign body being the cause.

I would urgently discuss the findings with the referring clinicians and suggest bronchoscopy to directly visualise the bronchus intermedius with a view to possible endoscopic retrieval of the obstructing object.

Diagnosis

Air trapping in right middle and lower lobes secondary to an aspirated peanut in the bronchus intermedius of a child.

Tips: Air trapping

Key points

The first challenge is to identify which area of the lung is normal and which is abnormal. Areas with air trapping will hardly change from inspiratory to expiratory films (see **Figure 1**).

The findings of air trapping on CT depend on the size of airway affected. It may manifest as mosaic attenuation if the obstruction affects small airways (there is a wide differential for this appearance including vascular and infiltrative disease) and may be compounded by hypoxic vasoconstriction in affected areas.

Differential diagnosis

Any partially obstructive lesion could be the cause (complete obstruction tends to lead to collapse of the subtending lung). Therefore in the small airways think of bronchiolitis, asthma, cystic fibrosis, chronic obstructive pulmonary disease, pneumonitis and sarcoidosis. Consider foreign bodies (particularly in children), tumours and mucus plugging in the larger airways (bronchial obstruction).

Foreign body aspiration

Aspiration of foreign bodies is a significant cause of morbidity and mortality and is most commonly seen in children. Before the age of 15 years, the angles of the mainstem bronchi at the carina are identical, hence foreign bodies are equally likely to pass down the left or right side. In adults, the right main bronchus is more vertical than the left, making it more likely that objects pass down this side. If not removed in a timely fashion, tracheo-oesophageal fistulation and mediastinitis can occur in addition to post-obstructive sequelae such as necrotising pneumonia and bronchiectasis.

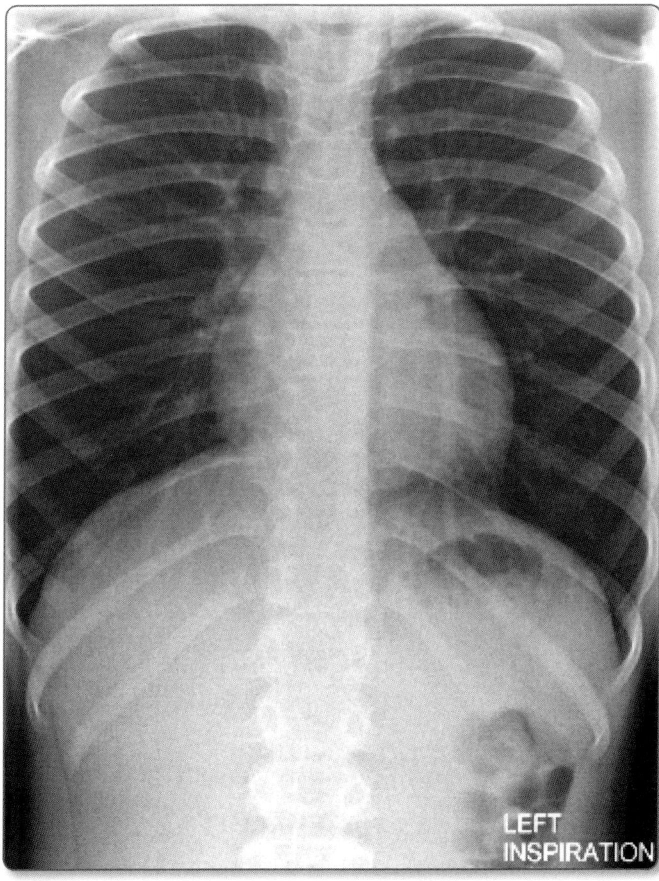

Figure 1 The inspiratory film from this case is normal.

Case 96

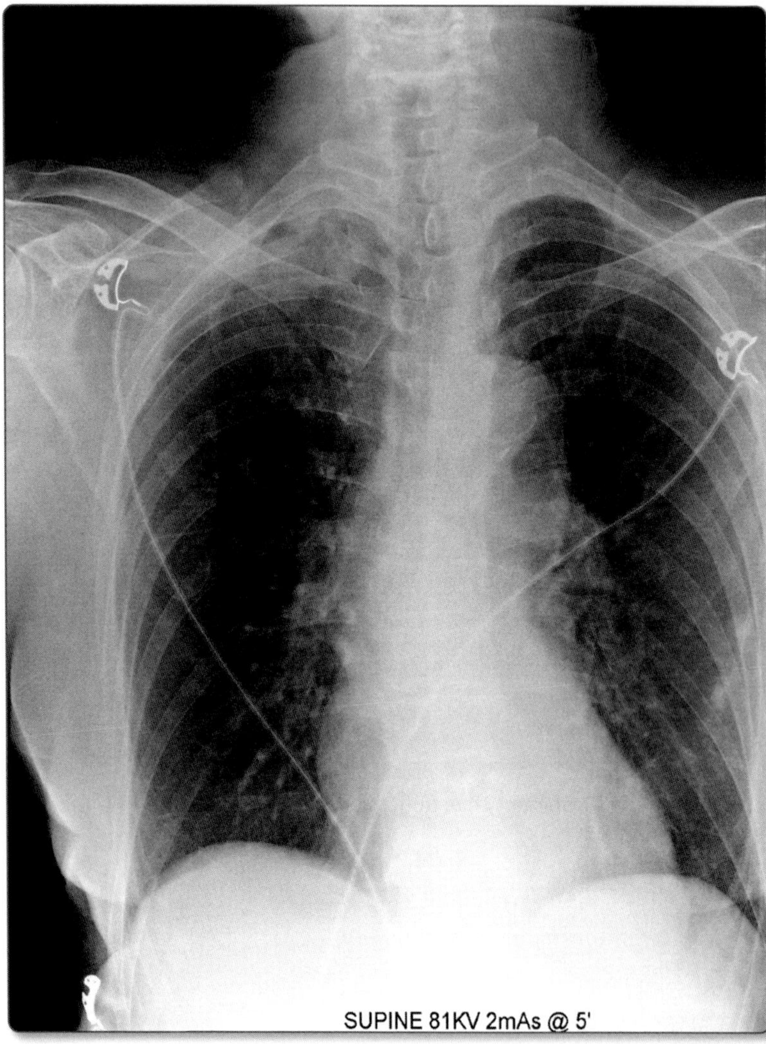

Suggested response

This is a supine chest radiograph of a skeletally mature patient. There is a mass at the right apex which is rounded inferiorly. The most superior extent of the mass is not clearly visualised. This is associated with erosion of the 3rd right rib posteriorly. No further masses are identified. The lungs are hyperinflated in keeping with a degree of chronic obstructive pulmonary disease. Accurate assessment of the hila is limited by the supine projection but I cannot see large volume lymphadenopathy.

This appearance is likely to represent a Pancoast tumour, especially if the patient has right arm or brachial plexus symptoms. If this is not a known diagnosis then I would recommend an urgent respiratory referral and further imaging with CT in the first instance, to further characterise and stage the lesion. MRI may also be indicated to delineate the extent of a superior sulcus tumour and assess for involvement of the brachial plexus.

Diagnosis

Right-sided Pancoast tumour.

Tips: An apical lung lesion

Key points and differential diagnosis

Consider the lateralisation of the lesion. If it is unilateral, possible differentials include benign pleural thickening, tumour, infection (e.g. tuberculosis) and effusion (look for 'pleural capping', particularly on supine radiographs). Look for ancillary findings of these differentials, for instance hilar enlargement, pulmonary and bony metastases. Causes of bilateral abnormalities include all of those listed for unilateral lesions and additionally progressive massive fibrosis (look for coexisting interstitial lung disease).

If there is bony destruction, the lesion is almost certainly neoplastic. There is a small possibility that it could be infective.

Pancoast tumour

Pancoast tumours, otherwise known as superior sulcus tumours, are usually non-small cell carcinomas and account for <5% of all lung cancers. They often present with clinical features relating to bony invasion or involvement of the sympathetic plexus (Horner's syndrome) or brachial plexus rather than respiratory disease. As such, MRI may be a more appropriate means of evaluation as it can delineate soft tissue, vascular and neural involvement. CT is generally more accurate at defining bony destruction **(Figure 1)**.

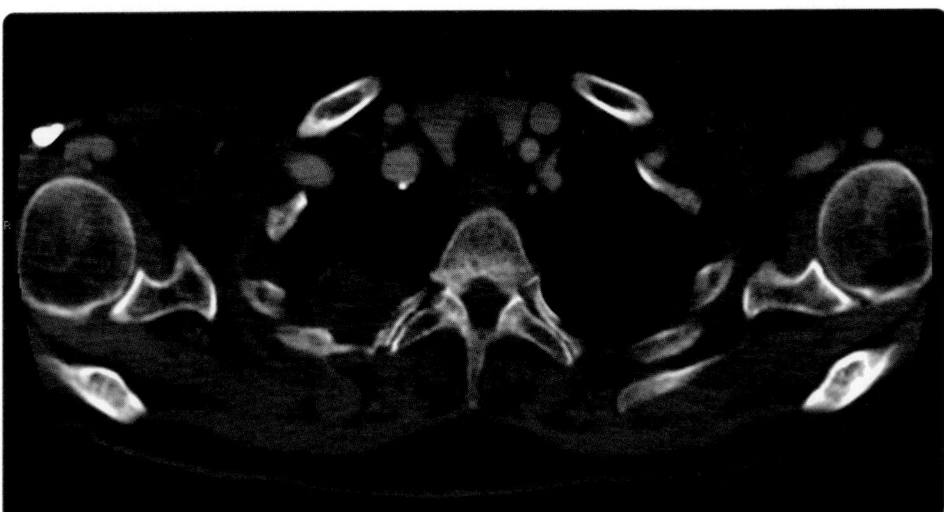

Figure 1 Axial CT on bony windows showing the right apical mass in this case, with rib destruction.

Case 97

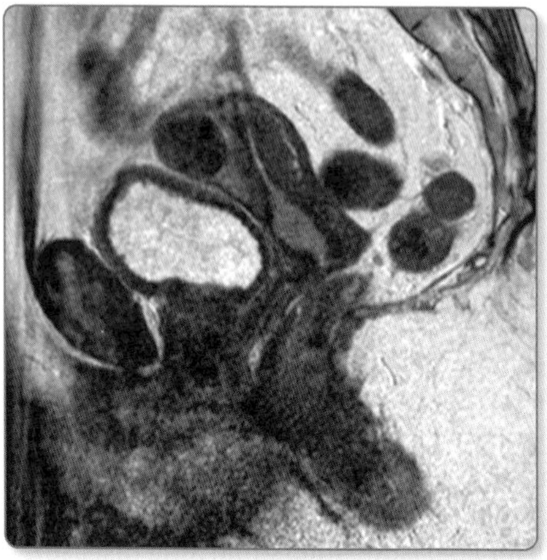

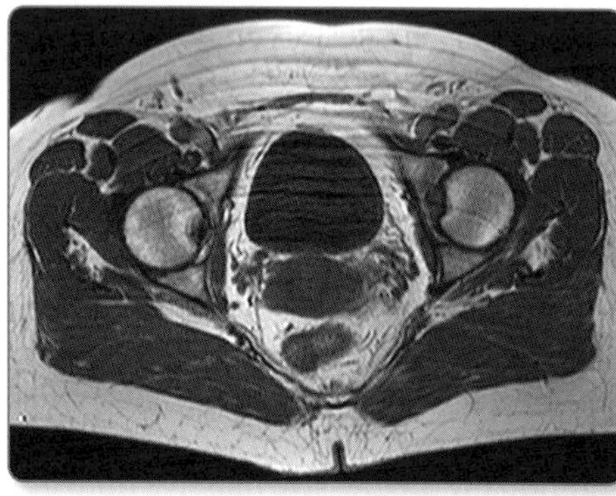

Suggested response

These are selected MRI images from a study of the pelvis in a female patient.

There is a soft tissue mass within the endocervical canal which exhibits high signal on T2-weighted imaging and which extends into the lower body of the uterus. The remainder of the uterine cavity at the fundus appears normal, implying that the cervical os is not obstructed. There is a further abnormality evident on the sagittal T2-weighted imaging, with a rounded mass which exhibits homogeneously low signal. Based on the available images this is most in keeping with an incidental fibroid.

No lymph nodes or adnexal masses are visible on these images although I would routinely review the whole study. The visualised bones are unremarkable.

It would be useful to correlate the findings with the patient's symptoms but the appearances are suggestive of a neoplastic process. I would suggest discussion of this case at the gynaecology multidisciplinary team meeting in the first instance. Further examination and biopsy are likely to be required.

Diagnosis

Cervical carcinoma visible in the endocervical canal [Grade 3 Federation of Gynaecology and Obstetrics (FIGO) 1b1].

Tips: MRI of the female pelvis

Key points and differential diagnosis

Specifically look at the adnexa, endometrium and cervix and always review the visualised bones for skeletal metastases. Also look for free pelvic fluid (although bear in mind that this may be a normal finding) and consider whether there is lymphadenopathy.

Ovarian lesions Dermoid cysts contain macroscopic fat and therefore return high signal on T1-weighted and T2-weighted imaging. Ovarian cysts and carcinomas have a spectrum of findings ranging from simple cysts to solid soft tissue lesions. For most part-solid part-cystic lesions, it is not possible to distinguish those which are benign from those which are malignant. Fibromas return low signal on both T1 and T2. Endometriomas are typically hyperintense on T1 and T2 (and can be differentiated from dermoid cysts by a fat suppression sequence; high signal persists in endometriomas but is suppressed in dermoid cysts).

Uterine lesions Endometrial carcinoma returns variable signal, but it is usually isointense to normal myometrium on T1 and heterogeneous on T2. Fibroids return low to intermediate signal on both T1 and T2 and often have a high signal rim on T2. In adenomyosis, there is a myometrial mass and widening of the junctional zone to >12 mm, with high intensity T2 spots or linear striations.

Cervical lesions Carcinomas return increased signal on T2. Nabothian cysts are extremely common and return a well-defined fluid signal.

Imaging of the female pelvis

Interpretation of images of the female pelvis, especially MRI scans, is a task for which a sound knowledge of anatomy is crucial. Confident identification of the various structures within the pelvis and knowledge of the signal characteristics of a range of pathologies will help you.

Case 98

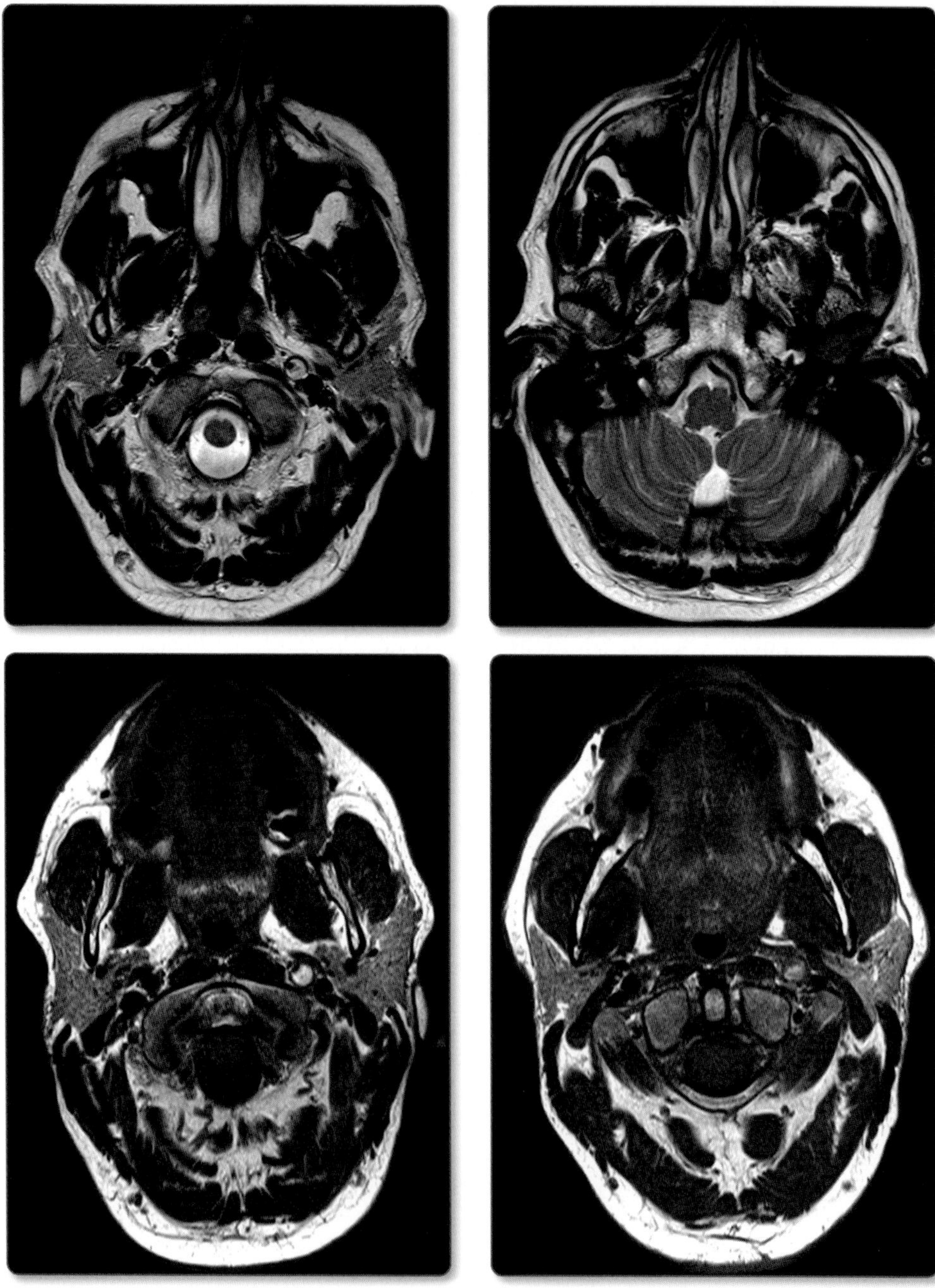

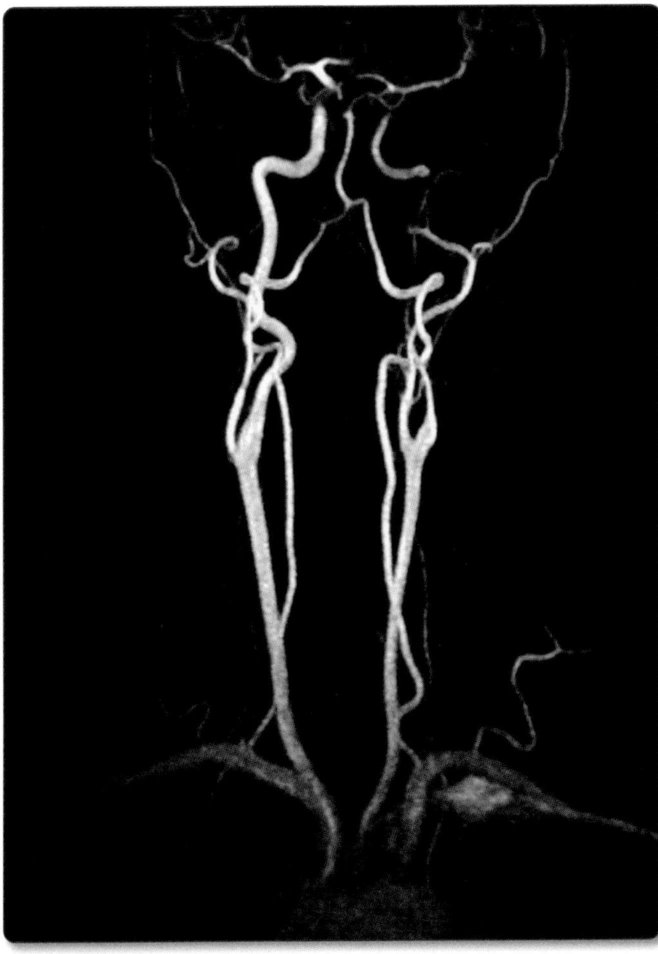

Suggested response

These are selected axial T1- and T2-weighted slices from an MRI scan through the neck, along with a coronally reformatted maximal intensity projection MR angiogram image. There is loss of the normal signal void in the left internal carotid artery, which instead returns predominantly high signal on both T1 and T2 images. This is most likely to reflect the presence of subacutely thrombosed blood products and the loss of normal flow within the vessel, with only a small area of flow void evident anteriorly in the vessel. This is consistent with severe stenosis. The left internal carotid artery is not clearly visualised in its entirety on the reformatted image. The other visible vessels, in particular the contralateral carotid arteries and both vertebral arteries, are unremarkable.

The findings are most in keeping with dissection of the left internal carotid artery. The presence of subacutely thrombosed blood products suggests that this is recent and I would discuss the findings urgently with the referring clinicians. It may also be appropriate to discuss this case with neuroradiologists with a view to considering whether intervention might be possible and appropriate.

Diagnosis

Left internal carotid artery dissection in a patient presenting with left-sided Horner's syndrome.

Tips: The loss of arterial flow voids

Key points

Be sure to examine the vertebral and carotid arteries along their entire courses, both extracranially and intracranially.

On MRI, signal characteristics from both T1 and T2 imaging can provide an approximation of the age of blood products. Be aware that low signal on both sequences may be seen both acutely (12–48 hours) and chronically (>1 month).

Look for ancillary features of arterial dissection on the imaging available. Extracranial neck vessel dissection is not infrequent in injuries resulting from craniocervical trauma, so look specifically for craniocervical fractures, high signal in the paravertebral muscles and ligaments or prevertebral swelling that may indicate an injury.

Collagen vascular disorders such as Marfan's syndrome and autosomal dominant polycystic kidney disease predispose to arterial dissection and are associated with intracranial 'berry' aneurysms, aortic aneurysms and cysts in other intra-abdominal viscera.

Carotid artery dissection

Dissection of the extracranial carotid arteries occurs more frequently than vertebral artery dissection and is a common cause of cerebral infarction in younger patients. So called 'spontaneous' carotid artery dissection is often a consequence of minor trauma (e.g. hyperextension when painting a ceiling), although true spontaneous dissection may be seen in those with collagen disorders that predispose to arterial wall defects (e.g. Ehlers–Danlos syndrome and Marfan's syndrome).

Carotid artery dissection is also seen in the context of acceleration-deceleration injuries that cause significant craniocervical trauma. Atraumatic carotid dissection may present with Horner's syndrome (as in this case) and/or with headache or neck pain. These features are followed by signs (sometimes transient) of retinal ischaemia or cerebral ischaemia (typically in the middle cerebral artery territory). MR angiography has largely replaced catheter angiography in the investigation of suspected carotid dissection and facilitates characterisation of intramural haematomas as well as visualisation of the intimal flap or double lumen.

Case 99

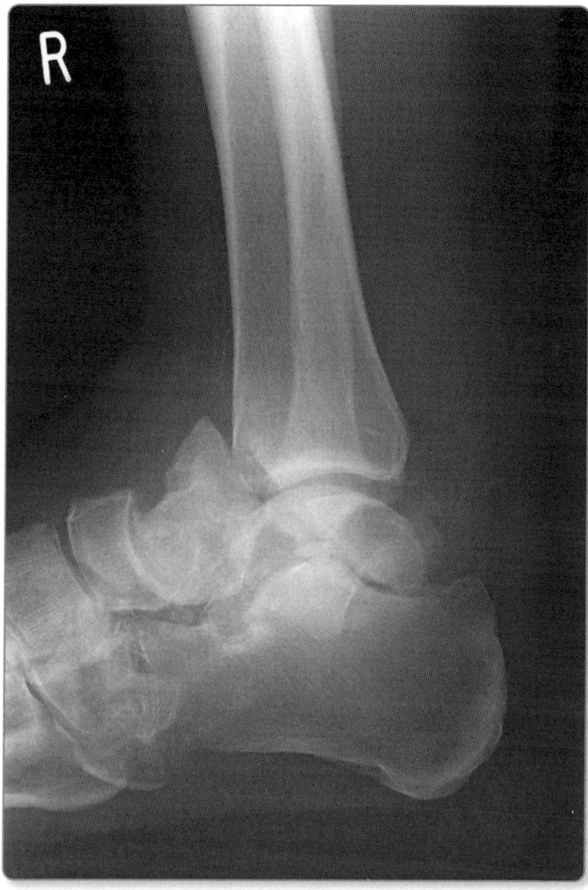

Suggested response

This is a lateral view of the right ankle of a skeletally mature patient. The ankle and hindfoot are grossly abnormal. There is a fracture/dislocation involving the talus with loss of congruity at the talonavicular joint in particular, although other joints are also malaligned. There also appears to be a fracture through the cuboid and there is bony fragmentation around the calcaneocuboid joint and what remains of the subtalar joint. There is some subchondral sclerosis but bone density is otherwise normal. Soft tissue calcification is evident posteriorly and there is also vascular calcification. If this patient is a diabetic or has known spinal cord abnormalities (e.g. syringomyelia), particularly if the presentation is with a warm and swollen but painless joint, then the most likely diagnosis is neuropathic arthropathy. The involvement of multiple joints in the ankle and foot makes septic arthritis less likely. If there is a history of severe trauma, then it is also possible that this represents an acute injury in a patient who also has vascular disease.

I would routinely review another orthogonal view and would discuss the case with the referring clinician, particularly to consider if there is a need for cross-sectional imaging to assess fracture pattern (CT) or for an infected collection (MRI).

Diagnosis

Elderly male diabetic patient with neuropathic arthropathy (Charcot's joint).

Tips: Joint destruction

When trying to differentiate between infection (septic arthritis or osteomyelitis) and neuropathic arthropathy, consider the features listed in **Table 1**.

Table 1 Differentiating infection from neuropathic arthropathy

Feature	Infection (septic arthritis or osteomyelitis)	Neuropathic arthropathy
Joint distribution	Usually monoarticular	Usually involves several joints
In the foot	More common in forefoot or hindfoot	More common in midfoot (characteristic pattern–talonavicular displacement)
Soft tissue involvement	Ulceration, sinus tract and fluid collection	Calcification
Age	More common in young	More common in elderly
Associated neuropathy	Not usually	Almost always (central or peripheral)

Key points

Look for the seven Ds of neuropathic arthropathy: distended joint, density increase, debris, dislocation, disorganisation, destruction and degeneration. Consider alternative (nondiabetic) causes of neuropathic arthropathy which, although rare in clinical practice, commonly arise in viva scenarios.

Spinal cord pathologies such as previous spinal injury or syringomyelia often affect the shoulder and may cause a 'mass' that mimics a chondrosarcoma. Spina bifida and myelomeningocele are the most common causes of this in childhood. With respect to other causes of joint destruction, congenital insensitivity to pain usually leads to damage of weight-bearing joints, syphilis is a potential cause of neuropathic joints in the lower extremity and spine and leprosy may give a 'licked candy cane' appearance to the metatarsals or phalanges.

Neuropathic arthropathy

Usually a manifestation of poorly controlled diabetes mellitus, neuropathic arthropathy has a range of causes which can present in different ways. All of these involve a neuropathic process, whether peripheral (e.g. neural trauma, leprosy and poliomyelitis) or central (typically relating to the spinal cord). Atrophic and hypertrophic patterns may be seen, with the atrophic pattern typically seen in nonweight bearing joints in the upper limb (e.g. neuropathic arthropathy of the shoulder in a patient with syringomyelia). Gross joint destruction is common to both.

Case 100

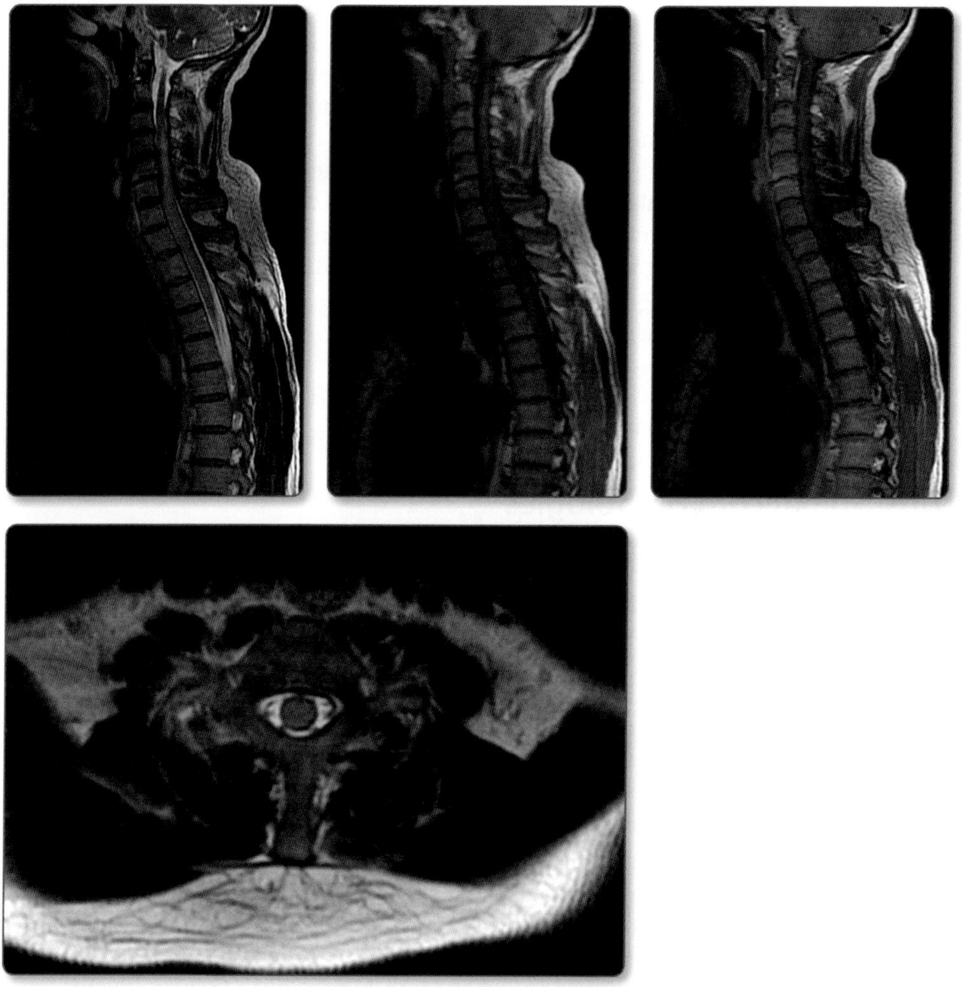

Suggested response

These are selected images from an MRI examination of the cervical and upper thoracic spine. An abnormality of the spinal cord is evident from the level of C3 to T4. The cord is expanded at these levels, with an intramedullary lesion. This is homogeneous, returns high signal relative to the remaining cord on T2 imaging and is predominantly isointense to the remaining cord on T1 imaging. No convincing contrast enhancement is identified.

Posterior disc/osteophyte bulges are evident in the mid cervical spine and the cord appears to be packed tightly within the vertebral canal, with no visible cerebrospinal fluid anterior or posterior to the spinal cord at these levels. I would routinely review the axial imaging at these levels to assess for spinal cord compression. Modic type 2 endplate changes are evident at C5/C6. The posterior fossa is unremarkable. There are no further positive findings.

If there was a gradual onset of neurological symptoms, I would favour a diagnosis of an intramedullary spinal cord tumour such as ependymoma, astrocytoma or haemangioblastoma, although the lack of enhancement makes these less likely, particularly haemangioblastoma. If the presentation was more acute, I would favour a diagnosis of a spinal cord infarct. The lack of enhancement also tends towards this diagnosis. If there is a history of trauma, I would also consider the possibility of haematoma. I would review the remaining images from the scan, including diffusion-weighted imaging if available, and would then discuss these findings with the referring clinician.

Diagnosis

Acute spinal cord infarction in a 51-year-old male.

Tips: Spinal cord pathologies

Key points

The localisation of a pathology is key to its diagnosis. Intramedullary lesions arise within the spinal cord, whereas intradural/extramedullary and extradural/extramedullary lesions arise from adjacent structures including neural tissues and bones. Expansion of the cord is suggestive of an intramedullary tumour, although acute spinal cord infarction and haematoma can also cause expansion. Intramedullary tumours are usually malignant and are most commonly ependymomas, astrocytomas or haemangioblastomas. Syringomyelia is of cerebrospinal fluid intensity and may signify pathology elsewhere within the spinal cord.

Indolent bony changes are a feature of many extramedullary pathologies, especially if they are longstanding, because they take time to develop, e.g. neural foraminal widening secondary to a longstanding neurofibroma. Widening of the interpedicular distance and vertebral scalloping may be seen with intramedullary tumours, particularly slow-growing ependymomas, but are not a feature of cord infarction.

Look for ancillary features on the available imaging that may suggest a particular diagnosis. Cysts or tumours in the pancreas or kidneys may suggest von Hippel–Lindau syndrome (haemangioblastoma). The posterior fossa is a key review area and a coexistent brain tumour may point to drop metastases or von Hippel–Lindau syndrome.

Tumours from outside the central nervous system (CNS) may metastasise to the spine. Lung carcinoma is the most common extra-CNS malignancy to metastasise to the spinal cord, so look at extraspinal tissues and particularly at any visible portion of the lungs.

Spinal cord infarction

Infarction of the spinal cord is rare, in part due to its rich blood supply. It typically presents with sudden onset of neurological symptoms, thus helping to distinguish it from other spinal cord pathologies such as tumours. Although it may be spontaneous, spinal cord infarction is well documented following such procedures as open aortic aneurysm repair or bronchial artery embolisation, in which the artery of Adamkiewicz (an anterior medullary artery) may inadvertently be occluded.

MRI is the imaging modality of choice, with cord expansion seen in the acute phase and often with intramedullary high signal on T2 images. Diffusion-weighted imaging also has a role to play, demonstrating restriction of diffusion.

Index

Note: Page numbers in *italic* refer to figures, respectively

R

U

V

W

Y

Z